PRAISE FOR *VEGAN FOR HER*

"*Vegan for Her* provides sensible guidance for women of all ages. Whether your focus is sports nutrition, eating to prevent cancer or heart disease, or simply understanding how a plant-based diet can meet your unique needs, this book is for you."
—REED MANGELS, PhD, RD, author of *The Everything Vegan Pregnancy Book* and coauthor of *Simply Vegan*

"This is an exceptional book for vegan and not-yet-vegan women everywhere. Ginny Messina has outdone herself when she created this ultimate go-to guide for women during all aspects of their lives and has made being healthy cool and easy."
—ANNIE SHANNON, coauthor of *Betty Goes Vegan*

"*Vegan for Her* is an excellent and articulate resource for every woman who wants to eat with compassion while protecting and enhancing her health."
—CAROL J. ADAMS, author of *The Sexual Politics of Meat* and *Living Among Meat Eaters*

"A fantastic science-based resource by one of the giants in plant-based nutrition."
—MICHAEL GREGER, MD, founder of NutritionFacts.org

PRAISE FOR *VEGAN FOR LIFE*

"Jack Norris and Ginny Messina have produced a highly readable, information-packed book about vegan nutrition. . . . I highly recommend *Vegan for Life*—for new vegans, established vegans, people curious about vegan diets. . . . It's essential reading!"
—*Vegetarian Journal*

"Packed with science yet never boring, Norris and Messina—both long-time vegans themselves—put their wealth of knowledge at your fingertips while putting to rest any nutritional issues that concern those aspiring to a plant based-diet. . . . No vegan myth goes unbusted. Overflowing with charts, meal and menu plans, interesting factoids, and separate chapters devoted to specific issues (pregnancy, children, athletes, etc.), *Vegan for Life* is a complete reference guide that deserves a spot in your library or kitchen." —*VegNews*

"Armed with this compendium and a vegan cookbook, novices will make an easy, healthy transition to meat, egg, and dairy-free meals, while practicing vegans can use it as a guide to the best food choices." —*Publishers Weekly*

"*Vegan for Life* is one of those books that you'll pull off the shelf for inspiration and consultation time after time." —Curled Up with a Good Book

"Simply amazing . . . displaces *Becoming Vegan* as the definitive vegan nutrition book." —*Reno Gazette-Journal*

"The most authoritative vegan nutrition book on the planet." —Vegan.com

"If you're an animal lover, this book may be helpful in helping you find a more compassionate way to eat." —*Portland Book Review*

"An interesting, easy-to-read, and extremely informative resource . . . *Vegan for Life* is a fantastic educational guide and resource for new or seasoned vegans alike. In addition, it's a great resource for dieticians who wish to promote aspects of a plant-based diet to clients, whether vegans or omnivores." —*Today's Dietitian*

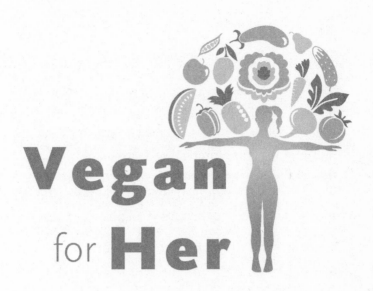

Vegan for **Her**

THE WOMAN'S GUIDE TO BEING HEALTHY AND FIT ON A PLANT-BASED DIET

VIRGINIA MESSINA, MPH, RD

WITH

JL FIELDS

DA CAPO LIFELONG
A Member of the Perseus Books Group

Da Capo
LIFE
LONG

Copyright © 2013 by Virginia Messina and JL Fields
Plant Plate copyright © 2013 by Virginia Messina and Ari Evergreen

Designed by Linda Mark
Set in 10.5 point Guardi LT Std by the Perseus Books Group

Cataloging-in-Publication data for this book is available from the Library of Congress.

First Da Capo Press edition 2013
ISBN 978-0-7382-1671-3 (paperback)
ISBN 978-0-7382-1672-0 (e-book)

Published by Da Capo Press
A Member of the Perseus Books Group
www.dacapopress.com

Note: The information in this book is true and complete to the best of our knowledge. This book is intended only as an informative guide for those wishing to know more about health issues. In no way is this book intended to replace, countermand, or conflict with the advice given to you by your own physician. The ultimate decision concerning care should be made between you and your doctor. We strongly recommend you follow his or her advice. Information in this book is general and is offered with no guarantees on the part of the authors or Da Capo Press. The authors and publisher disclaim all liability in connection with the use of this book. The names and identifying details of people associated with events described in this book have been changed. Any similarity to actual persons is coincidental.

Da Capo Press books are available at special discounts for bulk purchases in the U.S. by corporations, institutions, and other organizations. For more information, please contact the Special Markets Department at the Perseus Books Group, 2300 Chestnut Street, Suite 200, Philadelphia, PA, 19103, or call (800) 810-4145, ext. 5000, or e-mail special.markets@perseusbooks.com.

10 9 8 7 6 5 4 3

To a goat in Africa, to a calf on his way to the slaughterhouse—
for starting us on this journey toward a life of compassion.

CONTENTS

PART FOUR: RECIPES

INTRODUCTION

Trading in animal foods for plant-based meals is one of the most powerful decisions you can make. For starters, a menu built around plant foods is very likely to put you on the road toward better health. Plant-based diets can lower your risk for heart disease, diabetes, hypertension, and cancer. This way of eating has a lot of history behind it, too. The healthiest diet patterns in the world—like traditional Mediterranean and Japanese diets—are plant-based, including only small amounts of meat, fish, and poultry. Those who opt for vegetarian diets, which include no meat, poultry, or fish, may reap even greater benefits.

But being vegan is a little bit different. It takes choices beyond health and, in fact, beyond food. When you go vegan, you embrace a way of eating and living that brings big-picture kinds of benefits. It's a chance to take care of yourself and, in the process, give a little bit of care to the rest of the world. There is truly no other lifestyle choice that delivers as many benefits or makes the same kind of impact.

The word *vegan* was coined nearly seventy years ago in England by Donald Watson, who said it was "a way of living that seeks to exclude, as far as possible and practicable, all forms of exploitation of, and cruelty to, animals for food, clothing and any other purpose." Although he wasn't the first to address the choice to forgo animal products, he was the first to give it a name. The Vegan Society, which he founded with a small group of like-minded individuals in

1944, is still active in England, and people all over the world are choosing a vegan lifestyle for their health, for the environment, and for the animals.

A Book for Vegan Women

I wrote this book for vegan women because women's nutrient requirements and health concerns are unique.

Vegan for Her provides specific guidance about food choices that work against a range of health concerns and that address the distinctive nutrition needs of women. It's all from a vegan perspective, of course, highlighting areas where a vegan diet gives you a definite edge, and directing you to vegan-specific solutions to nutrition problems. I'll talk about how to eat to lower your risk for breast cancer, diabetes, and heart disease; manage hunger and eat intuitively; protect your skin and brain as you get older; boost your mood; and deal with PMS, cramps, infertility, and painful conditions like arthritis and migraine headaches. Some of these conditions are obviously unique to women; others are more common among women or they affect women in unique ways.

My goal is to help you make the best choices possible based on what we know about nutrition science right now. And "best" choices are ones that help you incorporate more healthy plant foods into your meals in ways that are practical and realistic for you. It means finding foods that fit your schedule, the needs of your family and others in your life, and include the foods you love.

I asked vegan lifestyle coach and educator JL Fields to provide the recipes for this book because I love the joyful approach she brings to vegan cooking and lifestyle. I also appreciate—and know you will, too—that her recipes are super-easy and practical without ever sacrificing flavor and health. They've been thoroughly tested by a diverse team of vegans, including some who are brand-new to vegan cooking.

JL also contributed a chapter on how to take your veganism beyond the plate—that is, how to build a vegan wardrobe, find cruelty-free

Omnivore, Vegetarian, Vegan— What's the Difference?

In this book, I use the terms *omnivore* and *meat-eater* interchangeably, even though, technically, they don't mean exactly the same thing. From a biological standpoint, humans are omnivores—or really, herbivorous omnivores. That is, we can eat, digest, and metabolize a wide range of plant and animal foods but we do best on a diet that emphasizes plants. And while we couldn't survive on a diet of 100 percent meat, we are able to thrive on an all-plant diet if we choose.

Here are some other terms I use throughout this book to describe different eating patterns.

Plant-based: A diet that is built around plant foods; it may or may not include small or moderate amounts of animal foods. Traditional Mediterranean and Japanese diets are plant-based diets. So are vegetarian, vegan, semi-vegetarian, and raw foods diets. Some of what we know about vegan nutrition is actually drawn from research on other types of plant-based diets.

Semi-vegetarian: A little bit of a fuzzy term since it means so many things. This is usually a person who eats mostly a vegetarian diet but occasionally consumes some meat. Some people who describe themselves as semi-vegetarians actually eat chicken and fish fairly regularly but avoid red meat.

Lacto-ovo vegetarian: One type of plant-based diet that eliminates meat but includes dairy foods and eggs. When I use the term *vegetarian* in this book, it refers to lacto-ovo vegetarians. In many research studies, lacto-ovo vegetarians and vegans are grouped together and simply referred to as vegetarians.

Vegan: A lifestyle or ethic that seeks to avoid all animal products for food, clothing, and personal care. However, many people who eat a vegan diet but don't exclude animal products for other uses call themselves vegans. This book is for both groups. When I use the term *vegan*, I'm talking about a vegan diet—that is, a diet that includes no meat, fish, poultry, dairy foods, or eggs. JL will look at the broader implications of veganism in Chapter 17.

Raw foods diet: It's just what it sounds like—a diet that includes no cooked foods. Raw foods diets are usually vegan and they include fruits, vegetables, nuts, seeds, and sprouted grains and legumes.

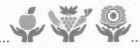

products for your home, and—if you choose—how to seek out opportunities for vegan activism.

MY JOURNEY TO LIVING THE VEGAN LIFE

Vegan diets weren't much on my radar when I was in college and then graduate school, studying to become a public health nutritionist in the 1970s. I knew a few vegetarians but had never met a vegan and it certainly wasn't an issue that came up in my studies. Once I became a registered dietitian and obtained my master's in public health, I settled into a job in a small rural clinic in southwest Michigan, working with migrant farm workers, low-income elderly people, and pregnant teens. I was also newly married and experiencing a newfound enjoyment in cooking in my miniscule apartment kitchen. Part of that experience involved exploring the wonderful vegetarian cookbooks that were starting to become popular.

As I experimented with meatless cuisine, I found myself coming face-to-face with the reasons for choosing a diet that didn't include animal flesh. One of my first vegetarian cookbooks was *Laurel's Kitchen*, and I credit it with opening my eyes to the reality of meat—that the slab of flesh on my plate was once a living, breathing creature. It was the dedication in that cookbook—which was to a "glossy black calf on his way to the slaughterhouse many years ago"—that caused the little lightbulb above my head to click on. I suddenly knew that I didn't want to eat meat any longer—that it didn't fit with how I felt about animals.

I found ways to use my interest in vegetarianism as I pursued my career in dietetics. While teaching nutrition to dietetic students at Central Michigan University, I made sure that they understood the core principles behind plant-based nutrition. As the director of nutrition services for a large medical clinic in Washington, D.C., I was able to help clients who wanted to control chronic diseases with plant-based diets. But the next big step in my understanding of what it means to eat compassionately came when I took a job with the

Physicians Committee for Responsible Medicine (PCRM), a vegan advocacy nonprofit group in Washington, D.C. That's when I really learned about the cost of meat, egg, and dairy production in terms of animal suffering and environmental devastation. It was a turning point for me both personally and professionally. I went vegan over a period of several months, and I knew that I wanted to dedicate my work to helping others adopt and thrive on a vegan diet.

WHY VEGAN?

Everyone knows that chickens make great moms. They cluck and fuss all day long over their eggs and then over their fuzzy little hatchlings. It's where we got the term *mother hen*, after all. Hens on egg farms never even get to see those babies, though. They sit in cramped cages, dropping their precious eggs onto a conveyer belt. Or if they're "free-range," they spend their entire lives in crowded windowless sheds.

It's the same on dairy farms. Cows give birth every year; they have to in order to continue producing milk. But that milk is for profit, not for nourishing their own babies, so the calves are separated from their mothers within hours of birth. The males, often still on wobbly newborn legs, are sold at auction to be raised in veal crates or for beef. On pig farms, breeder pigs get to see their babies and even nurse them, but they do so through the bars of a tiny crate. Some of them never leave that crate until they are too old to produce any more piglets and are trucked off to the slaughterhouse.

It's hard to reconcile those kinds of stories with the cozy ones we all grew up with—where animal families live happily on farms and baby animals play in fields and are fed and kept warm by their mothers. But the reality of modern farming is this: continuous exploitation of female reproduction, so that mother animals can produce babies, eggs, and milk, all for human consumption. They are forced to do it over and over until they are too tired or sick to be profitable and then they are sent to slaughter. These are the lives of female animals whether farms are owned by a corporation or a family, and it's true even in the production of organic eggs, dairy, and meat.

The natural lives and needs of these animals may not be exactly like ours, but no one denies that animals form deep bonds and that they are capable of suffering and of mourning. We know that, just like us, female animals will do anything to protect their babies. And that many of these animals, often forced to live in total isolation, are highly sociable, thriving in the company of their own kind.

In a world that values animal foods, these cruelties can't be avoided. It's a heartbreaking problem, but the solution is a simple one. Stop supporting the production of animal foods. We do it by going vegan, and, happily, it is increasingly easy and fun to do so. The wonderful bonus is a smaller carbon footprint—animal food production gobbles up a lot of natural resources and land—and for most of us, a much healthier diet.

GOING VEGAN: IT'S AN ADVENTURE

Whether you've already eliminated animal foods from your diet, or are just taking a few tentative steps, being vegan is truly an adventure. Knowledge about plant-based nutrition and vegan cooking, along with an explosion of new vegan products—as well as a society that keeps getting more and more vegan-friendly—makes veganism a more realistic choice with every passing day. But, even those of us who are experienced experts in living the vegan life know that there are sometimes hurdles and challenges. Most of us don't live in a vegan bubble for one thing. We might have meat-eating families and friends, or work in a nonvegan office. If you live in a small town like I do, you might not even know many other vegans.

In addition to providing you with the information you need to eat and live as healthfully as possible, I hope that this book will draw you into a community with other vegan women. We are such a diverse bunch—we look different from one another, have different political and religious beliefs, and often our vegan lifestyle is overlaid with traditions from our own families and cultural patterns. That's why JL and I established the VeganForHer.com community, a place where we cut through—or really celebrate—those differences in order to support and learn from each other. You'll find lots of resources there to augment and update what is in this book, and you'll be able to bring your questions on vegan nutrition, cooking, and lifestyle to JL and me. Most important, you'll find a community of women who choose to eat and live with purpose and compassion.

I hope this book will give you confidence about the ease and benefits of being vegan at every stage of your life, and that the information here will draw you closer to a diet and lifestyle that reflects your own spirit of generosity and compassion.

How to Use This Book

I expect that some readers will dip into the chapters of this book that are relevant to their needs, rather than read it cover to cover. If you aren't planning to have a baby, you probably don't have much interest in a diet to boost your fertility or support a pregnancy. If you're more a casual exerciser than an athlete, you may not wish to spend time learning about sports nutrition.

That's fine since most of the chapters of this book stand alone. Please be sure to read Chapters 2 through 5, no matter what, though. They provide important background about healthy eating that underscores much of the information on chronic diseases and the aging process. You'll see that I frequently refer back to the concepts in these chapters as they relate to cancer, heart disease, fertility, aging, depression, and even sports nutrition. Chapter 4 provides a little bit of explanation about the kinds of research I looked at in pulling together the information for this book. And the "Soyfoods and Estrogen" discussion on pages 57–63 is another little bit of foundational information that I'll build on throughout this book since it relates to questions about fertility, menopause, breast cancer, and the health of your bones, heart, and skin.

— continues —

— continued —

I think most readers will find Chapter 1 to be helpful, as well. It's aimed at those who are just getting started with vegan eating, but longtime vegans may find some fresh and useful ideas here. In particular, if you have ever struggled with staying vegan, be sure to look at the tips to help you ensure long-term success on pages 10–13.

In Chapter 9, I've shared some new perspectives on weight management and I'd encourage you to take a look at those even if you aren't trying to lose weight. It's material that brings a somewhat different view to the relationship between veganism and weight-loss diets and that also challenges some commonly held beliefs about body size, health, and dieting. Chapters 10 through 13 discuss health issues that are important to all women—how to slow the aging process, and reduce risk for breast cancer, heart disease, and osteoporosis.

Likewise, Chapter 16 shares some tips for boosting mood that you will find useful whether you suffer from chronic depression, have an occasional bout of the blues, or find that your spirit of compassion creates challenges in a world that isn't always kind. And finally, you won't want to miss JL's Chapter 17 with fun and inspiring tips for taking your veganism beyond the plate.

And if you have questions or thoughts about the material in this book, don't forget to swing by and join us at the VeganForHer.com community.

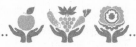

PART ONE
Going Vegan

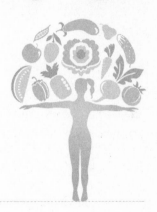

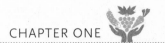

CHAPTER ONE

GOING VEGAN:
AN EASY TRANSITION

t's possible that nobody talks about food—and talks about it quite so enthusiastically—as vegans. That's because vegan food is so much fun. It's true that part of the fun sometimes lies in the unique challenges of eating an all-plant diet. Like creating the perfect birthday cake or putting together a drop-dead fabulous cocktail party without animal foods. But, vegan diets are popular, and the culinary world and food industry are completely on board. The growth of vegan foods—in stores and in restaurants—and the amount of information about vegan cuisine and cooking are nothing short of phenomenal. There are so many new foods and recipes to explore, which makes being vegan both a joy and an incredible adventure.

If you're new to veganism, the information here will help you get started. More experienced vegans may pick up a few ideas for pulling together satisfying vegan meals with minimal fuss, too. Don't worry if you don't like to cook or don't have a kitchen filled with expensive appliances. Vegan meals don't have to be fancy. JL's recipes are super-easy, and you'll also find plenty of ideas for meals that truly don't require any cooking skills at all. Basically, if you can steam vegetables, bake a potato, and open a can, you can be vegan. And if you want to do a little more prep than that, you still don't need more than a few pots and pans, a cutting board, and a food processor or blender.

PROGRESS, NOT PERFECTION

As you make changes toward more plant-based eating, you'll most likely find yourself tripped up now and again by unanticipated or challenging situations. The barriers aren't insurmountable, but they are definitely there. They tend to crop up mostly around social situations and travel—areas where food is not always within your control. You might find yourself faltering, too, when you are just too busy to come up with a meal that isn't familiar and easy, or when cravings for old favorites grab hold of you.

That's why this chapter is about transitioning, not diving in to become the perfect vegan overnight. Some people do that—and maybe you will in fact be one of them—but for most, going vegan is a process of learning, exploring, and experimenting. If you let yourself relax into that so that you enjoy and have fun with it, you're more likely to succeed at making long-term significant changes. Make those changes at your own pace and in your own way. These tips are ideas to keep you moving in the direction of a more vegan lifestyle.

ADD PLANT FOODS FIRST

When I counseled people with heart disease and diabetes, my patients were always surprised (and pleasantly so) that I didn't start them off with a long list of forbidden foods. Instead, I asked them to start by adding larger amounts of healthier foods to their diet. That's a process that works well for any kind of diet change and it's especially helpful when you're taking first steps toward a vegan diet.

Instead of anticipating a big empty space in the middle of your meal, keep filling your plate with more and more plant foods until there's no room for meat. You might start by eating more of the foods that are familiar and that you already like—plenty of fruit, vegetables, nuts and seeds, whole grains, and potatoes. Then, begin exploring new plant foods like beans and tofu and experimenting with simple substitutions like plant milks and veggie meats. You'll find that it's easy to reduce your intake of favorite foods ones you've discovered new favorites.

LEARN TO LOVE LEGUMES

Cooked beans and soyfoods are protein-powered mainstays of vegan eating. You don't need to eat huge amounts of them, but they play an important role in vegan diets. Depending on your family and your cultural background you may or may not be familiar with beans. When I was a kid, these foods made only the most infrequent appearances in our family meals. I saw baked beans at 4th of July picnics and lentil soup at my grandmother's house (and refused to eat either one). And I never even heard of tofu until I was an adult. Little would I have imagined that these foods would one day be on the menu for me every day.

An easy way to become familiar with beans is to explore the cuisines of other cultures where they are a dietary staple. White beans simmered with tomatoes, herbs, garlic, and olive oil are a Sicilian delicacy. Hummus from the Mideast, curried lentils from India, and re-fried beans from Mexico are dishes that combine tradition with some of the healthiest foods in the world.

You can soak and cook beans from scratch or simply open a can. In many cultures, bean preparation is simple. Dress up canned or cooked beans by adding spicy salsa and fresh or frozen corn kernels, or stir in a jar of curry or barbecue sauce. It's that easy to create healthy bean-based dishes. JL's recipes for Chik'n Lentil Noodle Soup (page 267), Adzuki Bean Potato Salad (page 258), and Mediterranean Beans with Greens (page 266) are great recipes to start with if you're new to bean preparation.

Legumes are more than beans, though. The diverse world of soy-foods provides additional opportunities to broaden your culinary horizons. Tofu is about the most versatile food on earth. It's bland and porous—soaking up whatever flavors it's cooked with—which means it is at home in soothing custards and sweetly decadent desserts as well as spicy and savory entrees. You can stir-fry it with noodles and vegetables for Asian-style entrees, slather it with barbe-cue sauce and toss it on the grill for an all-American picnic, or puree it with fruit to make a protein-rich smoothie. It makes a great break-fast scramble or quiche, too.

Tempeh, a fermented soy product that is a staple of Indonesian cooking, is another story altogether. Its flavor is robust and some-what mushroomlike. With its tender chewy texture, it's wonderful on the grill with herbed lemon marinade or cooked in coconut milk with curry powder. Or chop it with onions, celery, and vegan mayonnaise for a sandwich spread. For some fun and fast ways to introduce soyfoods into your menus, try the recipes for Easy Tofu Pumpkin Soup (page 271), Tempeh Patties (page 282), and Silky Strawberry Smoothie (page 250).

MAKE EASY EXCHANGES

You've seen veggie burgers in the store, but did you know that there are vegan versions of Italian sausages, chorizo, bologna, pulled pork, Pepper Jack cheese, Havarti cheese, mayonnaise, cream cheese, sour cream, ice cream sandwiches, and egg salad? Some require a trip to a natural foods market, but many are available right in your local gro-cery store. They are all available by mail order, too.

These foods make vegan meals convenient, fun, and familiar. Even as eating more vegan meals expands your food horizons and in-troduces more healthy plant foods into your diet, it really is nice to know that you can still have bagels with cream cheese on Sunday morning or apple pie à la mode for a special dessert.

Table 1-1: Simple Substitutions for Fast Vegan Meals	
Instead of . . .	**Try . . .**
Parmesan cheese	¼ cup walnuts + 2 tablespoons nutritional yeast + dash of salt ground to coarse powder in the food processor
An egg (for baking)	• 1 tablespoon ground flaxseed in 3 tablespoons water; let sit until thick • 1 tablespoon full-fat soy flour + 3 tablespoons water • ¼ cup soft tofu pureed with 2 teaspoons cornstarch • 6 ounces club soda (works well in cakes)
Buttermilk	2 tablespoons vinegar or lemon juice stirred into 1 cup soymilk; let stand to separate
Cream	Soak raw cashews in water to cover for 2 to 8 hours. Drain and puree in food processor. Add water to get desired consistency.
Ham or bacon in soup or beans	A few drops of liquid smoke
Meat in chili, spaghetti sauce, or sloppy Joes	Veggie ground meat
Chicken broth	Vegetable broth
Bacon in beans or crumbled on salads	Bacon bits, commercial tempeh bacon, homemade tempeh or soy curl bacon
Meat "cutlets"	Store-bought or homemade seitan cutlets

With these foods, going vegan doesn't necessarily mean starting from scratch—tossing out your old recipes and replacing them with new meals. Many of your favorite recipes could be just a step or two away from being vegan. Once you are a little bit familiar with legumes, soyfoods, plant milks, and the vast array of vegan specialty products, you'll see how easy it is to tweak favorite dishes to produce meals that don't taste all that different from what you're used to. Some examples:

- Make coleslaw or potato salad with vegan mayonnaise.
- Leave the ham out of lentil soup and give it a dash of flavor with liquid smoke.
- Use meatless ground "beef" in spaghetti sauce or on tacos.
- Top burritos with guacamole and shredded soy cheese.
- Stuff manicotti shells with a blend of silken tofu and vegan cream cheese.
- Take the beef out of your favorite chili recipe and replace it with lots of chopped vegetables for a healthier version.
- Pile homemade pizza high with grilled vegetables and, if you like, vegan pepperoni.

THINK OUTSIDE THE BOX

Granted—we're so used to building meals around meat and dairy foods that eating vegan already feels pretty far "outside the box." But your meals will become even easier if you let go of a few "rules." Who says fruit and cereal are for breakfast and vegetables and soups are for dinner? In Japan, the traditional breakfast is miso soup with vegetables and tofu. Vegetables typically appear in Chinese breakfasts, too, and beans are often on the morning menu in Mexico.

Getting too stuck in habits and tradition creates barriers to easy meal planning. When you're in a hurry, the fastest way to make breakfast is to heat up some leftovers from last night's dinner. Likewise, oatmeal makes a good afternoon snack—or dinner if you prefer. Apple slices spread with peanut or almond butter is a meal or snack for any time of day. So is a baked potato topped with hummus, or a few tablespoons of peanut butter mixed into a bowl of rice and topped with shredded carrots for a treat with Asian flair. Just eat healthy foods that you enjoy—whenever and however you like.

ADD WHAT'S MISSING

If you feel that something is lacking in your vegan menus and you can't quite put your finger on it, it's possible that you are missing *umami*. Described as the fifth taste (in addition to salt, sweet, bitter, and sour), umami is a flavor imparted by high levels of the amino acid glutamate in certain foods. Animal products—especially certain cheeses and fish—are packed with it. Umami was discovered more than 100 years ago, but scientists are only now beginning to explore how and why it makes certain foods so satisfying. It may be an innate preference or could be due to early experience (breast milk is high in glutamate and therefore in umami).

Fortunately, it's perfectly easy to add umami to your vegan meals, because there are plenty of plant foods and condiments that are loaded with it. Foods that provide umami include ripe and sun-dried tomatoes, ketchup, wine, tamari (soy sauce), miso (fermented soybean paste), dried sea vegetables, Marmite, nutritional yeast, dried mushrooms, olives, balsamic vinegar, sauerkraut, umeboshi plums, and umeboshi vinegar. Here are a few quick ways to add umami to foods. If some of these foods are new to you, check out "Vegan Pantry Staples" on pages 245–248. (Note: if you suffer from migraines or have fibromyalgia, please see my comments on umami on page 206.)

- Add a few drops of umeboshi vinegar (sometimes also called ume plum vinegar) to cooked vegetables. Look for it in the Asian section of the grocery store, and go easy on it; unlike other types of vinegar, umeboshi is very high in sodium.
- Sprinkle nutritional yeast over beans.
- Blend together oil-packed sundried tomatoes with white beans for an umami-rich sandwich spread or dip.
- Toss pasta with tapenade—a pâté made from olives.
- Add a dash of red wine, miso, or marmite (yeast paste) to bean soups.

Start Out Strong

There is no right or wrong way to transition to a vegan diet. You might want to just cut down on the amounts of animal products in your meals—aiming to use these foods more condiment-style rather than as the star of the mealtime show. Eventually, you can move toward cutting these foods out entirely as you learn to cook and plan meals without them. Another option is to simply start eating more vegan meals, gradually replacing your usual meals with more and more vegan ones as you gather new recipe ideas and explore new foods.

But many people opt to cut out types of animal foods, one at a time, and they often start with red meat. I'd like to suggest a slightly different approach. Dropping meat from chickens and turkeys from your diet has an immediate and significant impact on animal welfare. Because these animals are smaller than cows and pigs, eating just four ounces of chicken meat per week translates to 50 birds per year. And while all animals suffer in the agriculture industry, conditions for chickens and turkeys are the worst. These intelligent animals are also exempt from the Humane Slaughter Act, which means there are no laws in place to monitor the ways in which they are killed. So, if you want to make a big impact right from the start—and especially if you know that going vegan is going to be a gradual process for you—think about getting birds off your plate. It's a powerful step toward reducing animal cruelty.

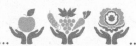

ENSURE LONG-TERM SUCCESS

We've all heard stories of people who give a vegan diet a shot and then go back to eating animal products. They say they didn't feel well or found it too hard to come up with satisfying meals or found social situations too difficult. Or maybe they didn't get what they expected from a vegan diet. When these people are high-profile celebrities, it can create an unfortunate image for vegan diets.

It's too bad because with a little bit of planning, some realistic ex-pectations, and some basic knowledge, anyone can make a successful long-term commitment to being vegan. Here are some guidelines to help you make sure that a vegan diet works for you.

Be Smart About Nutrition

I'll summarize the most important things you need to know about nutrition in Chapter 2. It's good to become familiar with the guide-lines (and they're easy) as you begin your vegan journey to make sure you have all your bases covered. You won't feel well if you aren't get-ting enough vitamin B_{12}, vitamin D, and iron. It's not hard to get them, but you need to know how.

Moderate Your Expectations and Celebrate the Benefits of Veganism

Boosting your intake of whole plant foods and cutting back on animal foods is almost guaranteed to make your diet healthier, especially if you've been eating fairly typical American meals up to now. It's a great way to take control of your blood pressure and cholesterol and to lower your risk for heart disease. You might see your skin getting clearer and you may shed some weight. But so far, nutrition scientists haven't identified the diet that makes you bulletproof against disease. Vegans may be less likely to develop chronic diseases, but a vegan diet isn't a promise that you'll never experience any health problems. It's not even a promise that you'll get skinny.

There are a few promises that a vegan diet can make, though. In ad-dition to any health benefits you may experience, eating more plants and fewer animal products will shrink your carbon footprint and lighten the load that your diet and lifestyle place on the planet. And it will remove your contribution to some of the worst cruelty to animals on earth. There is *no other diet* that can promise all of these things.

Find Support

One small study found that people who successfully limit animal prod-ucts for the long term are more likely to be involved with vegetarian groups.[1] Local vegetarian groups often hold social events that revolve around great vegetarian food. It can be a great way to meet others who share your vegan interests. But even if you aren't looking for vegetarian social events, you can find support in discussion groups online or on Facebook and Twitter. It really can help to know other vegans and vegetarians, to be able to talk through challenging situations, and to share recipes and food ideas. Don't forget to visit the VeganForHer.com community, too.

Opt for Convenience When You Need It

Every morsel of food you put into your mouth does not have to be cooked from scratch or be unprocessed perfection. Many people refer to veggie meats and cheeses as "transition foods," that help people go vegan. That suggests that you should drop these foods from your diet once you've made that transition. But the fact is that many vegans continue to eat these foods.

Whole plant foods don't have to be laborious, of course. It's no big deal to bake a potato or toss together a salad. Beans are far easier to cook than most people imagine. But sometimes you really do need to reach for a veggie burger or even a frozen microwave meal. It's okay to do that. When your diet is mostly whole plant foods, a little convenience won't hurt you.

Be Prepared

No matter how committed you are to eating a vegan diet, you might find yourself wavering when you're hungry and vegan choices aren't readily available. It's helpful to keep a few convenience items on hand for those extra-busy days. Batch cooking—making big quantities of food over the weekend to eat all week—is a time-honored approach of busy people that works just as well for vegans as for omnivores. It doesn't have to be fancy, either. Just cook up a couple of big pots of whole grains and beans to be quickly seasoned for soups, burritos, and salads during the week.

But the real challenges aren't in your kitchen; they're everywhere else. Many vegans have survived parties on a meal of margaritas, guacamole, and cherry tomatoes. It's not the end of the world, but it's not that much fun, either. The best way to make sure you'll have something to eat is to ask your host if you can contribute to the spread. When you show up with a platter of Brazil Nut and Almond Pâté (page 262) spread on French bread rounds, sundried tomatoes, and hummus with pita triangles, you won't feel at all left out (and you'll be very popular, too!).

Pack your purse with snacks for shopping, work, or meetings. In a pinch, you can make a meal of an apple, granola bar, and mixed nuts. Or pack a peanut butter and banana sandwich.

Remember Progress, Not Perfection

You may stumble sometimes in your commitment to a vegan diet. It might be a piece of nonvegan cake at your grandmother's ninetieth birthday party, or a nonvegan meal grabbed at the cafeteria on a day when you forgot to bring lunch and are up-to-your ears at work. Know that what you do most of the time is what matters and that the idea is to keep moving forward. Don't let little mistakes and slip-ups derail your efforts. Dietary and lifestyle changes take practice and knowledge. If you're learning, and moving forward, then you deserve to feel proud!

Easy Vegan Meals

10 GREAT BREAKFASTS FOR VEGANS
- Oatmeal with chopped apples and walnuts
- Scrambled tofu
- "Ice Cream" for Breakfast (page 249)
- Cereal with soymilk or almond milk

— continues —

— continued —

- Miso soup
- Toast with almond butter
- Fruit smoothie
- French toast using an egg substitute, see page 7
- Veggie pancakes (fold shredded carrots and zucchini into pancake batter)
- Bagel with tempeh bacon

10 GREAT LUNCH IDEAS

- Hummus wrap
- Spinach Bow Tie Pasta Salad (page 293)
- Peanut butter and banana sandwich
- Instant soup cup
- Soy Curl Paprikash Sandwich (page 279)
- Bean burrito topped with vegan sour cream
- Spinach salad with white beans, walnuts, and tahini dressing
- Quinoa or brown rice tossed with shredded carrots and chopped almonds with lemon vinaigrette
- Chickpea Salad Sandwich (page 278)
- Tofu Tacos (page 284)

10 EASY VEGAN DINNERS

- Pasta with tomato sauce and veggie ground "beef"
- Baked potato topped with barbecued tempeh
- Black-Eyed Pea and Collard Green Pizza (page 290)
- "Meaty" Lentil and Veggie Mac (page 293)
- Pizza topped with grilled vegetables
- Veggie burger and salad
- Tofu stir-fry with vegetables and noodles
- Baked beans, sweet potato, and braised kale
- Lentil soup with spinach
- Steamed vegetables topped with spicy peanut sauce

— continued —

10 HEALTHY VEGAN SNACKS

- Toast with Banana Butter (page 302)
- Trail mix
- Whole wheat bagel with vegan cream cheese
- Dark chocolate
- Whole-grain muffin
- Popcorn with nutritional yeast
- Frozen juice bar
- Vegan ice cream with chopped figs
- Salsa with baked corn chips
- Granola bar

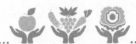

Three Days of Easy Menus to Ease the Transition

DAY ONE

Breakfast	Lunch	Dinner
Cereal with soymilk	Peanut butter and banana sandwich	Pasta with tomato sauce
Fortified orange juice	Raw vegetables	Steamed vegetables
Coffee or tea		
Snack	**Snack**	
Trail mix	Instant cup of soup (or homemade soup)	
Fruit		

— continues —

Three Days of Easy Menus to Ease the Transition   *– continued –*

DAY TWO

Breakfast	Lunch	Dinner
Whole wheat toast with almond butter	Veggie burger on whole wheat roll	Baked beans
Fruit	Chopped raw vegetables topped with **Sesame Tahini Dressing (page 259)**	Baked sweet potatoes
Snack		Vegetables sautéed with garlic and olive oil
Fortified orange juice	**Snack**	
½ whole wheat bagel with vegan cream cheese	Piece of dark chocolate	

DAY THREE

Breakfast	Lunch	Dinner
Oatmeal with chopped apples and walnuts	Bean burrito with guacamole	**"Meaty" Lentil and Veggie Mac (page 293)**
Fortified orange juice	Orange	Tossed salad with vinaigrette dressing
Snack	**Snack**	Steamed vegetables
Raw vegetables with hummus	Fruit smoothie made with frozen fruit and silken tofu	

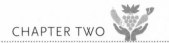

CHAPTER TWO

VEGAN NUTRITION: A PRIMER

If there's a learning curve with vegan nutrition, it's only because most of us don't have family or cultural habits to fall back on. Once you're in the swing of vegan meal planning, though, it all becomes second nature. The information in this chapter covers the fundamentals of planning healthy vegan diets. I'll expand on some of it in later chapters where some of these nutrients have special roles.

SEVEN GUIDELINES FOR PLANNING HEALTHY VEGAN DIETS

The basics of healthy vegan menus can be summarized as seven simple guidelines: eat legumes, eat lots of fruits and vegetables, choose whole grains, opt for healthy fats, choose calcium-rich foods, take appropriate supplements, and, finally, don't obsess over every bite of food. Let's look at these recommendations to see how they promote balanced and nutritious vegan diets.

1. Eat Legumes

Legumes are much more than beans. This group of foods includes peanuts (yes, they're legumes!) and peanut butter, and soyfoods such as tofu, tempeh, soymilk, veggie meats, textured vegetable protein, soy curls, and soy yogurt. And, of course, legumes also include cooked dried beans, peas, and lentils. These foods are important sources of protein in vegan diets, and in particular they are good sources of the essential amino acid lysine.

Amino acids are the building blocks of protein. Cells constantly take up amino acids from the blood to create new proteins, such as hormones, enzymes, muscle, and bone. Humans can make some of these amino acids, but nine of them—the essential amino acids—must be obtained from food. While all legumes, grains, nuts, seeds, and vegetables have all nine of the essential amino acids, legumes are the only plant foods that provide lots of lysine. If your diet falls short on legumes, you might not get enough of this essential amino acid. So aim for at least three servings of legumes every day. Even if you're just starting to add legumes to your diet, it's not nearly as difficult as you might think to work three servings into your daily menus, as you can see in table 2-1.

Table 2-1   Legumes in Vegan Diets
Include at least 3 servings of beans, peanuts, or soyfoods in your diet every day.

One serving of legumes =	Easy ideas for including legumes in meals:
½ cup of cooked beans, peas, or lentils	PB & J sandwich
½ cup of tofu or tempeh	Scrambled tofu
¼ cup of peanuts or soynuts	Veggie burger
2 tablespoons of peanut butter	Barbecued tempeh
1 cup of soymilk	Hummus wrap
1 ounce of veggie meats	Lentil soup
	Vegetables with peanut sauce
	Salad topped with toasted soynuts
	Bean burrito
	Taco with veggie "ground beef"

2. Eat Lots of Fruits and Vegetables

Diets high in vegetables may lower risk for a number of chronic diseases and may be helpful for weight control, too. Vegetables are incredibly nutrient dense, which means that they have very high nutritional value with low calorie content. They also contain thousands of plant chemicals—phytochemicals—that may have important health benefits. Frozen vegetables are sometimes more affordable and convenient, and they are just as good for you as their fresh counterparts.

Fruits aren't quite as nutrient dense as vegetables because they are higher in calories, but they are still packed with good nutrition and lots of phytochemicals. Their sweet flavor makes them useful in healthy desserts, and they can also add a nice contrasting element to more savory dishes. Aim for at least five servings of vegetables every day—½ cup of cooked or 1 cup of raw is a serving—and at least three of fruit. Be sure to include servings of dark green leafy vegetables or those that are deep orange in color. These foods—pumpkin, carrots, winter squashes, collard greens, kale, and spinach—are all excellent sources of beta-carotene, the compound that is converted in the body to vitamin A.

Vitamin C Improves Iron Nutrition

Fruits and vegetables that are rich in vitamin C are important for everyone, but they play an especially important role in vegan diets because they enhance iron absorption from plant foods. Women need nearly twice as much iron as men since significant amounts are lost through menstruation. The heavier your period, the more iron you lose, so younger women may have higher needs than those approaching menopause, a time when periods often (but not always) get lighter. Women taking birth control pills tend to have better iron status since their periods are generally light. In contrast, using an IUD for birth control can increase bleeding and may raise your iron needs.

Plant foods are rich in iron, and vegans typically have high iron in-takes. However, iron from legumes, grains, nuts, and seeds is bound to phytate, a naturally occurring compound that reduces mineral ab-sorption. Vitamin C can break the bond between iron and phytate, though, freeing the iron and increasing its absorption.

The effects of vitamin C can be rather dramatic, increasing iron absorption as much as fourfold in a single meal. You have to eat the iron-rich food and vitamin C–rich food at the same time, so it's im-portant to aim for vitamin C–rich foods at as many meals as possible. Good sources of vitamin C include citrus fruits, strawberries, green leafy vegetables, bell peppers, cabbage, broccoli, and cauliflower. (See Table 2-2) If you're eating these foods often, you shouldn't have any trouble absorbing enough iron. But, if you feel like you might be iron deficient—symptoms are fatigue, shortness of breath, and increased susceptibility to infections—ask your health-care provider to order a blood test.

3. Opt for Whole Grains

Whole grains are rich in minerals such as iron, zinc, and magnesium, all of which are stripped away from foods when grains are refined. Iron is usually added back, but other minerals aren't. Whole grains are also much higher in fiber and in a host of disease-fighting phyto-chemicals.

It doesn't mean you can *never* eat refined grains. It's okay to enjoy a piece of ciabatta bread or regular pasta at your favorite Italian restau-rant or to have a piece of cake made with white flour. Choose whole grains most of the time and enjoy refined ones occasionally if you like.

The way grains are prepared also affects their nutrition. For exam-ple, zinc absorption can be low from whole grains because, like iron, it's affected by phytates. But incorporating whole-grain flour into leavened breads enhances zinc absorption, because the leavening action of yeast or sourdough makes zinc more available. Zinc is also well absorbed from sprouted grains.

Table 2-2 Eat These Foods Together to Enhance Iron Absorption

Foods Rich in Iron	Foods Rich in Vitamin C
Almonds	Broccoli
Beet greens	Brussels sprouts
Black beans	Cabbage
Black-eyed peas	Cauliflower
Blackstrap molasses	Collard greens
Bran flakes	Grapefruit
Cashews	Guava
Dark chocolate	Kale
Garbanzo beans	Kiwifruit
Lentils	Oranges
Navy beans	Peppers
Peanuts	Strawberries
Peas	Tomatoes
Prune juice	
Pumpkin	
Sea vegetables such as dulse, nori, and kelp	
Soybeans	
Spinach	
Sunflower seeds	
Swiss chard	
Tofu	
Tomato juice	
Wheat germ	

Pair iron- and vitamin C–rich foods in meals to improve iron absorption:

- Lentil soup with spinach and tomatoes
- Bran flakes topped with sliced strawberries
- Baked beans with tomato sauce
- Strawberries dipped in dark chocolate
- Kiwi and orange segments sprinkled with toasted sunflower seeds
- Southern-style black-eyed peas with braised collard greens
- Stir-fried cabbage, broccoli, and tofu

4. Eat Healthy Fats

Some of the healthiest populations in the world have historically eaten plant-based diets that are relatively high in fat. Certain higher-fat foods like nuts and seeds are especially valuable in vegan diets. They're good sources of zinc, essential fats, and phytochemicals that reduce risk for chronic disease. Nuts are especially rich in the amino acid arginine, which is converted in the body to nitric oxide, a compound that keeps blood vessels relaxed and improves blood flow.

It's not surprising that women who include nuts in their diets are less likely to develop heart disease.[1,2] The big surprise is that, despite their high fat content, nuts may also help with weight control.[3,4] I'll talk more about this in Chapter 9. Aim to include a serving or two of nuts or seeds in your diet every day. A serving is ¼ cup of nuts, 2 tablespoons of nut or seed butter, or 2 tablespoons of seeds.

Avocados, which are actually a fruit, are another higher-fat food that can fit into healthy eating patterns. Used in Mexican cooking for more than twelve thousand years, they are rich in monounsaturated fats, the type that may help lower heart disease risk. They also provide lots of fiber and small amounts of vitamins and minerals.

While vegetable oils should be used sparingly, it doesn't mean that you need to eliminate them entirely. A teaspoon or two of oil can enhance flavors of foods and improve nutrient absorption, and, as I'll talk about in Chapter 12, olive oil may have some unique heart-healthy benefits. I'll also talk about coconut oil in that chapter since it's a fat that is increasingly popular in vegan diets. Since the jury is still out on how it affects heart disease risk, I recommend that you cook with coconut oil occasionally, rather than regularly.

Omega-3 Fats

Nuts, seeds, and oils also provide essential fatty acids to the diet, which are important nutrients. One, called linoleic acid (LA), is abundant in most diets. The other, an omega-3 fat called alpha-linolenic acid (ALA), is found in appreciable amounts in only a handful of plant foods. People who avoid all higher-fat foods run the risk of not meeting needs for this essential fat. Although you don't need much, it's important to include at least one of the following foods in your daily diet to meet needs for this essential nutrient. You can get enough ALA from any of the following:

1 tablespoon walnut or canola oil
1 tablespoon ground flaxseeds
1 teaspoon flaxseed oil
2 teaspoons hempseed oil
1½ teaspoons chia seeds
5 walnut halves
3/8 cup soynuts

Another group of omega-3 fats—called DHA and EPA—are not essential nutrients, but most experts think it's a good idea to include them in your diet. Also referred to as long-chain omega-3 fats, DHA and EPA are found in fatty fish and in fish oils; they're the reason fish oil supplements are so popular. They are thought to promote both heart and neurological health, and I'll be talking more about them in the chapters ahead. Technically, we can make all that we need of these two fats from their "parent" fat which is ALA—the essential omega-3 fat. It's possible that many people don't produce enough DHA and EPA, however.

One problem is that diets high in omega-6 fats, which are abundant in safflower, sunflower, corn, and soybean oils, may suppress the synthesis of DHA and EPA. So, a popular strategy for maximizing DHA and EPA production is to reduce use of those oils, choosing instead to use olive, canola, and nut oils. However, whether this truly helps in the production of DHA and EPA isn't clear. What is clear is that vegans and vegetarians have lower blood levels of DHA and EPA

Healthy Fats Primer

Linoleic Acid (LA): An essential omega-6 fat found in grains, seeds, nuts, and oils, especially safflower, sunflower, corn, and soy oil. Most vegans get plenty of this fat.

Alpha-linolenic acid (ALA): An essential omega-3 fat found in flaxseeds, chia seeds, hemp seeds, walnuts, canola oil, and soyfoods. Vegan diets can fall short if they don't include small amounts of these higher-fat foods.

DHA (docosahexanoic acid) and **EPA (eicosapentanoic acid):** Long-chain omega-3 fats found in fatty fish and algae. Some sea vegetables also provide small amounts of EPA. These fats are not considered essential in the diet since they can be synthesized from the essential fat ALA, but it's unclear how efficient the synthesis is. Vegans can consume supplements of these fats derived from algae.

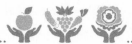

than people who eat fish.[5] To be on the safe side, I recommend taking a small supplement of these fats, about 200 to 300 milligrams of DHA and EPA combined (you can get both in one pill; check the label to make sure it contains both) several times a week. The DHA and EPA in vegan supplements come from algae, which is the exact same place that fish get theirs.

Avoid Bad Fats

As important as it is to emphasize healthy fats in your diet, it's just as important to minimize your intake of unhealthy fats. **Saturated fat,** the type found in meat and dairy foods, raises blood cholesterol and may contribute to risk for cancer and heart disease as well. It's not something you need to pay too much attention to, since most plant foods are naturally low in saturated fats.

Trans fats are also disease-promoting. While animal foods contain small amounts of trans fats, most come from processed foods where they are a common ingredient because they are stable and don't get rancid. Because they raise blood cholesterol and promote inflammation (I talk more about this in Chapter 3), trans fats are bad news all around and should be avoided. No more than 1 percent of your total calories—about 1 gram for every 1,000 calories you consume—should come from trans fats. Although food labels list trans fat content, this doesn't provide a foolproof way to avoid these fats. By law, anything less than ½ gram of trans fat can be noted as "0" grams. So you might be eating foods with small amounts of trans fats, and those small amounts could add up to 2 or 3 grams per day pretty quickly.

The easiest way to keep trans fats out of your diet is to look for the words "partially hydrogenated" oil on the ingredient label. That's a clue that the food contains at least some trans fat and should be avoided. Fortunately, trans fat intake is on the decline among Americans since they've been removed from many commercial foods.

5. Choose Plenty of Calcium-Rich Foods

Make sure you identify several calcium-rich foods that you enjoy and like to eat on a regular basis. I recommend six small servings per day of foods that are either naturally rich in calcium or that are fortified with it. That sounds like a lot, but these are foods that you're likely to be eating anyway—vegetables, plant milks, fortified juice, and tofu. And a calcium-rich serving of any of these foods is just ½ cup, or 2 tablespoons in the case of almond butter and tahini. While leafy greens are a great source of calcium, certain ones—spinach, Swiss chard, and beet greens—aren't included on this list because their calcium is too poorly absorbed. And tofu is a good source of calcium only when it includes the ingredient "calcium-sulfate," so look for that on the label.

6. Don't Shun Supplements

Supplemental sources of vitamin D and iodine can be important in helping some vegans meet needs. And in the case of vitamin B_{12}, supplements (or fortified foods) are absolutely necessary.

Vitamin B_{12}

Low intakes of this nutrient may raise risk for depression, memory loss, and heart disease.[6-8] An acute deficiency causes anemia and can do permanent damage to nerves. Plant foods don't contain vitamin B_{12} so vegans need to get it from either supplements or fortified foods. While you may see claims on the internet that fermented foods and sea vegetables provide vitamin B_{12}, what they actually contain is a compound that looks like B_{12} but doesn't have any vitamin activity. A daily supplement of 25 micrograms of vitamin B_{12} is the fastest and easiest way to cover your needs.

Iodine

Healthy thyroid function depends upon the right balance—not too much and not too little—of the mineral iodine. The most important sources of iodine for people in the United States are dairy foods and iodized salt. Dairy products aren't naturally rich in iodine; they contain it only because it's in the cows' feed and also because it leaches into milk from cleaning solutions used on dairy farms.

The iodine content of plant foods varies widely since it depends on how much is in the soil. The farther food is grown from the ocean, the less likely it is to be rich in iodine. Without knowing exactly how much iodine is in your diet, it's a good idea to give yourself a little insurance by using ¼ teaspoon of iodized salt on your food throughout the day or taking a small supplement of iodine—around 75 micrograms several times a week. The salt that is added to processed foods by manufacturers is usually not iodized. You could also consume a small serving of sea vegetables several times a week, since these foods tend to be rich in iodine—although as for land plants, the amounts aren't always consistent or reliable.

Vitamin D

All people, not just vegans, should consider a supplement of vitamin D. Vitamin D isn't strictly a nutrient since we evolved to get all we need when our skin is exposed to sunlight. That worked just fine when all humans lived near the equator, but in our modern world, the situation has become a little bit more complex. To make enough vitamin D, you'll need to expose your arms and legs to the sun several times a week for 10 to 30 minutes (the darker your skin, the more sun you need), during midday on a day when sunburn is possible. That's definitely not going to work in Duluth in December. To compound the problem, smog interferes with vitamin D synthesis, and so does sunscreen. Sun exposure also damages skin.

Since we didn't evolve to get vitamin D from our diet, it's not too surprising that there is so little in foods. A few fatty fish are the only natural sources, along with eggs from chickens who consume feed that is enriched with vitamin D. Foods like cow's milk are often fortified with vitamin D, but they usually don't contain enough to meet needs. Given that neither sun exposure nor foods are reliable sources of vitamin D, your best bet is a supplement. Most supplements contain vitamin D_3 (cholicalciferol), which is derived from animals, but vitamin D_2 (ergocalciferol) is a vegan option that is increasingly available. The RDA for vitamin D is 600 IUs.

7. Limit Processed Foods—But You Don't Have to Eliminate Them

Plant foods are beautifully complex packages of health-promoting compounds—not just nutrients, but thousands of phytochemicals. When we start to break these foods down, something will always get lost in the process. It's hard to replace the benefits of what gets lost, too, since many of these compounds work together to promote health. That's why whole plant foods should make up the bulk of your diet. But, gently processed foods have long played roles in cultural diets where people enjoy excellent health. For example, tofu, made by coagulating the liquid squeezed from soybeans (kind of like the way cheese is made) has been an important part of Asian diets for at least 1,000 years. Olive oil, a part of healthy Mediterranean diets for thousands of years, is the liquid squeezed from olives.

All of these foods can help vegans meet nutrient needs and create appealing meals. Processed foods such as fortified juices and plant milks can also help vegans meet nutrient needs. Veggie meats and cheeses should play a smaller role in your diet, but they sometimes make vegan diets more realistic for busy people, while foods like vegan ice cream are fun treats.

VEGAN NUTRITION IN A NUTSHELL: THE PLANT PLATE

You can put these recommendations into practice by planning menus around the Plant Plate (see page 30). It's a food guide especially for vegans, aimed at helping you plan a daily menu that meets nutrient needs.

Don't stress over it too much, though. It's the way you eat most of the time that matters, so if you miss a serving of legumes now and then, or fall a little short on your calcium-rich foods once in a while, it's not a big deal. And keep in mind that these are minimums. Almost all women will need more food to meet their calorie needs than what is specified in the Plant Plate.

Because foods containing calcium are everywhere in this guide, there is no "calcium group." Instead, calcium-rich foods from each group appear on the perimeter of the plate. As you make your choices from the Plant Plate groups, make sure you're including plenty of these foods from the perimeter. I've also included an optional group of plant milks made from almonds, hempseed, coconut, and rice. These foods—unlike soymilk, which is a legume—are generally low in nutrition and don't really fit into any of the food groups. Almond milk doesn't contain enough almonds to count as a serving of nuts, and rice milk doesn't have enough rice to be a grain. But, because most are fortified with calcium, these milks provide excellent ways to help you meet calcium needs. Hempseed milk has the additional advantage of providing some of the essential omega-3 fatty acid ALA.

You'll see a few other items on the side of the plate—a little shake of iodized salt, a B_{12} supplement, and a reminder to make sure you're meeting needs for ALA, the essential fatty acid. Add a vitamin D supplement if you aren't getting adequate sunshine.

Finally, vegetable oils are another optional menu choice. You don't need them in your diet, but it's fine to include them if you wish.

The Plant Plate

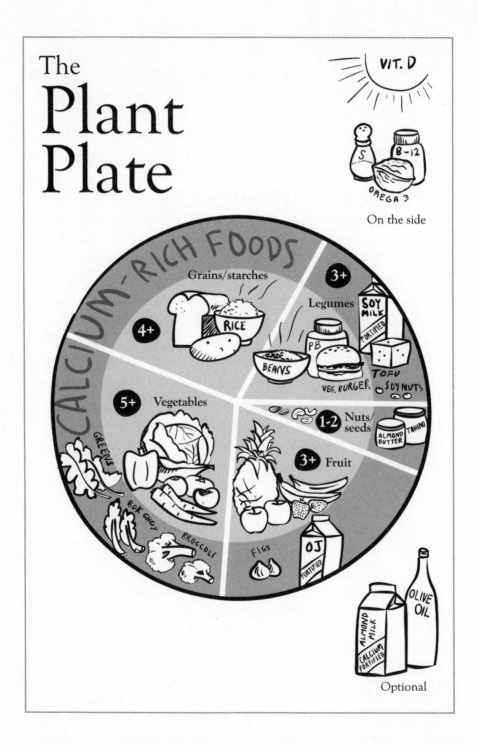

VIT. D

S
B-12

OMEGA 3

On the side

CALCIUM-RICH FOODS

Grains/starches

4+ RICE

3+ Legumes

SOY MILK
FORTIFIED
PB
BEANS
VEG. BURGER
TOFU
SOY NUTS

5+ Vegetables

GREENS
BOK CHOY
BROCCOLI

1-2 Nuts/seeds

ALMOND BUTTER
TAHINI

3+ Fruit

FIGS
OJ
FORTIFIED

ALMOND MILK
CALCIUM FORTIFIED

OLIVE OIL

Optional

USING THE PLANT PLATE

Food Group	Serving Sizes	Aim to include plenty of these calcium-rich foods among your choices from the Plant Plate groups.
WHOLE GRAINS and STARCHY VEGETABLES At least 4 servings per day	½ cup cooked cereal, pasta, rice, or other grain; 1 ounce ready-to-eat cereal; 1 slice bread; ½ cup white or sweet potato	Calcium-fortified cereal
LEGUMES & SOYFOODS At least 3 servings per day	½ cup cooked beans, tofu, tempeh; 1 ounce veggie meat; 1 cup fortified soymilk; 2 tablespoons peanut butter; ¼ cup peanuts or soynuts	Tempeh, calcium-set tofu, soybeans, soynuts, fortified soymilk
NUTS & SEEDS 1 to 2 servings per day	¼ cup whole nuts; 2 table-spoons seeds; 2 table-spoons nut or seed butter	Almonds or almond butter, tahini
VEGETABLES: At least 5 servings per day	½ cup cooked vegetable; 1 cup raw vegetable; ½ cup vegetable juice	Bok choy, broccoli, collard greens, Chinese cabbage, kale, mustard greens, okra, calcium-fortified tomato juice
FRUITS At least 3 servings per day	1 medium fresh fruit; ½ cup cooked or cut-up fruit; ½ cup fruit juice; ¼ cup dried fruit	Calcium fortified fruit juice, dried figs

ON THE SIDE

ALA (omega-3 fat)	1 tablespoon walnut or canola oil or ground flaxseeds; 1 teaspoon flaxseed oil; 2 teaspoons hempseed oil; 5 walnut halves; 1 ½ teaspoons chia seeds; ⅜ cup soynuts
Vitamin B$_{12}$	Daily supplement providing 25 micrograms
Vitamin D	Sunshine or supplement providing 600 IUs per day
Iodine	¼ teaspoon iodized salt or a supplement providing 75 micrograms of iodine 2 to 3 times per week

OPTIONAL

Vegetable oils	Be moderate with your intake—2 to 3 teaspoons per day. Choose extra-virgin olive oil most of the time
Fortified plant milks	A great way to get calcium

To summarize, use the Plant Plate to guide you toward a diet built around these core principles:

1. Eat legumes—at least three servings per day.
2. Eat at least eight servings per day of fruits and vegetables. Emphasize vegetables over fruits. Include dark green leafy vegetables and bright orange vegetables for vitamin A, and plenty of vitamin C–rich choices.
3. Emphasize whole grains over refined, and, if you like them, include some whole-grain bread and some sprouted grains in meals.
4. Choose moderate amounts of healthy higher-fat foods like nuts. Make sure you're getting enough of the essential fat ALA by including flaxseeds, walnuts, or one of the vegetable oils that provides this nutrient and consider an algae-derived supplement of DHA/EPA.
5. Make sure you are getting plenty of calcium by choosing leafy green vegetables, calcium-set tofu, soynuts, tempeh, fortified plant milks or yogurt, fortified juice, dried figs, almonds, or tahini.
6. Don't shun supplements. You absolutely need to take a supplement of vitamin B_{12} unless you are certain that your diet contains enough from fortified foods. Sea vegetables and fermented foods are *not* reliable sources of this nutrient. If you don't get adequate sun exposure, take a vitamin D supplement. And, if you don't use a few shakes of iodized salt on your food every day, a supplement of iodine can be a good idea.
7. Keep the focus on whole plant foods, but allow a little flexibility in your food choices where needed. Gently processed foods can be helpful for meeting nutrient needs and they can make your healthy vegan diet easier to stick with for the long term.

NUTRIENT NEEDS CHANGE AS YOU AGE

There's a little bit of a challenge to achieving healthy diets in later years since calorie needs often drop while certain nutrient needs increase. Even if you are eating and exercising the same way you did in your thirties, hormone changes can cause shifts in body composition that result in lower calorie requirements as you approach your fifties.

It's due in part to muscle loss, a common problem in aging. Since muscle burns calories and fat doesn't, your needs can drop by as much as 200 to 300 calories per day even if your actual weight stays the same.

Some loss of muscle is a normal part of aging, but excessive loss—called sarcopenia—can turn healthy older people into frail older people. As many as one-third of American women over the age of sixty have sarcopenia, which can interfere with quality of life in significant ways.[9] Loss of muscle makes it harder to do even simple daily tasks. It also causes bone loss and can raise risk for falls and broken bones. Incorporating more protein into meals and doing regular weight-bearing exercise can prevent muscle loss or even reverse it.[10,11]

The RDA for protein doesn't change for older people, but many experts think that needs are indeed higher. It's possible that protein is used less efficiently as we age, and the current RDA may not be enough to protect muscle mass in older women.[12-16] Packing additional protein into fewer calories may take a little more effort on a vegan diet, but there is an advantage to getting protein from plant foods. Compared to animal proteins, plant-derived protein may help preserve function of the aging kidney.[17] Getting more protein from plants—and eating lots of fruits and vegetables—also helps keep blood more alkaline, which may preserve muscles.[11]

Along with muscle loss, you're likely to lose bone content as you approach your fifties. Bone loss is greatest in the first five years following menopause, so it's a particularly important time to adopt bone-protective health habits. Higher protein intake and weight training are both important, and so, of course, are nutrients like calcium and vitamin D. Daily calcium needs jump from 1,000 to 1,200 milligrams after menopause. You can meet needs from plant foods that are naturally rich in this nutrient, but fortified foods—or supplements if you find yourself falling short—can help a lot.

Vitamin D needs increase after the age of seventy, too. If you depend on sunshine for vitamin D, you'll need more of it since vitamin D synthesis slows down with age. Too little vitamin D is bad for your bones and could also be linked to depression and chronic diseases like cancer, hypertension, and fibromyalgia. To protect the health of your skin, it makes better sense to slather on sunscreen and opt for a vitamin D supplement.

Nutritional Advantages for Older Vegans

Iron requirements drop dramatically after menopause since women no longer lose iron through monthly periods. It's still important to make sure you get enough, but getting too much probably isn't good. High stores of iron are associated with a higher risk for chronic diseases like heart disease and cancer. When researchers looked at iron stores in postmenopausal women in Korea, they found that vegetarians had lower stores and that this appeared to protect against metabolic syndrome—a cluster of risk factors for heart disease. Even when the vegetarian women were overweight, their lower iron stores were protective.[18]

Older vegans may also have a distinct advantage regarding vitamin B_{12}. Aging brings on digestive changes that make it harder to absorb the B_{12} that occurs naturally in animal foods. These changes don't have any impact on vitamin B_{12} that's found in supplements or fortified foods, though. As a result, people who are depending on meat and milk for their vitamin B_{12} may be worse off than vegans who are getting all of their vitamin B_{12} from supplements. Many omnivores don't realize that they should be taking supplements, so they might be at higher risk for some age-related changes like memory loss, depression, hearing loss, and insomnia that are sometimes due to poor vitamin B_{12} status. Since smart vegans are already taking supplements when they hit their fifties, it's not something they need to worry about.

HIGHER PROTEIN MENUS FOR DIFFERENT CALORIE LEVELS

Most vegan women will achieve adequate protein intake by eating a variety of whole plant foods that includes three servings of legumes per day. It's not necessary to eat foods in certain combinations to get adequate protein as was once thought. There are many times in a woman's life when higher protein intake might be desirable. A little more protein may be important for women over the age of fifty, or for those who have diabetes, or for women engaged in rigorous exercise. Since protein can help to control hunger, a small increase in protein can be a good approach for women who are trying to prevent weight gain or reduce their weight.

To get more protein in your diet:

- Replace one to two servings of grains or other starchy foods in your daily menu with legumes.
- If you don't already eat them, consider adding some soyfoods or seitan to your diet, since they are especially high in protein (although all legumes are protein-rich).
- Choose soymilk over other plant milks since almond, coconut, and hempseed milks tend to be low in protein.
- Choose protein-rich grains and starchy foods. Pasta, quinoa, and potatoes have considerably more protein than rice and barley.
- When you use nuts in recipes or for snacks, opt for the most protein-rich ones, which are pistachios and almonds.
- Make the most of your vegetable choices. Broccoli, corn, and spinach are among the most protein-rich vegetables.

The following menus are based on the Plant Plate, with extra legume servings, making them a little bit higher in protein than the average

Plant Plate Guidelines 1,500–1,600 Calories

SAMPLE MENU 1

4 Grains/starches   2 Fruits
4 Legumes   1 Fat
1 Nut/seed   1 Discretionary food
7 Vegetables

Breakfast	Lunch	Dinner
½ cup oatmeal with chopped apple, walnuts, cinnamon 1 cup soymilk **Snack** Raw vegetables with ¼ cup guacamole	Black bean burrito on whole wheat tortilla Salad with vinaigrette dressing (about 1 teaspoon olive oil) **Snack** ½ cup white beans pureed with sundried tomatoes on whole wheat crackers	Tempeh burger (see **Tempeh Patties [page 282]**) ½ cup brown rice 2 cups kale cooked in vegetable broth Red wine

SAMPLE MENU 2

Breakfast	Lunch	Dinner
½ cup scrambled tofu in 1 teaspoon oil 1 slice whole-grain toast ½ cup calcium-fortified orange juice **Snack** Corn muffin Green tea	1 cup white bean soup with chopped tomatoes and spinach Salad with **Tangy Tomato Dressing (page 261)** **Snack** ½ cup coconut milk yogurt with ½ cup sliced strawberries	Baked sweet potato ½ cup baked beans 2 cups steamed broccoli and cauliflower tossed with 2 tablespoons chopped walnuts Small ice cream sandwich

vegan diet. They give you an idea of what slightly higher protein intakes look like over a range of three different daily caloric intakes.

Each menu includes a "discretionary calories" item where you can plug in a treat or a glass of wine or whatever you like. I assumed that these extras would provide around 150 calories.

Plant Plate Guidelines 1,800–1,900 Calories

SAMPLE MENU 1

5 Grains/starches   2 Fruits
5 Legumes   2 Fats
2 Nuts/seeds   1 Discretionary food
7 Vegetables

Breakfast	Lunch	Dinner
1 cup muesli with 1 tablespoon ground flaxseeds 1 cup soymilk **Snack** Sprouted grain crackers with 2 tablespoons almond butter	2 cups vegetable soup with 1 tablespoon vegan parmesan cheese ½ cup **Red Hummus (page 263)** in whole wheat tortilla **Snack** ¼ cup roasted soynuts	1 cup black beans Baked potato with 2 tablespoons vegan sour cream 2 cups collard greens braised in vegetable broth Oatmeal cookie

SAMPLE MENU 2

Breakfast	Lunch	Dinner
Apple slices with 2 tablespoons peanut butter Bran muffin **Snack** ½ cup toasted chickpeas	**Soy Curl Paprikash Sandwich (page 279)** **Snack** Raw vegetables with ½ cup hummus	1 cup pasta 2 cups broccoli, spring peas, and summer squash cooked in 1 teaspoon olive oil ½ cup white beans 1 tablespoon pine nuts Red wine

Plant Plate Guidelines 2,000–2,100 Calories

SAMPLE MENU 1

6 Grains/starches
6 Legumes
2 Nuts/seeds
7 Vegetables

2 Fruits
2 Fats
1 Discretionary food

Breakfast

2 ounces tempeh bacon strips (try Fakin' Bacon)

2 slices whole wheat toast

Sliced tomatoes and optional shredded vegan cheese

Melon wedges

Snack

Bran muffin

Lunch

1 cup black bean soup

Shredded cabbage and orange segments with tahini dressing

Snack

Popcorn sprinkled with 1 tablespoon flaxseed

Dinner

1 cup quinoa

½ cup baked tofu

¼ cup peanut sauce

2 cups mixed greens braised in vegetable broth

SAMPLE MENU 2

Breakfast

1 cup brown rice baked in 1 cup soymilk with cinnamon and 2 tablespoons walnuts

½ cup calcium-fortified orange juice

Snack

Carrot sticks with 2 tablespoons peanut butter

Lunch

2 small (6-inch) whole wheat pita pockets with ½ cup white bean hummus

Shredded zucchini, chopped tomato

Snack

½ cup soy yogurt with ½ cup blueberries

Dinner

4 ounces tempeh baked in barbecue sauce

Salad with vinaigrette (1 teaspoon olive oil)

Sweet potato

2 cups cabbage braised in vegetable broth

GOOD NUTRITION IS MORE THAN NUTRIENTS

The Plant Plate and seven guidelines for healthy eating are really all you need to know in order to make sure your vegan diet is balanced and you're meeting nutrient needs. When it comes to reducing your risk for chronic diseases like heart disease, breast cancer, and depression, as well as addressing some of the special needs of the life cycle stages, other diet-related issues come into play, however. In the next chapter I'm going to look at some of the issues that lie at the center of many different concerns in women's health. You'll see that the types of carbohydrates and fats you include in your diet can have a big effect on health, and that there is much more to plant foods than their nutrient content.

CHAPTER THREE

BEYOND NUTRIENTS:
ONE HEALTHY DIET

The chapters ahead deal with diverse issues that affect women's lives—everything from infertility to heart disease to depression. As dissimilar as those concerns are, you're going to notice a recurring theme running through many of these topics. That's because the diet that protects the health of your heart is also the one that can clear up your skin, help you get pregnant, lower your blood pressure even if you're overweight, and protect against age-related cognitive decline.

Three particular conditions—insulin resistance, chronic inflammation, and oxidative damage—underscore many of the issues that are central to women's health. All three conditions are intricately related, usually occurring together and sharing common causes. I want to briefly describe each of them in this chapter. You'll see that, as complex as they are, their remedy is fairly simple.

INSULIN RESISTANCE

Carbohydrates from pasta, apples, brown rice, white bread, and that spoonful of sugar you put in your coffee this morning all share the same fate. They are broken down in the intestines to yield glucose, the sugar that serves as the body's main fuel.

Right after a meal, as nutrients are absorbed into the bloodstream, blood glucose levels start to rise. When the pancreas senses that glucose levels are increasing, it secretes insulin, the hormone needed to escort glucose into cells. Once glucose has passed through the cell membrane, it can be burned for energy. Then, as blood glucose levels drop, insulin production drops, too.

Although all carbohydrates turn into glucose, there is a big difference in how quickly they are digested, absorbed, and enter the bloodstream. Certain carbs, especially those in processed and refined foods, get dumped rapidly into the bloodstream, causing a fast surge of glucose followed by a burst of insulin. If this happens repeatedly—that is, if you are always eating these rapidly digested carbs—your body's cells are constantly exposed to high levels of insulin. They may react by becoming resistant to the effects of insulin, refusing to respond to its efforts to supply them with glucose. When insulin can't do its job, blood glucose levels get higher and higher. So do levels of insulin as the pancreas kicks into high gear, pumping out more and more of it, in a desperate attempt to move glucose into cells. The result is that blood glucose and insulin levels both remain elevated.

This is insulin resistance, also called insulin insensitivity. It's often a precursor to diabetes and is linked to heart disease, obesity, cancer, infertility, and even acne.

Some people have a genetic makeup that predisposes them to insulin resistance. It's also more common in people who are overweight. It's not clear, though, whether it's the cause or consequence of obesity, since insulin resistance itself promotes weight gain.[1]

You may think that cutting back on carbs is the way to prevent insulin resistance, but that's not the case. For one thing, despite a higher carbohydrate intake, vegetarians are actually less likely to have insulin resistance than omnivores.[2-4] This may be because vegetarian diets are often built around slowly digested carbohydrates.[5,6]

Slow Carbs

In 1981 Canadian researcher Dr. David Jenkins coined the term "glycemic index," or GI, as a way of comparing how quickly carbohydrate from different foods appears in the blood as glucose. Foods that cause a rapid elevation in blood glucose have a high GI, which may promote insulin resistance over time. Low-GI foods release their glucose more gradually, producing a gentle and sustained elevation in blood glucose. After a meal of these low-GI "slow carbs," glucose stays in the blood longer, feeding cells at a more even pace, and eliciting a slow and steady release of insulin.

The fiber content of foods is part of the reason for different GI responses. Other factors that affect GI include the way the starch is

Table 3-1: Building Diets Around Slow Carbs	
Choose these foods . . .	**More often than these . . .**
Pumpernickel, oat, and sourdough bread, and bread made from whole, cracked, or sprouted grains that have not been ground into flour	Breads made from flour
Sweet potatoes	White potatoes
Whole potatoes cooked in their skin	Mashed potatoes
Oats, pasta, and barley	Brown or white rice
Whole-grain cereals such as oatmeal, muesli, or shredded wheat	Ready-to-eat or instant cereals
Whole raw fruits	Juice or cooked or dried fruits
Raw or lightly steamed vegetables	Canned or thoroughly cooked vegetables
Regular full-fat soymilk	"Lite" or reduced-fat soymilk
Beans cooked from scratch	Canned beans

Adapted from *Vegan for Life*, Norris and Messina, 2011

configured (something that only food chemists can determine) and the way a food is processed or prepared. Mashing and pureeing foods increases the GI and so does prolonged cooking.

You don't need to know the GI of every food you eat in order to build your diet around slow carbs. A few substitutions along with attention to cooking practices are all it takes. (See Table 3-1) Flavoring foods with acidic ingredients such as lemon juice, vinegar, and tomato sauce will also reduce the overall GI of a meal.

INFLAMMATION

Redness, swelling, and tenderness are signs of inflammation, which is part of the body's immune response to injury. This reaction, which is aimed at healing, is temporary and beneficial. Sometimes the immune system goes into overdrive, however, causing chronic low-grade inflammation throughout the body. Unlike the acute inflammation that occurs around an injury, you can't feel this more subtle type. You wouldn't know you had it unless you had certain pro-inflammatory compounds measured in your blood or urine.

Inflammation is thought to be a common, quiet condition underlying heart disease, diabetes, obesity, cancer, and Alzheimer's disease. It's often seen along with insulin resistance and tends to be more common in people who are overweight.[7] Again, though, it's not clear which comes first—the fat tissue or the inflammation since lean people can have inflammation, too.[8]

People eating plant-based diets, including vegetarians and those who follow Mediterranean-style diets, have lower blood levels of pro-inflammatory compounds.[9–12] Foods linked to lower inflammation include fruits and vegetables, nuts, dark chocolate, and moderate (but not excessive) alcohol.[8] Exercise, diets built around slow carbs, and stress management all reduce inflammation.[13,14] So might the omega-3 fatty acids DHA and EPA.[15]

It has long been believed that the omega-6 fat linoleic acid—which is one of the essential fats—promotes inflammation. Found primarily in corn, safflower, sunflower, and soy oils, it may promote formation of pro-inflammatory compounds. It may also interfere with the production of the omega-3 fats DHA and EPA, both of which reduce inflammation. These effects have been questioned recently, though, and it's not clear that linoleic-rich oils have any effect on inflammation. While it's always a good idea to use vegetable oils with a light hand, there doesn't seem to be any reason to completely avoid oils that are high in these omega-6 fats.[16]

Smoking, stress, high cholesterol, elevated blood glucose, and trans fats all promote inflammation.[17,18] Another cause of chronic inflammation is oxidative stress.

OXIDATIVE STRESS AND ANTIOXIDANTS

As your cells burn glucose for energy, they produce damaging oxygen-containing compounds called free radicals. Free radicals have a short life span—about one-millionth of a second—but it's enough time for them to attack cells and impair their function. When these unstable oxygen molecules attack fats, protein, or your cells' genetic material, it sets off a chain reaction of cellular damage leading to a condition known as oxidative stress. Oxidative stress can speed the aging process and contribute to heart disease, diabetes, and cancer.[19–21] It also promotes inflammation.[8]

It's not possible to completely stop free radical production because it's a consequence of normal metabolism. However, it's possible to greatly limit exposure to external factors that contribute to oxidative stress. These include smoking, air pollution, ultraviolet light, and "pro-oxidants" in the diet (like excessive iron). High blood glucose levels also promote oxidative stress, which means that eating more slow carbs can reduce oxidative damage.[22]

The body has its own system that works to neutralize free radicals. But, plant foods, especially fruits and vegetables, are also rich in antioxidant compounds that work directly to put a stop to free radical damage. Nutrients such as vitamin C, vitamin E, and beta-carotene are powerful antioxidants. So are many phytochemicals. There may be as many as 100,000 phytochemicals in plants, including thousands of compounds with antioxidant activity. Animal foods contain antioxidants, too, but their content pales in comparison to plants. In a recent report on the antioxidant content of more than 3,100 foods, researchers noted that the average antioxidant content of plant foods is about sixty-four times higher than the average content of meats, eggs, and dairy foods.[23]

Advanced Glycation End Products (AGEs)

When diets high in refined carbohydrates dump glucose into the blood, insulin resistance and oxidative stress aren't the only things that can happen. Elevated blood glucose also promotes the formation of advanced glycation end products, or AGEs. These compounds can change the way proteins function. For example, AGEs may affect collagen, the main protein in skin, making it less elastic and leading to premature aging.

Although most of the research on AGEs has focused on people with diabetes or has been research in animals, there is good reason to believe that AGEs promote inflammation and oxidation and that they might raise risk for heart disease, Alzheimer's disease, and muscle loss in older people.[24-30]

Foods also contain preformed AGEs,[31] which are especially abundant in meat and foods that are grilled, broiled, roasted, or fried. Choosing moist cooking methods like steaming helps to prevent AGE formation. If you grill or bake foods, using acidic marinades like those made from lemon juice, vinegar, or tomatoes may also reduce AGE formation. Plant foods have much lower AGE contents, maybe because their high antioxidant content prevents AGE formation.[32-34]

A Simple Approach to Healthy Eating

Insulin resistance, inflammation, oxidative damage, and AGE formation are complex processes with potentially far-reaching effects. But they are so tightly intertwined that the best diet for controlling all of these issues can be boiled down to a handful of recommendations. In the chapters ahead, I'll talk about these concepts as they relate to specific health conditions. You might want to bookmark this page, because you'll see that I send you back to these core concepts regarding healthy food choices often.

- Eat a diet rich in antioxidants, found in abundance in plant foods, especially vegetables and fruits. Antioxidants reduce free radical damage, help protect against AGE formation, and reduce inflammation.
- Build menus around low GI foods—the slow carbs that produce a gradual and steady release of glucose to the blood. Moderate and sustained blood glucose levels reduce oxidative stress and help to prevent insulin resistance, inflammation, and AGE formation.
- Choose healthy sources of fats, those from nuts, seeds, and vegetable oils. Avoid trans fats.
- Cook foods with acidic ingredients like lemon juice, tomatoes, or vinegar. This slows the release of glucose into the blood and also prevents AGE formation.
- Use more moist cooking methods such as steaming to prevent AGE formation.
- Include exercise in your routine since it's associated with improved insulin sensitivity, reduced inflammation, and possibly lower AGE formation.[35]

Table 3-2: Underlying Health Issues Have Common Causes

	Causes	Prevention
Insulin Resistance A condition in which cells fail to respond to the actions of insulin and are unable to absorb glucose from the blood. It's characterized by high blood levels of glucose and insulin.	Elevated blood glucose Inflammation	Slow carbs Weight loss Exercise
Chronic Inflammation Abnormal, sustained, and systemic inflammation that can raise risk for chronic disease.	Elevated blood glucose Smoking Stress Trans fats Oxidative stress Advanced glycation end products (AGEs)	Slow carbs Exercise Stress management Long-chain omega-3 fats (DHA and EPA) Antioxidant-rich diet
Oxidative Stress An imbalance that occurs when free radicals overwhelm the ability of antioxidants and the body's internal antioxidant system to neutralize their harmful oxidizing effects.	Elevated blood glucose Normal metabolism and energy production Smoking Pollution	Slow carbs Antioxidant-rich diet

PART TWO

Healthy Eating for All the Times of a Woman's Life

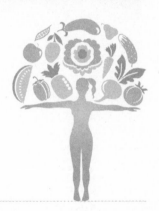

CHAPTER FOUR

Understanding Research on Vegan Diets and Women's Health

The medical database is packed with studies on women's health and with research on plant-based diets. They all contribute to our understanding about diet and health, but every study has limitations and there are always conflicting findings. Consequently, we can't draw conclusions based on any single study. It's the whole picture that matters—the totality of the evidence—not individual studies.

We need to also consider that some types of studies carry more weight than others. You may wonder why certain studies that are often mentioned in popular vegan resources aren't included in this book. It's because sometimes studies that are popular or that garner the most media attention turn out to be weaker types of research. In this book, I've tried to emphasize findings from the most robust and scientifically credible studies and to build recommendations around evidence that has the most solid support.

Best Evidence: Intervention Studies

In **intervention** (clinical) studies researchers divide study participants into two or more groups and have the groups consume different diets (or take a different supplement). Then they measure a specific outcome such as weight loss, or cholesterol levels, or bone density.

The gold standard for nutrition research is a type of intervention study called a randomized clinical trial or RCT. In these studies, subjects are randomly assigned to different treatment groups, and the treatment is compared to a placebo or to a control group. These studies are expensive, so they usually have a small number of subjects and last for a relatively short period of time. They aren't very practical for diseases that develop over a period of many years.

GOOD EVIDENCE: PROSPECTIVE STUDIES

Observational or epidemiologic studies contribute to understanding about diet and health but they carry less weight than intervention studies. However, in some cases, where it's difficult to conduct intervention studies—regarding diet and cancer, for example—observational studies are the basis for most of what we know.

Of the different types of epidemiologic research, **prospective** studies are the strongest. Subjects fill out questionnaires about their diets at the beginning of the study. Then the researchers follow their health over a long period of time. They're especially useful for looking at diseases that develop over the long term. A number of prospective studies are following large groups of meat eaters, vegetarians, and vegans, and comparing their disease rates over many years.

Case-control (also called **retrospective**) studies are a type of epidemiologic research that provides somewhat weaker evidence than prospective studies. In a case-control study, people with a particular disease are matched to a similar group of people who don't have this disease. Researchers ask the subjects about past lifestyle and dietary habits and look for differences. This approach is subject to "recall bias," in that people may "remember" their past diet lifestyle habits differently depending on whether they have a disease or not.

WEAKEST EVIDENCE: ECOLOGICAL, ANIMAL, AND IN VITRO STUDIES

An even weaker type of observational study is **ecological** research. In these studies, researchers don't look at the health of individuals. They pool information from different populations and compare the averages. Ecological studies generate information for further research, but they can't be used to draw conclusions about diet and health. In Chapter 13 I'll talk about ecological research on bone health and show how the studies have actually led us completely in the wrong direction.

Animal studies are much less expensive than human studies, and they provide relatively quick results. They also allow for the study of toxic compounds that can't legally be tested in humans. However, animals are metabolically, physiologically, and anatomically different from humans, so the findings from animal research are often poor predictors of what will happen in humans.

In vitro ("in glass") studies look at effects of dietary components on cells grown in a petri dish. They have obvious limitations, since cells don't replicate the complexity of living organisms. Nevertheless, because in vitro studies are very inexpensive and they produce very quick results, they are widely used. They are obviously also more humane

What Is a Meta-Analysis?

One way to make use of studies that have small numbers of subjects is to combine them into a meta-analysis. This type of study pools data from subjects in similar studies. A meta-analysis of randomized clinical trials provides stronger evidence than one that combines data from prospective studies. But in both cases, the results have greater strength than any of the individual studies included in the analysis.

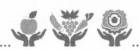

than animal studies and can be useful for looking at relationships that can't easily be studied in humans.

Most of the information in this book is based on the most credible types of research—that is, intervention studies and prospective observational studies.

Important Ongoing Studies on Vegetarian Health and Women's Health

There isn't much research looking directly at diet and health in vegan women. For this book, I've used findings from research in all different kinds of study populations, looking for diet and health relationships that are relevant to vegans. There are some large ongoing studies that include vegan populations, however, as well as smaller intervention studies that have used vegan diets. We also have a number of prospective studies that directly examine effects of diet on women's health. These are a few of the studies you'll see mentioned in this book. They have all generated findings that are important in guiding us toward making dietary recommendations for vegan women.

Prospective Studies That Include Findings on Vegetarian Health

European Prospective Investigation into Cancer EPIC-Oxford: Established in 1993 in the United Kingdom, its main objective is to look at the relationship of diet to cancer risk, although it is also evaluating effects on other chronic diseases. Of the 65,000 subjects, more than one-third are vegetarian and around 4 percent are vegan.

Adventist Health Study (AHS): This has been the only large study on health of vegetarians in the United States. The subjects are all members of the Seventh-Day Adventist Church living in California. Of the 34,192 subjects, 29 percent are vegetarian and around 7 percent are vegan. The study started out as a cancer investigation and then added a component to look at heart disease.

The Adventist Health Study-2 (AHS-2): Started in 2002, this second AHS study has enrolled approximately 96,000 subjects from all fifty states in the United States. About 28 percent of the subjects are lacto-ovo vegetarian, and 8 percent are vegan. With more than 7,500 vegans, this study promises to be a wonderful source of information about vegan health. It will also look at effects of individual food choices on cancer, heart disease, Alzheimer's disease, and other conditions and try to determine the impact of heredity versus lifestyle on health.

Smaller studies like the **Heidelberg Study** in Germany and the **Oxford Vegetarian Study** in England have also produced information about the health of vegetarians.

Prospective Studies Focusing on Women's Health

The studies below have not looked specifically at vegan women, but a number of them have provided important information on diet and plant foods that can be useful in guiding food choices for all women.

Nurses' Health Study: This study began in 1976 to investigate the potential long-term consequences of oral contraceptives. It enrolled 122,000 married female registered nurses ages twenty to fifty-five. In 1980, the researchers started collecting dietary data, and since then, this study has produced many findings about diet and health. You'll see it mentioned often in this book. While the prevention of cancer is still a primary focus, the study has also produced landmark data on cardiovascular disease, diabetes, and many other conditions.

Nurses' Health Study II: The primary motivation for developing the Nurses' Health Study II was to study oral contraceptives, diet, and lifestyle in a population younger than the original Nurses' Health Study cohort. It has enrolled 116,686 female nurses. A third population is currently being enrolled for the Nurses' Health Study III.

Iowa Women's Health Study (IWHS): This study began in 1986 with 41,836 postmenopausal women aged 55 to 69. Its aims include determining how body fat distribution, diet, and other lifestyle factors affect chronic disease risk.

Shanghai Women's Health Study (SWHS): This large ongoing study includes 75,000 women from Shanghai, China, who were between the ages of forty and seventy when they were enrolled into the study. Findings are providing information about diet and lifestyle effects on cancer and heart disease as well as other diseases. It's been an especially good source of information about the effects of soy-foods on the health of women.

Shanghai Breast Cancer Survival Study: Subjects of the SBCSS include 5,042 women living in urban Shanghai who were newly diagnosed with breast cancer between the ages of twenty-five and seventy-four. Its goal is to identify lifestyle and genetic predicators for breast cancer prognosis and survival.

The Women's Health Initiative Observation Study: Subjects are 93,676 women between the ages of fifty and seventy-nine. The study is examining the relationship between lifestyle, health, and risk factors and chronic disease over a period of eight to twelve years.

Intervention Studies on Women's Health

The National Institutes of Health established the **Women's Health Initiative Clinical Trial (WHI)** to address causes of death, disability, and impaired quality of life in postmenopausal women. It enrolled 68,131 women between the ages of fifty and seventy-nine, to look at effects of hormone therapy and diet on chronic disease.

Two studies have looked specifically at effects of dietary change on breast cancer survival. The **Women's Intervention Nutrition Study (WINS)** looked at effects of a low-fat diet on disease-free survival in women who were diagnosed with early-stage breast cancer between the ages of forty-eight and seventy-eight years. The **Women's Healthy Eating and Living Study (WHELS)** assessed the effects of a diet rich in fruits, vegetables, and fiber and low in fat on breast cancer prognosis in both pre- and postmenopausal women.

Many other studies contribute to knowledge about plant-based diets in women, some of them looking at cultural patterns like Mediterranean diets. All of this research comes together to help us paint a picture of optimal diets for vegan women.

CHAPTER FIVE

DIET AND HORMONES THROUGHOUT A WOMAN'S LIFE

One hundred years ago, the time between puberty and menopause lasted about twenty-eight years. Today, women can expect to have their periods for ten years longer than their great-grandmothers did as the age of a girl's first period continues to decline, and women reach menopause much later. And with increasing life span, you can expect to spend many more years in the postmenopause phase of your life, too.

In this chapter, I'll share some findings about the interplay between food choices and hormonal changes that can affect PMS, menstrual cramps, and menopausal symptoms. Soyfoods are of particular interest to women's health because they contain estrogen-like compounds called isoflavones. So, I'm going to start with some background on soy, which is relevant to this chapter and also to many of the other topics I'll be discussing.

SOYFOODS AND ESTROGEN: UNDERSTANDING THE CONNECTION

Soyfoods got their start in China more than 1,500 years ago and they have been a part of Asian diets ever since. In Japan, babies are often eating miso soup and tofu—two foods that play starring roles in traditional Japanese cuisine—well before their first birthdays. In China, soymilk and tofu are the most popular soyfoods. And, in Indonesia, the fermented soybean cake tempeh is a widely used traditional food, still produced the way it's been made for a couple of hundred years, by wrapping the beans in banana leaves and allowing them to ferment.

In addition to traditional Asian foods, soybeans have also been used to produce an array of veggie meats and cheeses, desserts, and convenience products for western vegetarians. All of these foods, traditional or newfangled, can make it easier and more fun than ever to be vegan.

Although soyfoods have been around for centuries, the interest in their potential health benefits is fairly new. In the 1980s nutrition scientists began considering the possible health benefits of soyfoods because they are uniquely rich sources of compounds called isoflavones. Soybeans and the foods made from them—like tofu, tempeh, and soymilk—are the only commonly consumed foods that provide isoflavones in nutritionally relevant amounts. If you don't eat soyfoods, your intake of isoflavones is negligible. Average isoflavone intake among older people in Japan and places like Shanghai, China, is between 30 and 50 milligrams per day (one serving of traditional soyfoods has about 25 milligrams of isoflavones), but in Western countries, it's typically no more than 3 milligrams.

Isoflavones Aren't Estrogen

Isoflavones are commonly referred to as phytoestrogens, or plant estrogens. It's not a very precise way of describing them, however, because isoflavones and estrogen are chemically different and have different effects in the body.

Estrogen, the female sex hormone, promotes secondary sex characteristics like breast development and regulates the menstrual cycle and reproduction. The onset of puberty in girls is the result of increased estrogen production, and many of the changes seen in menopause are due to estrogen decline.

Estrogen also enhances bone formation and protects heart health by raising levels of the good HDL-cholesterol and lowering levels of harmful LDL-cholesterol (more about this in Chapter 12). In contrast to those benefits, estrogen can promote growth of certain types of breast tumors.

Isoflavones have been found to have *some* of the same effects as estrogen, but not all of them. In fact, in some cases, isoflavones don't act like estrogen at all. So why don't these plant estrogens—which chemically look similar to the hormone estrogen—always have the same effects? The answer, at least in part, is linked to a monumental discovery made in 1996. It was a finding that completely changed the way scientists view estrogen and molecules that are similar to it.

To produce a biological response, estrogen needs to attach to receptors in cells. The existence of these receptors has been known for more than fifty years. But it wasn't until 1996 that researchers realized that there were actually two different types of receptors. The newly discovered one was dubbed estrogen receptor beta (ER β) and the original receptor is now called estrogen receptor alpha (ER α).

Some tissues have only one of these types of receptors. Most have both, but the relative number of the two different receptors varies greatly among tissues. This can affect how a given tissue or organ responds to estrogen and to estrogen-like compounds. And it explains much of the difference between estrogen and isoflavones. Isoflavones can attach to estrogen receptors, but they have a strong preference for ER β. In contrast, the hormone estrogen attaches to both types of receptors equally.

So, in theory, cells that have only or mostly ER α have a greater response to estrogen than to isoflavones. It might explain, for example, why isoflavones haven't been found to reduce bone loss in postmenopausal women even though estrogen clearly does. ER α is the main type of receptor in bones, so isoflavones are less likely to have an effect.

So isoflavones are not the same as estrogen at all. Instead, they are what scientists call *selective estrogen receptor modulators*, or SERMs. That is, because they prefer ER β, they are "selective" in how and where they exert their effects. The upshot of all this is that isoflavones sometimes act like estrogen, but they also sometimes have anti-estrogenic effects. They also have effects that have nothing to do with estrogen—for or against. And in some tissues that are affected by estrogen, isoflavones just plain have no effect at all.

Table 5-1: How Estrogen and Isoflavones Compare		
	Estrogens	**Isoflavones**
BACKGROUND		
Where they are produced	In the ovaries in premenopausal women, the placenta in pregnancy, and in fat tissue in men and postmenopausal women.	In hundreds of plants; among commonly consumed foods, soybeans are the richest source.
Types	Estradiol, estrone, and estriol. Estradiol is the most potent form of estrogen and is the dominant form in younger women.	The predominant isoflavone in soybeans is genistein. Two others are daidzein and glycitein.
How they work	Bind to estrogen receptors in cells.	Bind to estrogen receptors in cells.
Receptor preferences	Bind with equal affinity to ER α and ER ß. These two types of receptors can have different (and sometimes opposite) effects.	Preferentially bind to ER ß. Tissues that have more ER ß may respond more to isoflavones than tissues that have more ER α.
General effects throughout the body	Estrogenic effects in all tissues that have estrogen receptors.	Can have estrogenic effects, anti-estrogenic effects, or no effects. Isoflavones are SERMs (selective estrogen receptor modulators).

— *continues* —

Table 5-1: How Estrogen and Isoflavones Compare — *continued* —		
	Estrogens	**Isoflavones**
CLINICAL EFFECTS		
Hot flashes	Reduce frequency and severity.	Reduce frequency and severity.
Endometrial tissue	Stimulate cell proliferation and increase uterine cancer risk.	No effect.
Bone loss	Reduce bone loss and fracture risk.	Mixed results, but seem to have no effects on bone.
Heart	Improve health of cells lining the blood vessels.	Improve health of cells lining the blood vessels.
Breast cancer	Effects of estrogen on breast cancer risk are unclear.	May reduce breast cancer risk if consumed early in life. May reduce recurrence in women who have been diagnosed with breast cancer.
Skin	Preliminary research suggests a reduction in wrinkles.	Preliminary research suggests a reduction in wrinkles.
Cognitive function	May be beneficial in early postmenopause.	May be beneficial in early postmenopause but benefits appear to be limited.
Triglycerides	Increases levels.	No effect or reduces levels.

Certain drugs used to treat osteoporosis and breast cancer are also SERMs. For example, the osteoporosis drug raloxifene has estrogenic effects on the bone, which helps prevent bone breakdown. But it has anti-estrogenic effects in the breast and also in the uterus, lowering cancer risk in both organs.

The discovery that soy isoflavones are SERMs has been an exciting one because it suggests that soy could mimic estrogen in helpful ways—by reducing hot flashes or lowering risk for heart disease, for example—without the harmful effects that estrogen has in other tissues. As a result, the effects of soy isoflavones on breast tissue, heart health, cognitive function, bone health, and menopausal symptoms have been important topics of research over the past three decades.

The research in all of these areas is still evolving, but the one thing that has become clear is that *isoflavones are not estrogen*. And we can't predict how isoflavones will act in the body based on how estrogen acts. To learn about the effects of isoflavones, we have to study isoflavones, not estrogen.

How Much Soy to Eat

The amount of isoflavones in traditional soyfoods correlates fairly well with the amount of protein. For every gram of protein in a soyfood, there are about 3½ milligrams of isoflavones. This isn't the case for many processed foods, though. As much as 80 percent of the isoflavones are lost when protein is isolated from soybeans. These isolated and concentrated soy protein products are used in many veggie meats and protein bars. As a result, these more modern soyfoods or soy protein–fortified foods are often low in isoflavones.

Guidance for how much soy to eat comes from Asia where these foods are a usual part of diets. People in Japan and certain locations in China eat about 1½ servings of soyfoods per day.[1,2] Studies show that those eating larger amounts—two to three servings—have lower disease rates compared to people who eat little soy. So one to three servings of soyfoods per day is a reasonable amount. Choose traditional soyfoods made from the whole soybean most often. In addition to losing most of their isoflavones, veggie meats and other more modern soyfoods are sometimes very high in sodium and much lower in fiber and nutrients. Throughout Asia, the most commonly consumed soyfoods are miso, tofu, and soymilk. Tempeh also plays an important role in Indonesian meals.

Table 5-2: Isoflavone Content of Soyfoods	
	Milligrams of Isoflavones
Soy protein concentrate (a common ingredient in veggie meats)	3.5–28.6
Miso, 1 tablespoon	6.4
Soymilk, 1 cup	11.6
Edamame (green, immature soybeans), ½ cup	17.7
Tofu, regular, ½ cup	29.3
Tofu, firm, ½ cup	31.5
Soy flour, defatted, ¼ cup	32.8
Tofu, silken, ½ cup	34.6
Tempeh, ½ cup	36.1
Soy flour, full fat, ¼ cup	37.4
Soybeans, ½ cup cooked	47
Soynuts, ¼ cup	55

THE MYSTERIOUS MENSTRUAL CYCLE

Is it just a coincidence that your menstrual cycle and the moon follow a similar pattern? One popular theory is that, because we evolved from marine creatures who lived with the flow of lunar-regulated tides, our reproductive cycle adapted to that influence. The theory doesn't hold up very well, though, when you consider that other mammals have menstrual cycles ranging from 4 to 60 days.

Before its biological basis was understood, and, in part because of its lunarlike pattern, there was a real mystique around the menstrual cycle. Now we understand that menstruation is part of a tightly controlled, cyclical series of changes revolving around monthly release of an egg and hormone-driven effects that prepare your body for conception.

Many women experience some distinct symptoms as levels of hormones ebb and flow throughout the month. And, the decline in estrogen production that signals menopause can bring on its own unique set of physical and emotional experiences.

Premenstrual Syndrome and Cramps

The days before your period can be a time of intense discomfort characterized by bloating, breast tenderness, headaches, backache, mood swings, and craving for sweets. And getting your period may not bring much relief if you suffer from cramps.

Changes in hormone levels are thought to affect neurotransmitters—chemicals that transmit messages between nerve cells—in ways that give rise to some symptoms of PMS. For example, levels of the neurotransmitter serotonin may drop before your period, affecting mood and sometimes creating a desire for carbohydrate-rich foods, especially sugary ones. That's one reason why low-dose antidepressants that target serotonin are sometimes used to treat severe symptoms of PMS.

One group of study subjects found that both PMS symptoms and cramps eased when they followed a low-fat vegan diet.[3] This could have something to do with the higher fiber content of plant-based meals, which may help modulate estrogen levels.[4,5] Vegan women also tend to have high intakes of magnesium compared to both lacto-ovo vegetarians and meat-eaters, and supplements of this mineral are sometimes helpful in alleviating PMS symptoms.[6] Vitamin B_6, found in beans, bananas, potatoes, spinach, sweet potatoes, and avocadoes, might also have some beneficial effects.[7] Finally, it's possible that soyfoods could help with PMS symptoms, although there isn't much research in this area.[8]

Omega-3 fats—the ones that vegans get from algae-derived supplements of DHA and EPA—might help reduce painful cramps through their anti-inflammatory effects. Getting enough of these fatty acids along with adequate vitamin B_{12} seems to be especially effective.[9] Calcium supplements—1,000 to 1,200 milligrams a day—can be effective in reducing symptoms of both PMS and cramps.[10]

Although herbs have a long history of use for menstrual problems in folk medicine, the science isn't especially supportive. Despite more than sixty studies on effects of different herbal remedies on PMS, the only one that shows any promise is chasteberry.[11] There also isn't much evidence for benefits of restricting caffeine, sugar, or salt.

If you suffer from PMS or from debilitating cramps, any of these ideas are worth trying:

For cramps:

- Consider a calcium supplement providing around 1,000 milligrams per day.
- Take a daily supplement providing 500 milligrams of DHA/EPA from algae.
- Make sure you get adequate vitamin B_{12} by taking a daily supplement providing around 25 micrograms.

For PMS symptoms:

- Try supplements of calcium (1,000 milligrams per day) and magnesium (200 to 400 milligrams a day).
- Talk to your health-care provider about vitamin B_6 supplements since the levels that have been shown to be effective (up to 100 milligrams) are much higher than the RDA.
- Eat a couple of servings of soyfoods if you aren't doing so already. The evidence is sparse for a beneficial effect, but some women may get relief from these foods. (Veggie meats and foods made from isolated soy protein are typically low in the isoflavones that may be helpful, so choose whole soyfoods like tofu, tempeh, soymilk, and soy curls.)
- Sip on some soothing chasteberry tea. (Note, however, that this herb can blunt your libido—thus the name *chaste*berry.)
- Even though one study showed that high-glycemic index foods—the kinds that rapidly dump sugar into your bloodstream—

relieved symptoms of PMS, you will probably feel better in general throughout the month, and will certainly do more to protect your health, by eating a diet based on slow carbs.[12] But if you want a soothing sweet before your period, then by all means, go ahead and have it.

POLYCYSTIC OVARY SYNDROME (PCOS)

Polycystic ovary syndrome, which affects as many as 10 percent of all women, is a group of symptoms related to hormone imbalance and overproduction of male hormones. Women normally produce male sex hormones like testosterone, but in small, well-regulated amounts. In PCOS, production of these hormones goes into overdrive. The result is irregular periods or a lack of menstruation and often excess facial and body hair along with acne. PCOS, which is a common cause of infertility, is characterized by enlarged ovaries filled with cysts, which is where the syndrome gets its name.

Three characteristics—irregular menstruation, symptoms of excess male hormone production, and polycystic ovaries—form the "PCOS triad," although many women with PCOS don't exhibit all three. In fact, because there is a range of severity in symptoms, many women may not know that they have PCOS until they find themselves unable to conceive.

Between 50 to 70 percent of women with PCOS are insulin resistant, which means that they have high blood levels of both glucose and insulin as I talked about in Chapter 3. Elevated insulin levels may stimulate the ovaries to produce excess male hormones while higher glucose levels promote inflammation, which is also common in women with PCOS.[13] Drugs used to treat diabetes can improve insulin sensitivity and promote ovulation in some women with PCOS. For women who aren't trying to become pregnant, certain types of birth control pills can be very effective in reducing testosterone levels.

Many women with PCOS carry excess weight around their midsection and weight loss is often effective in reducing symptoms of

PCOS and improving fertility for these women. But it can be a challenge to shed that weight for women with PCOS. Insulin resistance promotes weight gain and higher levels of male hormones can increase appetite. It's often more realistic to aim for small reductions in weight, and, fortunately, losing just 5 percent of your body weight can reap real benefits. It can improve insulin sensitivity, lower testosterone levels, improve ovulation, clear up acne, and reduce facial and body hair.[14,15] This means that if you weigh 170 pounds, dropping 8 to 9 pounds could reverse many of the symptoms of PCOS.

Eating more soy might also be beneficial, although there is only scant research on the relationship of soyfoods to PCOS. Iranian women with PCOS who consumed isoflavone supplements—about the same amount of isoflavones that you would get from a cup of soymilk or one-half cup of tofu—experienced beneficial changes in hormone levels.[16] In contrast, an isoflavone supplement equal to about 1½ servings of soy per day didn't affect hormone levels in Italian women, but it did improve their cholesterol levels.[17] That's important since women with PCOS are at higher risk for heart disease.

It's even possible that the type of bacteria residing in your intestines—which is affected by diet—could affect symptoms of PCOS. Unhealthy diets that are rich in saturated fat and refined sugars can reduce the growth of beneficial bacteria—called Bifidobacteria and Lactobaccilus—while favoring the growth of harmful bacteria that may promote insulin resistance and inflammation.[18] The best way to reduce harmful bacteria colonies is to crowd them out by feeding the beneficial bacteria a diet that helps them grow and thrive. In particular, good bacteria love the sugars in beans. In fact, if eating beans gives you gas, you can take some comfort in knowing that it's the result of happy, healthy bacteria breaking down the carbohydrates in legumes. These are sugars that humans can't digest, so they travel intact to your colon where bacteria use them for food. You can also give your good bacteria population a boost by eating yogurt made from soy, almond, or coconut milk that contains live bacterial cultures.

The same diet that improves ovulation in women experiencing infertility can also improve many of the symptoms of PCOS. So even if you aren't trying to get pregnant, the guidelines for increasing fertility in Chapter 6 can be helpful for women with PCOS.

Here are tips for reducing symptoms of PCOS:

- Build your diet around slow carbs to reduce insulin resistance.
- Feed the healthy bacteria in your gut by eating plenty of beans.
- Include soy, almond, or coconut milk yogurt in your diet to boost the healthy bacteria population.
- Avoid trans fats, which can promote inflammation.
- Include soyfoods like tofu, tempeh, soymilk, edamame, and soy curls in your diet.
- If your symptoms are severe, drug therapy or birth control pills can help.

DIET, HORMONES, AND HAIR LOSS

You have some 100,000 strands of hair on your head and it's normal to shed about 100 to 150 strands per day. So hair at the bottom of the tub after a shower is nothing to be alarmed about. Rapid weight loss can cause excessive hair loss, so if you went vegan to slim down and lost some hair in the bargain, you may be tempted to blame your vegan diet. But it's much more likely to be the weight loss, not the absence of animal foods.

Menopause is also a major cause of hair loss in women. Hair growth slows and the strands fall out more quickly with declining estrogen levels. In most women, this is self-limiting; your hair will thin and then just stay that way.

No matter your age, though, if you think your hair loss is excessive, talk first to a health-care provider, preferably a dermatologist. She'll probably want to run an "alopecia blood panel" to test iron status and thyroid function. If your iron stores are on the low end of normal—and they often are in vegans—that could be part of the explanation. Even when iron is adequate to prevent anemia, it may not be in that golden zone that promotes luxurious hair growth. Although the lower iron stores of vegan women are thought to protect against chronic disease, if they aren't supporting a healthy head of hair, it's possible that getting more iron could help.

The essential amino acid lysine is needed for optimal iron absorption, and vegan women who aren't eating plenty of legumes may not get enough. In one study, women who took a supplement providing 72 milligrams of iron plus 1½ to 2 grams of lysine every day saw their hair loss decrease by nearly half.[19] This is a high dose of iron, however, and it wouldn't be advisable to take this much unless you know your iron status is suboptimal. Talk to your healthcare provider first and get your iron status tested before taking a supplement.

Zinc deficiency may also result in hair loss. Poor zinc status isn't easy to measure, however, so it's important to make sure you're getting enough of this nutrient by including plenty of beans, nuts, and especially seeds in your diet. Nuts and seeds are also important sources of fat in vegan diets. Getting enough fat, especially enough essential fatty acids, is important for healthy hair.[20] Finally, if you aren't certain that you get enough sun exposure to make adequate vitamin D, be sure to take a supplement. In addition to keeping bones strong, vitamin D may be important for preventing hair loss.

A commercial vitamin and antioxidant product manufactured in Belgium claims to reduce hair loss and improve wrinkles. The company performed its own tests, the results of which were published in a medical journal in 2007.[21] This was a small but legitimate study, but, since it comes from the company that manufactures the product, you'll have to weigh the evidence based on that. Because it contains fish oil and shark cartilage, it's not vegan. You could come close to mimicking the pill by taking a multivitamin and mineral supplement, drinking a few cups of green tea, and taking 700 milligrams of borage seed oil, 150 milligrams of grape seed extract, and a vegan supplement providing 350 milligrams of DHA and EPA.

Oral Contraceptives and Vitamin B$_{12}$

Birth control pills have been associated with low levels of vitamin B$_{12}$ in some women, but the reasons aren't clear—especially since taking supplements of B$_{12}$ doesn't always correct the situation. The reason might be that these low B$_{12}$ levels don't actually reflect a deficiency.

Blood levels of vitamin B$_{12}$ aren't necessarily the best indicator of B$_{12}$ status anyway. It's far better to measure levels of two compounds—MMA and homocysteine—that require vitamin B$_{12}$ for their metabolism. In B$_{12}$ deficiency, blood levels of both of these compounds are elevated. But in birth control pill users, low blood levels of B$_{12}$ don't always translate to elevated MMA or homocysteine.

Researchers think this is because of changes in the proteins that transport B$_{12}$ in the blood. In women taking birth control pills, the changes affect blood levels of B$_{12}$ but not the amount of vitamin B$_{12}$ that is making its way to tissues.[22,23] So, despite the drop in measurable blood levels of vitamin B$_{12}$, actual vitamin status seems to be fine.

This doesn't mean it's impossible to develop a B$_{12}$ deficiency while using oral contraceptives. Low blood levels of vitamin B$_{12}$ should be checked out with further tests. But this isn't an issue for vegan women any more than for those who eat meat. If you are keeping up with your B$_{12}$ supplements, you aren't at any higher risk for vitamin B$_{12}$ deficiency than any other woman taking birth control pills.

Plant Foods for Clear Skin

Some new vegans report an unexpected benefit to adopting a more compassionate eating style: clear skin. As most of us remember painfully well, skin problems often erupt during puberty when rising hormone levels stimulate the glands in pores to produce more oil. For many women, the problem can recur decades later as they approach menopause. This time, it's due to declining estrogen levels which result in a higher ratio of testosterone to estrogen. It's the same problem seen in younger women with PCOS.

Skin breakouts can occur at any time in a woman's life, though, and diet may help—although not in the way that most people think. It's not fatty food or chocolate that brings on pimples. Instead, the main culprits seem to be insulin resistance and possibly dairy foods.

A high-glycemic index diet makes acne worse, while switching to a diet based on slow carbs can produce significant improvement.[24,25] In fact, in women with PCOS, drugs that improve insulin resistance can also produce clearer skin.[26]

The effect may have something to do with blood levels of a protein called *sex-hormone binding globulin* or SHBG. Higher blood levels of SHBG lead to lower levels of testosterone in women, and less acne. In one study, women had measurable increases in their SHBG levels when they followed a vegan diet through two menstrual cycles.[3,27]

Dropping dairy from your diet may help clear up your skin, too. Because it often comes from pregnant cows, milk contains a number of hormones, including some testosterone precursors that may promote skin breakouts.[28,29] Interestingly, skim milk seems to cause more skin breakouts than whole milk.[30] It might have something to do with changes in hormone ratios when fat is removed from milk. Milk is also often high in iodine, which may worsen acne.[31]

Vegans tend to get plenty of several nutrients like vitamins A and E that help prevent acne. You may want to give a little bit of extra attention to zinc, which is also important for healthy skin, by getting plenty of legumes, nuts, and seeds in meals.[32,33]

The good news is that you don't need to give up chocolate. Eating a dairy-free diet that is based on slow carbs and rich in vitamins and minerals seems to be the best approach to preventing skin breakouts. For skin creams that fight acne, look for those that contain salicylic acid, a beta-hydroxy acid (see page 149 for more information on this).

VEGAN DIETS AND MENOPAUSE

Today, the average age of menopause is fifty-one years and average life expectancy for women is eighty-one years. So you can expect to live more than a third of your life as a postmenopausal woman. In fact, maybe a little bit more than that since life expectancy might be longer for vegetarians.[34]

The term *menopause* actually refers to a single moment in time—defined as the point at which you haven't had a period for twelve months. The time leading up to menopause, when your period is likely to be irregular, plus the first year during which you don't have a period, is called perimenopause. Once you haven't had a period for a year, you are postmenopausal. Some of the symptoms typically referred to as "menopausal" symptoms—like hot flashes—actually occur during perimenopause and during your first postmenopausal years.

Some women breeze through menopause without encountering so much as a bump in the road. They are happy to be done with birth control, cramps, and PMS. They never suffer even one hot flash and don't know what all the fuss is about. For others, changes in hormones don't go unnoticed and menopause represents a little bit of a rocky transition to this next stage of life.

What Changes with "The Change?"

Menopause occurs because your ovaries have run out of eggs, which causes them to stop producing the hormones estrogen and progesterone. It's the drop in estrogen production that results in so many of the changes associated with menopause.

Without estrogen, skin loses collagen and moisture. Lower estrogen levels are also associated with poorer hair growth, dry eyes, muscle loss, bone loss, and sometimes poor sleep patterns. Since women continue to produce some testosterone (it's a male hormone, but women normally produce small amounts), the higher ratio of testosterone to estrogen in the body can cause facial hair growth and acne.

These are all natural consequences of estrogen decline. Other effects, the symptoms we associate with the perimenopausal years, like hot flashes, are by no means universal, though. They vary considerably within populations and across cultures. In the United States, as many as 55 percent of women report having hot flashes at some time during menopause (which means, of course, that nearly half of all women *don't* have them). In comparison, Japanese women seldom complain of hot flashes.[35] The more common symptoms in Japan are chilliness and shoulder stiffness. Hot flashes are also uncommon among Mayan women in Guatemala, even though their hormone levels are similar to those of U.S. women.[36]

Comparisons around the world also show that how menopause is defined and viewed varies greatly. In some indigenous cultures, the menopausal transition brings power and respect to women as they become spiritual elders and healers. Menopause is likely to be viewed differently in cultures where older people hold positions of prestige compared to more youth-oriented societies like ours.

But even though it's clear that culture and outlook affect how we experience menopause, the hormonal changes that take place can't be denied. It's possible that vegetarians and vegans have an advantage since their higher fiber diets might be associated with somewhat lower blood levels of estrogen prior to menopause.[4,5,37] While this could create a little bit of a smoother transition to menopause, it's a theory that hasn't been tested yet. And certainly, many vegan women do experience menopausal symptoms.

Cooling Hot Flashes

The hot flashes that some women experience—those out-of-nowhere bursts of heat that can cause your whole body to break out in a sweat—are a little bit of a mystery. It's not clear how estrogen relates to hot flashes and who is most susceptible to them.

Some women choose to take hormone therapy as a way to reduce menopausal side effects and ease into their postmenopausal years. While hormone therapy can be effective, it can also raise risk for heart attacks, stroke, and breast cancer if you wait for several years beyond menopause to begin it. It's also not advised to take hormone therapy beyond the age of sixty.

Many herbal and alternative remedies have been recommended for dealing with hot flashes, but unfortunately most haven't been studied very well. Some of the most popular, dong quai, evening primrose oil, and gingseng, haven't been shown to give any relief from hot flashes. Studies on black cohosh and St. John's wort aren't conclusive, so it's not clear whether they help or not. It's important to remember that any herb that affects health is essentially a druglike compound with potentially harmful side effects. Taking big doses of herbs, especially without knowing whether they really help, isn't a good idea. They can interact with medications as well.

Some women get relief from "paced breathing," which is a simple free remedy that is always on hand. Slow your breathing to six to eight breaths per minute, instead of the usual fifteen. Inhale deeply through your nose for 5 seconds and then exhale deeply for another 5 seconds, keeping your thoughts focused on your breath. If you practice meditation, this is an exercise that will feel familiar to you. Some women are able to stop hot flashes in their tracks with this technique.

Smoking appears to trigger hot flashes, and so do spicy foods, hot drinks, and caffeine, so you might find that avoiding any or all of these is helpful.

Soyfoods and Hot Flashes

The low incidence of hot flashes among Japanese women, including those living in the United States, has long been of interest to researchers.[38] While there could be a number of reasons for this, research has focused on soy isoflavones in Asian diets as at least part of the explanation. Since 1995, there have been more than fifty studies on the effects of isoflavones from different sources in alleviating hot flashes. Most have used supplements of isoflavones, because it makes it easier to standardize the treatment (and also to "blind" the subjects from knowing if they are in the treatment group or the placebo group), but some have also looked at effects of soyfoods.

One of the problems in studying effects of foods or supplements on hot flashes is that researchers can't easily measure hot flashes in the same way they can measure blood cholesterol or blood pressure or weight changes. They have to depend on women's reports of hot flash frequency and intensity, and these kinds of subjective observations are always prone to error. In addition, there is a considerable placebo effect when it comes to hot flashes. That is, simply being enrolled in a study is likely to reduce incidence of hot flashes—whether you are taking the intervention product or the fake placebo pill.

Because of these issues, along with the fact that many of the studies have been small, it's not surprising that the findings haven't been consistent. But it does appear that isoflavones are effective in relieving hot flashes.

In particular, supplements that contain more of one certain type of isoflavone—called genistein—seem to be most effective. This is also the predominant isoflavone in soyfoods. An analysis of seventeen clinical trials found that isoflavones were consistently helpful in women who suffered from hot flashes, reducing both the number and severity by approximately 50 percent.[39] Some of these trials used supplements that were low in genistein. Had the analysis included only studies that used genistein-rich isoflavone supplements, the results would have shown even bigger benefits.

The amount of isoflavones needed for relief of hot flashes seems to be about 50 milligrams, which would be provided by two servings of soyfoods per day. A serving of soy is ½ cup of tofu, tempeh, edamame, cooked soybeans, or soy curls, or 1 cup of soymilk.

BEYOND MENOPAUSE

Declining estrogen levels and other changes that occur around the time of menopause set changes in motion that continue throughout the decades. They affect skin health, cognitive function, and more. I'll talk about these issues in Chapter 10.

CHAPTER SIX

A Plant-Based Plan to Enhance Fertility

Almost 15 percent of women who are trying to have a baby experience difficulty in getting pregnant. Sometimes the reasons aren't known, but often the problem can be identified and fixed. A blocked fallopian tube or fibroids on the uterus can often be resolved with relatively minor surgery. Endometriosis is another common cause of infertility that can sometimes be surgically resolved. This benign but often painful condition involves abnormal growth of the endometrial tissue, which lines the uterus. Removal of excess tissue can relieve symptoms and sometimes improve fertility.

About 25 percent of all female fertility problems are related to hormone imbalances that interfere with ovulation. PCOS, which I talked about in Chapter 5, falls into this category. Insulin resistance is often an underlying problem in women who have trouble conceiving, whether or not they also have PCOS. While the ovaries normally produce small amounts of the male hormone testosterone, high blood levels of insulin can cause testosterone production to go into overdrive, ultimately preventing ovulation. So not surprisingly, a healthful diet that prevents insulin resistance and therefore lowers risk for chronic diseases is also a diet that may normalize ovulation and help you get pregnant. This is an eating pattern that is built around slow carbs, healthy fats, and nutrient-rich meals. Getting your nutrition from plants may provide some additional benefits.

EATING TO IMPROVE FERTILITY

Most of the suggestions that follow are aimed at improving ovulation, but some of them could also help prevent endometriosis. Following these guidelines doesn't guarantee a pregnancy, but it can definitely improve your chances of having a baby. In the Nurses' Health Study, women who followed a "fertility diet" pattern based on the guidelines below had a nearly 70 percent lower risk of experiencing infertility due to abnormal ovulation.[1]

Choose slow carbs: If you're trying to get pregnant, pay particular attention to the tips on pages 43–44 for choosing slow carbs as often as possible. These are the carbohydrate-rich foods that produce a gentle, gradual, and sustained release of glucose into the blood. It's hard to imagine that the key to reversing fertility could be as simple as choosing sweet potatoes over white mashed potatoes, but it really does seem to make a difference. In the Nurses' Health Study, women were more likely to experience infertility when their diets were high in carbohydrates with a high GI—the foods that dump glucose into blood causing both glucose and insulin levels to rise.[2] And according to research in Danish women, keeping blood glucose levels in a healthy range can improve efforts to conceive as much as twofold.[3]

Choose healthy fats: Everyone should avoid trans fats, but it might be especially important for women who are trying to get pregnant. These fats can provoke insulin resistance and may also be linked to a higher risk for endometriosis.[4,5] There is evidence that they might raise risk for miscarriage, too.[6] It's easy to remove these fats from your diet; just avoid any foods that have the words "partially hydrogenated" on the label.

In contrast, healthy plant fats might be helpful for women who are trying to get pregnant. Both types of omega-3 fats—the essential fatty acid ALA that comes from walnuts, flaxseeds, canola oil, and chia seeds, and the DHA and EPA that vegans get from algae-derived supplements—might lower risk for endometriosis.[1] And choosing more good fats like the ones found in olive and canola oils, avocado, and nuts could improve insulin sensitivity and reduce inflammation.[7]

Get enough protein, and get it from plants: This is a non-issue for vegans, of course, since we eat *only* plant protein. If you're transitioning to veganism, though, it's worth knowing that every time you replace a serving of meat with protein from plant foods, you could cut your risk of infertility by as much as half. In fact, replacing some of the carbohydrates in your diet with more protein-rich foods like beans might be helpful, too.[8]

Eat good sources of the B-vitamin folic acid: Taking a multivitamin supplement seems to improve fertility and it's possible that it is the folic acid in that supplement that makes the difference.[1] This B-vitamin is crucial for cell reproduction and for amino acid metabolism. Folate, the natural form of the vitamin, is abundant in leafy green vegetables, orange juice, and beans, which explains why vegans tend to have higher intakes than meat-eaters. Folic acid is the synthetic version of this vitamin, and it's more powerful than folate; 1 microgram of folic acid from a supplement is equal to 2 micrograms of food folate. Eating a diet high in this nutrient from both foods and supplements improves fertility. It's also crucial for development of the embryo in the very earliest days of pregnancy; too little folic acid in the diet is linked to serious birth defects including spina bifida. So, taking a folic acid supplement now can do double duty: it may help you get pregnant and will also protect your baby right from the first days of conception.

Get adequate iron from plant foods: There is some evidence that a diet rich in iron from plant foods (but not from animal foods) supports normal ovulation.[1] This could be another advantage for vegan women since all of our iron comes from plant foods. Vegans do need to give a little bit of attention to getting enough iron in their diet, though, or more precisely, to ensuring that iron is well absorbed. The best way to do this is to consume a good source of vitamin C at as many meals as possible. See Table 2-2 on page 21 for a refresher on good sources of iron and vitamin C.

Eat a diet rich in antioxidants: Women with PCOS, endometriosis, and unexplained infertility all have increased markers of oxidative stress in their blood.[9] This suggests damage from free radicals, the compounds that cause oxidative damage to cells. Not surprisingly, when researchers in Italy compared diets of women who had endometriosis to those who didn't, they found that eating green vegetables and fresh fruits lowered risk for this condition.[10] It's possible that antioxidants may improve fertility in general.[11]

Avoid sweet drinks: In the Nurses' Health Study, women who drank more than two servings of soda per day were 50 percent more likely to experience infertility.[12] The effect might be due to the fast rise in blood glucose that comes from highly sweetened beverages. This suggests that it could be a good idea to avoid all highly sweetened drinks, including juices.

Avoid alcohol: Heavy drinking interferes with conception and puts your baby at risk for birth defects. Whether moderate drinking impacts either conception or your baby's health in the first few weeks of pregnancy isn't known. This is an area where, with so much at stake, it's best to err very much on the side of caution. If you're trying to become pregnant, become a teetotaler first.

Aim for a healthy body weight: If you are underweight, adding a few pounds can improve your chances of getting pregnant.[13] Cutting down on physical activity could help, too, since excessive exercise can

Diet and Fertility: It's Not All About You

It takes two to make a baby, of course, and the health of your partner impacts your likelihood of conceiving. Think of the guidelines for enhancing female fertility as a family plan since most of them are likely to affect male reproductive health as well. For example, supplements of folic acid and zinc improve sperm counts in men being treated for infertility while alcohol and smoking lower sperm counts.[15–17] Because free radicals can cause sperm damage, a diet high in fruits and vegetables and other whole plant foods could enhance male fertility.[18]

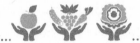

cause your body fat to get too low. (More moderate exercise is probably helpful for fertility, though.) If you are overweight and are having trouble getting pregnant, losing even a few pounds could help.[14]

VEGAN DIETS, SOYFOODS, AND FERTILITY

Although there isn't a great deal of research on this, it's possible that eating a plant-based diet gives you a little fertility edge.[19] Vegetarian women seem to have higher levels of SHBG, or sex hormone binding globulin, which helps to lower testosterone levels in women and may improve ovulation.[20] In fact, switching from a meat-containing diet to a vegan diet can increase SHBG levels.[21] One small study also found that vegetarian women had fewer ovulation disturbances than non-vegetarian women.[19]

The advantages of eating more plant foods were also seen in a group of women from Spain. The ones who ate a more Mediterranean diet—a plant-based pattern that lowers risk for many chronic diseases—

were less likely to have trouble getting pregnant.[22] And when you think about it, it makes a lot of sense in a body wisdom kind of way. Your body is most ready to support the growth and development of your child when you are healthy.

Since they are a source of isoflavones, which have effects that are sometimes similar to estrogen, soyfoods have naturally come under scrutiny for a possible relationship to fertility. Eating soyfoods had no effect on hormone levels in British vegans, vegetarians, and meat-eaters in the EPIC-Oxford study.[23] However, women who regularly eat soyfoods may experience a very slight increase in the length of their menstrual cycle of about one day.[24] This increase doesn't interfere with normal ovulation; it just delays it by a day or so. It may be a beneficial difference, too, since the slightly longer cycle may lower risk for breast cancer.[25] In Japan, where soyfoods are commonly consumed, women are at lower risk for breast cancer but don't experience any greater rates of infertility than Western women. In fact, Japanese women who eat the most soy have a lower risk for endometriosis.[26]

You might also be wondering whether it's okay for your male partner to consume soyfoods. A couple of highly publicized news reports focused on two men who developed signs of feminization—like lower testosterone levels—which were attributed to soyfoods. These men were consuming between fourteen and twenty servings of soyfoods per day. One of them, a nineteen-year-old vegan, was getting nearly all of his calories from soy. At those levels, it's certainly possible that soy isoflavones might have an effect on hormone levels.

In fact, many foods—including vegetables that you and your partner probably eat all of the time—can have negative effects on health when they are eaten in extreme quantities. For example, compounds in certain Chinese cabbages can affect thyroid function. They won't hurt you when you eat normal quantities of these foods, but one woman ended up in the emergency room after eating many pounds of bok choy every day.[27] Food is, after all, a great big complex stew containing thousands of chemicals. Some that are beneficial or benign at normal intakes become dangerous at high intakes.

Looking at what happens with more normal intakes of soy provides some reassurance. A meta-analysis published in 2009 that included thirty-two human intervention (clinical) studies found no effects of soy or soy isoflavone intake on hormone levels in men.[28] In fact, even in men who consume as much as two to three times the usual Japanese intake, there is no evidence of any effect on hormone levels.[29]

Clinical research also hasn't found any adverse effects on sperm or semen from eating soyfoods. For example, when British men consumed 40 milligrams of isoflavones per day—the amount in about one and one-half servings of soyfoods—for two months, there were no changes in their hormone levels or sperm counts or sperm quality.[30] Similarly, a Canadian study that compared men consuming diets supplemented with either milk protein or soy protein found no effects on sperm concentration.[31] Even when men consumed isoflavones in amounts that are many times the usual Asian intake, there were no effects.[32]

Interestingly, there is one case report of a situation where soy may have helped a couple conceive after struggling with infertility. The male partner, who had a low sperm concentration, took daily supplements of isoflavones for six months, which led to an increase in sperm quantity and quality, and a successful pregnancy.[33] That's not sufficient evidence to suggest that soyfoods cure male infertility, but it helps to bring some balance to the whole discussion.

People in Asia, where the birth rate is robust and healthy, would be surprised to know that Western vegetarians are concerned about the effects of soy on fertility. If you are eating soyfoods the way Asian people do—between one and three servings per day of traditional foods like tofu, soymilk, and tempeh—there is no reason to think that it will interfere with your efforts to have a baby.

HEALTHY PRE-PREGNANCY DIET

Up to half of all pregnancies are unplanned, and women often don't know they are pregnant for several weeks. If there is a chance that

Beans for Babies

It's just possible that beans are the ultimate fertility food. When you consider the recommendations for boosting your chances of getting pregnant, beans pretty much have it all. They are among the best plant sources of protein and are also packed with fiber—two things you want plenty of in your fertility diet. And that protein plus fiber makes them the ultimate slow-carb food. Beans are also rich in folate and iron, nutrients associated with improved fertility. The fact that they play a starring role in vegan diets shows just how it smart it is to build your ready-to-be pregnant diet around healthy vegan foods.

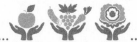

you could get pregnant, make your diet as healthy as possible right now. And there is no need for a whole separate set of recommendations, because the diet that gives you a little edge in conceiving is the same one that will see you through the early weeks of a healthy pregnancy. The most important things you can do are to ditch tobacco and alcohol and to start taking a supplement that provides 400 micrograms of folic acid. This is in addition to eating a diet that is rich in folate-containing foods like beans, orange juice, and leafy green vegetables. If you are underweight, you might want to try to put on a few pounds. If you are overweight, losing just a few pounds could reduce your risk of pregnancy complications. Aside from that, avoiding sodas (they're really never good for you anyway), getting active, and loading your diet with lots of good things—slow carbs, fruits and veggies, healthy plant proteins, and good-for-you fats—will help you give your baby-to-be the best start in life possible. And when that pregnancy test strip shows that there is a baby on board, turn to the next chapter for advice on how to eat well through your pregnancy.

CHAPTER SEVEN

GROWING NEW VEGANS: NUTRITION FOR PREGNANCY AND BREASTFEEDING

Your decision to stick with a vegan diet through your pregnancy might raise some eyebrows among friends and families, and maybe even health-care providers. Don't worry, though; the evidence is on your side. Well-nourished women give birth to healthy vegan babies who thrive on their mom's breast milk. There are definitely things you need to pay attention to. (That's true for meat-eating pregnant women, too.) But it's not at all difficult.

VEGAN WOMEN HAVE HEALTHY BABIES

Back in 1987, researchers looked at the medical records of 775 women who had babies while living in a vegan community in Tennessee. They found that a vegan diet had no effect on pregnancy weight gain or the birth weights of babies.[1] Both are important indicators of a healthy pregnancy. An earlier and smaller study in England also found that being vegan during pregnancy didn't affect birth weight of babies.[2]

In contrast to those findings, some women who follow low-calorie macrobiotic diets have given birth to small babies.[3,4] Macrobiotic diets are generally more restrictive than nonmacrobiotic vegan diets, which may explain the too-low-calorie intakes of these pregnant women. Adequate calories and weight gain are keys to a healthy pregnancy.

CALORIES FOR YOU AND YOUR BABY

You're eating for two, but that second person is a tiny one. You'll need around 340 extra calories a day beginning with the fourth month of pregnancy and will need to add another 100 calories to that beginning with the seventh month of pregnancy. It's not at all difficult to get those extra calories on a vegan diet. By adding just one cup of beans, ½ cup of brown rice, a piece of fruit, and a cup of cooked vegetables to your diet, you'd meet needs for the additional 450 calories needed in the last trimester.

Many women find that their appetite guides them toward a natural increase in food intake. If you're struggling to meet calorie needs and to maintain a healthy weight gain it can help to eat more frequently—many small meals throughout the day instead of three big ones—and to take advantage of foods that are higher in calories like nut butters, trail mix, dried fruits, and foods cooked with a little bit of vegetable oil. Liquids like juices, smoothies, and shakes can make it easy to incorporate extra calories into meals also. It's fine to indulge a little bit, too, with some higher-calorie treats—especially if you choose healthier versions like fruit crisps, or muffins made with whole grains—but it's also important to remember that you'll need to pack lots of extra nutrition into those 350 to 450 calories every day.

GOOD NUTRITION FOR A HEALTHY VEGAN PREGNANCY

While calorie needs increase by about 15 to 20 percent in pregnancy, needs for some nutrients rise by as much as 30 to 50 percent. You need considerably more protein, folic acid and other B vitamins, iodine, iron, and zinc in pregnancy, so it's crucial to choose good sources of these foods. In some cases, as you'll see below, supplements are recommended to meet needs. Be sure to talk with your health-care provider about which supplements are right for you since high doses of certain nutrients can be harmful.

Protein

Your baby needs protein to grow muscles, skin, and bones and for formation of compounds such as hormones and enzymes. Some of the protein in your diet will also go toward changes that support pregnancy, like an increase in blood volume and expansion of your uterus. As a result, protein needs increase in pregnancy by 25 grams per day, which is an increase of roughly 50 percent more than needs of a nonpregnant woman. It's possible that requirements are somewhat higher for vegan women because plant protein is digested slightly less well than animal protein. It's a small difference, though, and it's easy to meet protein needs of pregnancy on a vegan diet. Depending on body size, most pregnant vegan women need between 75 and 85 grams of protein per day.

Protein-rich foods and snacks to emphasize in your menus include beans, hummus, peanut butter, tofu (try silken tofu in smoothies or soups), and veggie meats. Opt for more protein-rich grains like quinoa and oats in place of rice. In a pinch, a protein bar can be a good on-the-go snack.

Table 7-1: Protein Superstars for Pregnancy	
Legumes	All legumes—beans, peanuts, and soyfoods—are good sources of protein. Certain soyfoods, like tempeh and firm tofu, are especially protein-rich.
Grains and starchy foods	Quinoa, oats, potatoes
Nuts	Almonds and almond butter, cashews, pistachios, walnuts
Vegetables	Broccoli, spinach

Iron

Iron needs also increase by about 50 percent in pregnancy. Your baby needs iron for growth and will also store iron to be used during the first few months outside the womb. Iron is also needed to make hemoglobin, the blood component that carries oxygen to all your cells and to your baby. In fact, your blood volume will expand by nearly 50 percent to accommodate the oxygen needs of pregnancy. Since your baby gets first dibs on the iron in your diet, inadequate intake raises your risk for anemia.

A couple of things work in favor of iron status in pregnancy. Lack of menstruation conserves iron, while absorption of non-heme iron, the kind found in plant foods, is much more efficient in pregnancy. But, because iron is less available from plant foods compared to meat, needs can be quite a bit higher for vegans. The RDA for non-vegetarian pregnant women is 27 milligrams, but it may be closer to 50 milligrams for pregnant vegans.

The truth is that it's hard to meet the iron needs of pregnancy whether you eat meat or not. Most pregnant women benefit from iron supplements and they are routinely prescribed regardless of a pregnant woman's diet. Most prenatal supplements include iron and the amount your health-care provider recommends will be based on your iron status.

Even with supplementation, it's still important to consume an iron-rich diet and to aim for a small serving of a vitamin C–rich food at every meal to improve iron absorption. Refer back to the list on page 21 for some tips on matching up iron and vitamin C sources.

Zinc

Pregnant women need 11 milligrams of zinc per day, and it's possible that vegans require more. It's the same as the situation for iron; absorption of this mineral is lower from plant foods compared to animal foods. You might remember from Chapter 2 that the zinc in sprouted grains is well absorbed. But because of food safety issues, pregnant women should avoid sprouts since they can be a source of bacterial contamination. Including some whole grain bread in your diet is a good way to get plenty of well-absorbed zinc, since leavening frees up zinc for absorption. (Breads made from white flour and other refined grains are typically low in zinc, though.) Other good sources of zinc include wheat germ, legumes, peanut butter, and tahini. For some additional insurance, make sure that your prenatal supplement contains zinc.

Calcium

While you'll be supplying all of the calcium needed to build your baby's skeleton, dietary requirements for this mineral don't increase when you are pregnant. This is because absorption of dietary calcium increases dramatically with pregnancy. If you were meeting calcium needs before you became pregnant, chances are that you'll continue to do so. If you think your diet may have fallen short, take a look at the calcium sources in the Plant Plate and make sure you're consuming at least 6 servings a day of these foods.

Vitamin D

Although requirements for vitamin D also don't change with pregnancy, getting enough is important. Take a supplement of vitamin D unless you are absolutely certain that you are making enough from sun exposure. Even people living in sunny climates can sometimes fall short on this nutrient.

Vitamin B$_{12}$

Smart vegans are already taking vitamin B$_{12}$ supplements or regularly eating foods that are fortified with this essential nutrient. If you've been lax about it, now is definitely the time to get on track. A lack of vitamin B$_{12}$ can have serious consequences for your baby. Although your prenatal supplement probably contains vitamin B$_{12}$, it may not be enough for vegans. Look for a supplement that provides around 25 micrograms of vitamin B$_{12}$ and take it daily. It's best if you can crush or chew it to maximize absorption.

Folic Acid

Folate and folic acid are two forms of the same B vitamin. Folate is the form that occurs naturally in foods. The best sources are leafy green vegetables (the word *folate* is derived from "foliage"), but dried beans, oranges and orange juice, and peanuts are also great sources. Not surprisingly, vegans often have higher folate intakes than omnivores.

Folic acid is the synthetic form of the vitamin, used in supplements and fortified foods. Since 1998, it's been added to all enriched grain products like bread, pasta, and cereals in the United States, in an effort to make sure that pregnant women get enough. Adequate folic acid is absolutely crucial in the earliest stages of pregnancy—usually weeks before a woman even knows she is pregnant—to prevent serious neurological birth defects like spina bifida. It also may reduce risk for cleft palate and possibly for autism. The Centers for Disease Control and Prevention recommend that women who might become pregnant should take 400 micrograms of folic acid daily beginning a month before pregnancy.

But what about vegans whose diets are already high in foods that are rich sources of folate? Do they need supplements of folic acid? We don't know the answer to that question. We do know that folic acid supplements are extremely effective in preventing birth defects, but there haven't been any studies evaluating the effects of diets high in folate from foods. It's possible that, in some women, there are differences between the protective effects of the two types of the vitamin since folic acid is always well absorbed, while a number of factors, including genetic differences, affect absorption of food folate.[5]

Some concerns have been raised about a possible connection between folic acid supplements and cancer risk. But this research looked at people consuming large doses of folic acid or taking supplements over a number of years. The results don't appear to be relevant to women taking a daily supplement of 400 micrograms of folic acid throughout pregnancy. Based on the current research, benefits of folic acid supplements in pregnancy far outweigh any risks. These supplements are recommended for all pregnant women, including vegans who are getting plenty of folate from beans and leafy green vegetables.

Omega-3 Fats

DHA is the long chain omega-3 fat that is found in fatty fish and in vegan supplements derived from algae. It's important for development of your baby's vision and could play a role in cognitive development, too. Vegetarians who don't take DHA supplements typically have low blood levels of this fatty acid. The debate continues about whether this matters for pregnant vegans, but some research suggests that higher DHA intake during pregnancy is associated with slightly better development in infants.[6] Right now, many experts recommend that pregnant women take supplements providing 300 milligrams of DHA and EPA combined per day.[7] Vegan supplements derived from algae are a good choice for everyone since they are more sustainable than fish oil supplements. Because fish can be contaminated with mercury, vegan supplements of DHA and EPA are also a safer choice for pregnant women in particular.

Iodine

Essential for brain development, iodine is another mineral that needs a little attention in the diets of pregnant women. You may very well get plenty of it since vegetables take up iodine from the soil and sea vegetables also provide iodine. Because iodine content of these foods varies, however, it's a good idea to shake a little bit of iodized salt on your food or to make sure that your prenatal supplement contains 150 micrograms of iodine (the RDA for pregnant women is 220 micrograms). And while it's fine to consume sea vegetables, it's also a good idea to limit servings to no more than two to three per week. These foods can sometimes be excessive in iodine, which could cause harm to your baby.[8] Some women who consumed several servings of sea vegetables every day had iodine intakes that were well over 2,000 micrograms per day, which is more than twice the upper limit for safety.

Foods That Are Off the Menu for Pregnant Women

You probably already know that alcohol is out during pregnancy. Excessive drinking can cause a host of irreversible problems that are part of fetal alcohol syndrome. A safe level of alcohol consumption hasn't been established, so it is important to stop consuming alcohol as soon as you know you are pregnant and preferably as soon as you begin planning for a pregnancy.

Avoid raw sprouts and unpasteurized juices as well since there is always a risk of bacterial contamination of these foods. If you eat tofu, purchase the aseptically packaged type—the kind that is shelf stable and doesn't need to be refrigerated. Or, if you use refrigerated water-packed tofu, steam it for 15 minutes before using. This is just a little bit of extra precaution to be observed in pregnancy.

Small amounts of caffeine are okay, but it's best to limit your intake to one or two cups of coffee per day.

When You Are Too Sick to Eat

Morning sickness—fancily known as pregnancy hyperemesis and less fancily as NVP (nausea and vomiting of pregnancy)—plagues many women in the early months of pregnancy and sometimes well beyond those first few months. It can make your life miserable and also interfere with efforts to eat a nutritious diet.

You may not be able to eat everything in the food guide in this chapter when you are suffering from nausea, so eat whatever you can. Many women find that bland foods like baked potatoes, rice, pasta, graham crackers, and bread are well tolerated. Frozen grapes or fruit juice bars can help keep you from getting dehydrated. A snack of crackers or toast before you get out of bed in the morning can help stave off nausea, and so can eating small meals throughout the day. Take your prenatal supplements before going to sleep at night if they upset your stomach.

Ginger can relieve some of the symptoms, so you may want to snack on gingersnaps or sip ginger tea.[9] It's not clear whether acupuncture helps with morning sickness, but Sea-Bands, which are acupressure wrist bands marketed for sea sickness, have been used successfully by some women to reduce nausea.[10] Supplements of vitamin B_6 may improve symptoms of morning sickness, but be sure to talk to your health-care provider before adding supplements to your diet while you're pregnant.[11]

Pressure from the uterus on your stomach, along with changes to the muscles in your digestive tract can cause stomach acid to move into the esophagus, giving the burning sensation known as heartburn. Eating smaller and more frequent meals, staying upright after meals, and avoiding fatty and spicy foods can all help.

VEGAN BREASTFEEDING

Your baby is here! A beautiful—and hungry—little miracle. If you are breastfeeding, then your diet continues to be your infant's sole source of nutrition, at least for the first few months. You'll actually need more calories than you did when you were pregnant, since nursing a baby requires about 500 calories per day. Your baby needs those calories for growth, and it also takes a lot of energy for you to manufacture milk.

Some nutrient requirements stay the same after you've had your baby and started to breastfeed, while others drop. Requirements for vitamin A, vitamin C, and iodine are higher for breastfeeding moms than for pregnant women. Continuing with a prenatal supplement without the added iron (since iron needs decline dramatically in breastfeeding women until their period returns) can be a good way to make sure you're meeting basic needs. Make sure it includes iodine. In addition, choose plenty of dark green leafy and deep orange/yellow vegetables to get enough vitamin A along with lots of vitamin C–rich fruits and vegetables.

Although breast milk of vegans is lower in the omega-3 fat DHA, it is higher than what commercial infant formulas have historically contained, and infants have thrived on these formulas.[12,13] Some experts recommend that breastfeeding women take 300 micrograms of DHA/EPA per day.[7] Getting it from microalgae-derived pills is a good choice and is effective for raising the levels of DHA in breast milk.[14]

Nearly all of the stories about sick vegan infants that appear in the news have been due to poor vitamin B_{12} and vitamin D nutrition. It is absolutely crucial to continue with vitamin B_{12} supplements while you are breastfeeding. An alternative could be to give your baby a B_{12} supplement—but then *you'll* end up with a deficiency. You both need B_{12} and you both can get it from the supplement you take. While getting adequate vitamin D—from supplements, fortified foods, or sun exposure—continues to be important for you, your baby will also need supplemental vitamin D if he doesn't get adequate sun exposure. Breast milk is typically low in vitamin D regardless of your own vitamin D status. Be sure to talk to your health-care provider about vitamin D supplements before administering them to your baby. He or she will help you determine the right dosage and type.

If you are able to breast-feed, by all means take advantage of the opportunity to provide your baby with the food that is designed expressly to meet her needs. Your milk also provides antibodies to boost your infant's immune system. Breastfed infants are less likely to develop asthma or allergies and have a lifelong lower risk for diabetes, heart disease, and obesity. It's also good for *you* since breastfeeding can lower your lifetime risk for breast cancer. Breastfeeding is far more economical when you compare the cost of the little bit of extra food you need to the cost of formulas, bottles, and the paraphernalia associated with safe formula preparation. And as a vegan mom, you have a couple of additional advantages. Since cow's milk protein is a common cause of colic when it's passed to a baby through breast milk, your baby may have a lower risk for this problem. Breast milk of vegans also has lower levels of pesticide residue.[15]

If you are not breastfeeding your baby, be sure to choose a commercial formula according to your pediatrician's recommendations. Most vegan moms opt for soy infant formula. Use only a commercial formula that is produced specifically for babies since regular soymilk isn't sufficient nutrition for infants (and neither is regular cow's milk).

SOYFOODS FOR PREGNANT AND BREASTFEEDING WOMEN

Soyfoods have been a part of Asian diets for centuries and women in these countries don't stop eating them when they become pregnant. Not only are these foods important sources of nutrients for pregnant and breastfeeding women in some Asian countries, but tofu and other soyfoods are often among the earliest solid foods introduced to infants.

Throughout pregnancy, your baby is bathed in a sea of estrogen since amniotic fluid is very high in this hormone. Even though isoflavones from soyfoods are transferred to the fetus, they make only a small contribution overall to this estrogen environment. Since infants fed soy infant formula grow and develop normally, as do infants in Asia, it's clear that soy can be a part of healthy diets in pregnancy and while breastfeeding.

Soy, Vegetarian Diets, and Hyposadias

Hypospadias is a relatively common birth defect affecting less than one of every three hundred male babies. It involves a displacement of the urethra—the tube through which urine passes—in the penis. Hypospadias is usually easily repaired with no long-term consequences. A study in Great Britain published in 2000 found a higher incidence of hypospadias in boys whose mothers were vegetarian and a possibly higher incidence when their mothers consumed soymilk or soy-based veggie meats more than once per week.[16] However, the number of women who ate soy was very small in the study, making it hard to draw conclusions about any relationship of soyfoods to hypospadias. Also, because of changes that occur with processing, soy-based veggie meats are typically very low in isoflavones anyway. In fact, consumption of chickpeas, lentils, and dried beans—which don't contain isoflavones—was more strongly associated with hypospadias than consumption of soyfoods.

A much larger study published in 2012 found no relationship between vegetarian diets and hypospadias,[17] and a study in the Netherlands in 2004 found no association between soy intake and risk for hypospadias.[18]

PRACTICAL STEPS TOWARD MEETING NUTRIENT NEEDS OF PREGNANCY AND BREASTFEEDING

- It's easy to build healthy menus for pregnancy around the Plant Plate (page 31) with just a few additional servings from the food groups. By adding two servings each of grains and legumes, and a second serving of nuts, you should have no trouble meeting nutrient needs for pregnancy. If you can't eat nuts, add another serving of legumes. Here's what the Plant Plate looks like for pregnant women:

  Grains: 6 servings
  Legumes: 5 servings
  Nuts: 2 servings (or another serving of legumes)
  Vegetables: 5 servings
  Fruits: 2 servings
  Fats: 2 servings

- Don't forget to make sure that at least six of those servings are calcium-rich foods from the rim of the plate.
- Some pregnant women will need more food than this. If you aren't gaining adequate weight, you'll obviously need to increase servings from some of the groups a little bit. It's fine to

add some treats to your menus, too, especially if you're struggling with weight gain. Just make sure you add them to your daily quota of nutritious foods rather than replacing those foods with less nutrient-dense options.

- Include a good source of vitamin C in as many of your meals and snacks as possible.
- Supplements for pregnant women:

  > Vitamin B$_{12}$: 25 micrograms per day or 1,000 micrograms three times per week
  > A prenatal supplement that provides iron, folic acid, and iodine (unless you get adequate iodine from iodized salt) and vitamin D (unless you make enough from sun exposure)
  > DHA/EPA: 300 micrograms (DHA and EPA combined) from algae

BREASTFEEDING MOMS

- Choose plenty of vitamin A–rich vegetables since needs for this nutrient are high during breastfeeding. Good choices are carrots, winter squash, pumpkin, and leafy green vegetables.
- Give your diet a little calorie boost since you need slightly more calories while breastfeeding than you did when you were pregnant.
- Supplements for breastfeeding moms

  > Vitamin B$_{12}$: 25 micrograms daily or 1,000 micrograms three times per week
  > 300 milligrams of DHA/EPA
  > 150 milligrams of iodine unless you are consuming at least ¼ teaspoon of iodized salt per day
  > 600 to 1000 IUs of vitamin D

Sample Menus for Pregnant Women

DAY ONE

Breakfast	Lunch	Dinner
Bran flakes	Hummus wrap	Quinoa
1 cup soymilk	Raw red pepper strips	Steamed vegetables
Sliced banana	Fortified orange juice	**Cashew Cream Tofu (page 298)**
Snack	**Snack**	
1 cup instant lentil soup	Ice cream with figs	
Chopped tomatoes		

DAY TWO

Breakfast	Lunch	Dinner
Oatmeal	**Quinoa Daiya Burger (page 280)**	Pasta tossed with edamame
Chopped walnuts	Salad with lemon vinaigrette dressing	Bok choy sautéed in sesame oil
Fortified almond milk	Leftover quinoa	
Fortified orange juice		**Snack**
Snack		Apple with peanut butter
Kale smoothie (soymilk, kale, fruit)		
Graham crackers		

DAY THREE

Breakfast	Lunch	Dinner
Toast with peanut butter	**"Meaty" Lentil and Veggie Mac (page 293)**	Brown rice
Soymilk		Baked tofu
Strawberries	Kale sautéed in olive oil	Butternut squash
Snack		Green beans
Crackers and hummus	**Snack**	**Snack**
Fortified orange juice	Trail mix with nuts	Whole wheat English muffin with almond butter

— continues —

DAY FOUR		
Breakfast	**Lunch**	**Dinner**
Smoothie with banana, strawberries, silken tofu	**Chickpea salad sandwich (page 278)** with sliced tomatoes on whole wheat bread	Black beans topped with chopped tomatoes
Snack	Salad with chopped walnuts, vinaigrette	Baked sweet potato
Fortified orange juice		Sautéed collard greens
Toast with peanut butter	Vegan ice cream sandwich or frozen juice bar	

DAY FIVE		
Breakfast	**Lunch**	**Dinner**
Oatmeal with walnuts, chopped apple	Baked beans	**Creamy Vegetable Breakfast Casserole (page 252)**
Snack	Salad with **Cashew-Almond-Orange Dressing (page 260)**	Baked potato
Peanut butter and banana on whole-grain bread	Toast	**Snack**
	Snack	Bran muffin
	Fruit salad	Fortified juice

CHAPTER EIGHT

POWERED BY PLANTS: THE FEMALE VEGAN ATHLETE

A **balanced diet based on** the guidelines in Chapter 2 provides plenty of nutrition for your daily jog or Zumba class. But, if you run marathons, are a serious body builder, or are training to compete in any sport, you might need to give a little bit more attention to meeting nutrient needs. The issues of particular concern for female athletes—energy intake, protein, and iron—are important for active women whether they are vegan or not.

Unfortunately, research on female vegan athletes is virtually nonexistent. So we have to extrapolate a little bit from research on men and from findings in lacto-ovo vegetarians and meat-eaters. It's an imperfect approach that leaves us with a fair number of unanswered questions. What is clear is that elite female athletes can thrive and compete on vegan diets. The proof lies in the careers of plant-powered athletes like Olympic cyclist and runner Fiona Oakes, professional cyclist Christine Vardaros, high jumper Weia Reinboud, and ultramarathoner Catra Corbett. If they can do it, so can you.

VEGAN DIETS AND THE ANTIOXIDANT ADVANTAGE

We know that vegan diets can support elite athletes at least as well as diets that contain animal foods. Whether there are performance advantages for vegans isn't known, but in one area—related to antioxidants—there may be a distinct benefit to eating more plants.

Normal metabolism produces free radicals, the oxygen-containing compounds that can damage cells and increase disease risk. Since athletes burn up more fuel than the average person, they also produce more free radicals, which can promote injury to muscle proteins along with muscle fatigue.[1] In people who are well trained, the body's own antioxidant systems may gradually become more active in order to cope with the increase in free radical formation. In the more casual exerciser, or those just starting to train, keeping up with free radical damage may be harder. A higher intake of antioxidants—which is common in vegans—could speed recovery and reduce injuries.[2] Making sure that your diet contains plenty of fruits and vegetables is the best way to increase antioxidant intake, but the foods that lie at the center of vegan meals—whole grains and legumes—also provide compounds with antioxidant activity.

THE FEMALE ATHLETE TRIAD

Inadequate energy intake along with bone loss and amenorrhea (cessation of menstruation) describes what has become known as the female athlete triad. It's most common in sports that emphasize very lean figures like gymnastics, figure skating, and running, although it's also seen in women involved in other sports. For example, as many as 65 percent of young women who are long-distance runners may fail to menstruate normally.[3]

While eating disorders or restrained eating are a common part of the triad, it's also possible that some athletes may fall short of meeting calorie needs even when they aren't intentionally restricting food intake. Eating to satisfy appetite doesn't guarantee adequate calories for athletes since their higher energy needs don't necessarily translate to sufficient hunger.[4]

Some female athletes may engage in restrictive eating that doesn't quite meet the definition of an eating disorder and some might also experience disturbances like skipped or irregular periods, which fall short of amenorrhea. However, any female athlete who has one of the triad symptoms is likely to experience all three to some extent. That is, if you are missing periods, you can assume that you're also losing bone mass, and that you aren't eating enough. And while vigorous exercise is very good for protecting bone health, it is simply no match for the damaging effects of amenorrhea.[5]

Some early research suggested that vegetarian athletes were at higher risk for amenorrhea. These studies have limited value since the term *vegetarian* was very loosely defined (that is, many of the women described as vegetarian actually ate meat). The studies also depended on self-reporting of past menstrual problems and dietary habits—a type of experimental design that is very prone to error. It's certainly possible that some vegans could be at higher risk if they are eating diets that are extremely low in fat, but that's probably not a usual eating pattern for female athletes. The evidence suggests that overall, it's not a matter of what you eat, but how much you eat— whether you are meeting calorie needs.

It can be helpful to meet with a sports nutritionist to calculate your calorie needs and then set up an eating plan to make sure you meet those needs. For endurance athletes especially, it's also wise to keep track of your periods on a calendar. Missing three in a row is a sign that your food intake is probably falling short. The best way to return your period to a normal schedule is to increase calorie intake and body weight.[6] Even a small increase of about 10 percent of your usual calorie intake can make a difference. Some athletes may need to cut back on training, however, to reverse these symptoms. It's also extremely important to make sure you're eating a diet that supports bone health, as I'll talk about in Chapter 13.[7]

Meeting Energy Needs

In addition to its effects on bone and menstruation, inadequate calorie intake can cause injury and fatigue and make it difficult to maintain adequate muscle mass. Athletes need additional calories not just to support rigorous exercise but also to support recovery and repair. Getting enough energy also spares muscle protein that would otherwise be used for energy. For weight lifters, inadequate calorie intake can prevent muscle growth.

So how many calories do you need to stay healthy and competitive? That's not so easy to answer since it depends on your body size and muscle mass, your sport, and the intensity of activity. Because of these variables, needs of elite female athletes can be anywhere from 2,400 to 4,000 calories per day. It's possible that vegan women could have higher needs since their higher carbohydrate intake may cause a small increase in energy expenditure, but this would translate to only a very slight increase.[8,9]

Pinning down your exact calorie needs takes some calculating and some experimentation. You'll need to calculate the three different components of your energy needs: resting energy expenditure, daily activity, and energy expenditure for training.

1. Estimate your resting energy expenditure (REE)—the calories needed to support lungs, heart, brain activity, and other organs while you're at rest—using this formula:

     655 + (4.35 x weight in pounds) + (4.7 x height in inches) minus (4.7 x age in years)

2. Add your daily nontraining calorie needs by multiplying your REE (as calculated above) by one of the following factors:

     0.3 if you are sedentary throughout the day
     0.5 if you're moderately active, and on your feet through much of the day.
     0.7 if your work or daily activities keep you moving throughout the day.

3. Add in calories needed for training.

Table 8-1: Calories Needed for Activities	
Activity	Calories/minute/kilogram
Running 8 minutes per mile	0.22
Running 7 minutes per mile	0.24
Running 6 minutes per mile	0.28
Cycling 12 to 14 miles/hour	0.14
Cycling 14.1 to 16 miles/hour	0.18
Cycling 16.1 to 19 miles per hour	0.21
Weight training	0.5 to 1.0 depending on intensity
Swimming, moderate	0.14

Calculating Calorie Needs for Female Athletes

Here is an example of how to calculate needs for a female athlete. I'm using a forty-five-year-old woman who weighs 130 pounds (59 kilograms) and is 5'6" tall (67 inches). She has a sedentary desk job and runs 60 minutes per day at 7 miles per hour.

Resting energy expenditure = 655 + (4.35 x 130) + (4.7 x 67)–(4.7 x 45) =1,324 calories per day

Daily activity = 0.3 x 1324 = 397

Calories for exercise = 60 x 0.24 x 59 = 850

Total calories needed for day: 1324 + 397 + 850 = 2,571

Obviously, this depends on your sport and how much time you spend in training. It can vary with seasonal changes in your training, too. You'll find extensive tables on the internet that give estimated calories burned for different activities. Table 8-1 gives some examples of calorie needs for several different activities at different levels of intensity. Calories are calculated per minute of time spent exercising per kilogram of body weight. To find your body weight in kilograms, divide your weight in pounds by 2.2.

Although these formulas can help you reach a ballpark figure for calorie intake, you'll need to do a little experimenting to find out what's right for you.

MEETING PROTEIN NEEDS OF FEMALE ATHLETES

Vegans who get most of their protein from whole grains and legumes may have slightly higher needs compared to nonvegans since the protein in these foods is less well digested than animal foods. In their position statement on nutrition and athletic performance, the American College of Sports Medicine (ACSM), along with the dietetic associations of both the United States and Canada, recommended somewhat higher protein intakes for vegetarian athletes. Based on their recommendations, vegans participating in strength training require between 0.6 and 0.7 grams of protein per pound of body weight. Those involved in endurance sports need between 0.6 and 0.8 grams of protein per pound of body weight. (For comparison, the ACSM recommendations for nonvegetarians are 0.54 to 0.77 grams of protein per pound of body weight for strength athletes and 0.54 to 0.63 grams of protein per pound of body weight for endurance athletes.)

There are a couple of things to keep in mind about these recommendations, however. First, much of what we know about protein needs of athletes comes from research in men, and it's possible that requirements are lower for women.[10] Second, for both endurance and strength athletes, the higher ends of these ranges may be needed only when you first start training since protein metabolism becomes more efficient over time.[11]

But even at the lower end of recommendations, some vegan women could fall short, especially when just beginning a training program and also especially when a woman's calorie intake is toward the lower end of usual intakes for athletes. Athletes who are intentionally restricting calories to lose weight may also not get enough protein. A vegan athlete who weighs 130 pounds would need at least 78 grams of protein per day (0.6 x 130). Vegans typically consume about 11 percent of their calories from protein—or 27.5 grams of protein per 1,000 calories. So, at 2,400 calories per day, a vegan woman would get about 66 grams of protein, which is 15 percent below requirements. If her calorie intake was closer to 2,800, she wouldn't have any trouble meeting needs.

This doesn't mean it's difficult to meet protein needs for athletic performance on a vegan diet. In fact, the diet that I recommend, based on the Plant Plate, is fairly protein dense, providing around 14 to 15 percent of calories from protein. If you're following those guidelines, and being generous with servings of legumes, you'll meet protein needs with ease. If you shun beans and soyfoods and get most of your calories from grains, vegetables, fruits, and nuts, you could fall short. You can see the protein content of different plant foods in Appendix B.

CARBOHYDRATES FUEL INTENSE EXERCISE

Carbohydrate is the body's preferred fuel for intense exercise. It produces energy quickly and doesn't require as much oxygen to metabolize. However, glycogen supplies—the body's storage form of carbohydrate—are limited. When they're gone, the body turns to its stores of fat, which can lead to fatigue since fat is burned more slowly than carbohydrate. That's why high-carbohydrate diets are so valuable for athletes; they improve glycogen stores and allow you

Table 8-2: Approximate Carbohydrate Content of Vegan Foods	
Food	**Grams of carbohydrate**
Beans, peas, and lentils, ½ cup cooked	15–18
Bread, 1 slice	15
Rice, pasta, or other cooked grains, ½ cup	15
White or sweet potato, ½ cup cooked	15
Fruit, ½ cup	15
Carrots or winter squash, ½ cup cooked	7–8
Greens (kale, collard greens, spinach), ½ cup	2.5 to 5

to exercise longer. Aim for 2.7 to 3.2 grams of carbohydrate per pound of body weight.[12] If you're eating enough calories, it's easy to achieve this on a vegan diet since so many of the foods we eat—grains, legumes, and fruits—are rich in carbohydrates. Table 8-2 gives some examples of the carbohydrate content of plant foods.

FAT FUELS EXTENDED EXERCISE

While glycogen is important for shorter-term intensive exercise, fat is preferred for extended exercise performed at a lower intensity. Research in female athletes shows that small deposits of fat stored in muscles are ideal for this purpose.[13] It's possible that eating a diet that is too low in fat could compromise availability of these stores. In a study of eight female runners, eating a low-fat vegetarian diet made it difficult to replenish fat stores in muscles after exercise while a higher-fat intake allowed those stores to be replenished with ease.[14] Diets that dip below 15 percent of calories from fat are also associated with missed periods in female athletes.[15]

Your ideal fat intake depends to some degree on your calorie needs. If these are below 3,000 calories per day, you'll probably need to keep fat intake down to 20 to 25 percent of calories or it might be

Table 8-3: Approximate Fat Content of Vegan Foods	
Food	**Average amount of fat in grams**
Nuts, ¼ cup	17–20
Tofu, firm, ½ cup	11
Tempeh, ½ cup	9
Seeds, 2 tablespoons	8
Avocado, ¼ cup cubes	5.5
Vegetable oils, 1 teaspoon	5
Tofu, soft, ½ cup	4.5
Grains, ½ cup cooked	0.8–1.7
Leafy green vegetables, ½ cup cooked	0.2–0.35

difficult to meet needs for protein and carbohydrates. That's about 22 to 28 grams of fat per 1,000 calories. If you have a higher calorie intake, you can consume somewhat more fat. Table 8-3 shows amounts of fat in common vegan foods.

MEETING IRON NEEDS

Even marginal iron deficiency that doesn't cause outright anemia can impair athletic performance. Iron is central to the function of hemoglobin, which delivers oxygen to all the tissues of the body, and of myoglobin, which stores oxygen in muscles. It's also needed by enzymes involved in energy production.

Iron is normally lost through perspiration, menstruation, and through normal shedding of cells from the skin and intestinal tract. Athletes lose additional iron through sweat, red blood cell destruction due to physical impact from training, and sometimes from intestinal bleeding, which is not uncommon in some endurance athletes.

While iron needs don't increase for strength athletes, the ACSM recommends that all endurance athletes, especially distance runners, aim for iron intakes that are about 70 percent higher than the RDA. For premenopausal women, this is about 30 mg of iron per day.

It's possible that vegan and vegetarian female athletes have even higher needs than this, since iron isn't as well absorbed on vegan diets. These higher iron needs can present a little bit of a challenge; after all, many women, including those who eat meat, fall short of meeting the usual RDA of 18 milligrams per day. Fortunately, endurance athletes consume more calories, which should translate to a higher iron intake. Vegans also often have higher iron intakes than people who consume animal foods since plant foods are rich in iron.

As I talked about in Chapter 2, it's important for vegans to maximize iron absorption by consuming good sources of vitamin C at as many meals as possible. Although some endurance athletes choose to take iron supplements, there is no reason to do so unless your iron status is poor. The ACSM recommends that *all* women athletes be regularly screened to assess their iron status. Screening can be especially important for teen athletes and pregnant women.

SUPPLEMENTS FOR ATHLETES

Creatine

Creatine is found in muscle tissue where, as creatine phosphate, it's an important storage form of energy. Meat-eaters consume around 2 grams of creatine per day,[16] but there is little to no creatine in vegetarian or vegan diets. Even though we can synthesize it, vegetarians typically have lower creatine levels in their blood, urine, red blood cells, and muscle tissue.[17-19] Some studies have shown that vegetarians benefit more from creatine supplementation than meat-eaters, with greater increases in muscle mass and better performance.[17,19] The ACSM and the International Olympic Committee have stated that creatine is generally considered to be safe for adults and may have performance benefits. Common side-effects are cramping, nausea, diarrhea, and fluid retention.

Creatine is usually available as a vegan powder that can be mixed into carbohydrate-rich drinks like juice since carbohydrates increase its absorption. Look for pure creatine since added ingredients may not be vegan and won't add any benefits.

Carnitine

Carnitine is an amino acid needed to transport fat into the part of cells where it's burned for energy. Because of its role in fat metabolism, carnitine has been touted as a supplement for weight loss and for improving performance in endurance exercise. There is no real evidence that it does either.

This is another compound we can synthesize ourselves, but since it's not found in plant foods, vegetarians have lower blood levels, compared to meat-eaters, who consume about 100 to 300 milligrams of carnitine per day.[18,20,21]

Although supplements appear to be safe and there are vegan options available, there doesn't seem to be any benefit to vegans who take them. In fact, supplements of 120 milligrams per day don't appear to have much effect on blood levels of carnitine in vegans.[22]

Caffeine

Some people use caffeine to wake up in the morning while others use it to enhance mental or physical performance. It's effective in all of these situations. Caffeine has a positive effect on short-term cognitive function and also can improve athletic performance. If you like coffee, a couple of cups an hour or two before exercise may be beneficial. Too much caffeine can upset your stomach, though, and have side-effects such as rapid heart rate.

OPTIMAL EATING FOR FEMALE ATHLETES

Optimal athletic performance depends on a good balance of protein, fat, and carbohydrates, and it's not at all difficult to achieve that balance on a vegan diet. The menus on pages 112–113 provide some examples of food patterns for athletes at different calorie intakes. Keep in mind, though, that needs are very individual, depending on your training schedule, body size, and body composition. In these menus, a serving of "discretionary calories" is a glass of wine or beer or a dessert providing around 150 calories.

Sample Menus for Vegan Athletes

MENU 1   2,400 CALORIES–90 GRAMS PROTEIN

6 Grains	5 Fruits
6 Legumes	3 Fats
2 Nuts	1 Discretionary food
8 Vegetables	

Breakfast

1 cup oatmeal with ½ cup chopped apple and 2 tablespoons chopped walnuts

1 slice whole-grain bread with 2 tablespoons peanut butter

1 cup calcium-fortified orange juice

Snack

Raw vegetables with ½ cup hummus

Lunch

Large whole wheat flour tortilla topped with 1 cup black beans, 1 cup raw chopped vegetables, ¼ cup guacamole, salsa

½ cup fruit salad

Snack

1 cup vegetable soup

Dinner

1 cup quinoa

1 cup curried lentils with 2 tablespoons almonds

2 cups kale sautéed in 2 teaspoons olive oil

Baked pear

Red wine

MENU 2 3,000 CALORIES—115 GRAMS PROTEIN

9 Grains   6 Fruits
9 Legumes   4 Fats
2 Nuts   1 Discretionary food
8 Vegetables

Breakfast

1 cup bran flakes with 1 cup soymilk and ¼ cup chopped walnuts

1 cup strawberries

Snack

1 slice toast with ½ cup scrambled tofu

Apple

Lunch

1 cup brown rice

1 cup black beans plus ½ cup tomatoes

Salad (2 cups greens and raw vegetables) with 1 tablespoon oil and vinegar dressing

Banana

Snack

Whole wheat pita bread

½ cup hummus

Raw carrots

Dinner

Large baked potato

2 cups lentil soup

1½ cups kale sautéed in 2 teaspoons olive oil

½ cup fruit salad

8 ounces beer (or 6 ounces apple juice)

Snack

Low-fat granola bar

½ cup orange juice

PART THREE

Lifelong Health for Vegan Women

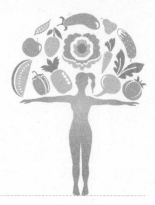

CHAPTER NINE

HEALTH AND HAPPINESS BEYOND THE SCALE

On any given day, more than 50 percent of Americans—most of them women—are on a weight-loss diet. And for most, it's not a first attempt to shed some pounds.

With all the focus on weight management—a multibillion dollar industry built around books, programs, and products—you'd think we'd be a nation of svelte citizens. Instead, we've developed a culture of chronic dieting with little success. More than four-fifths of those who lose weight end up gaining most or all of it back within five years.

Dieting itself can carry health risks since losing and regaining weight could leave you less healthy than you'd be if you had never lost the weight to begin with. There is also a considerable psychological and emotional cost to chronic dieting. Dropping pounds can become successively more difficult and the failure to keep those pounds off can be depressing and demoralizing. That's especially true in a culture where many people believe that being overweight or obese is all about a lack of willpower, or is simply a failure to make responsible lifestyle choices.

To the contrary, the science shows that weight is far more complex than anyone realized fifty years, or even a decade ago. We live in a fattening world and our genetics produce different responses to that.

This chapter doesn't offer the one true method for permanent weight loss, because no one knows what that method is, if it exists at all. Instead, I'm going to talk about some advantages that plant-based diets have whether you'd like to shed a few pounds or are looking to improve your health at your current weight. I'm also going to explore some questions about who should be trying to lose weight. In the end, my hope is that you'll choose to eat in a way that supports your health and happiness and that you will embrace the benefits of your vegan diet that go beyond body size.

THE CAUSES OF OBESITY

At its simplest, weight is a matter of energy balance. Take in more energy than you need and the excess calories are stored as fat. When you consume fewer calories than required, your body turns to burning up its own fat deposits for energy. That explanation is deceptive, though, because weight control turns out to be far more complex than what a simple mathematical equation can describe.

The Obesogenic Environment

Obesity has risen dramatically in the United States since 1980 and it's certainly not because our genes have changed or we have suddenly become more gluttonous. What has changed is the food environment and the fact that Americans have unlimited access to cheap, good-tasting, high-calorie food. Energy-rich snack foods and sweetened drinks are sold almost everywhere and are easier to find and much less expensive than healthy foods like fruits, vegetables, and whole grains. Government subsidies also keep prices of high-calorie animal products low, making it easier for families to build meals around these foods and for restaurants to sell large portions.

The worst of these changes are those that target eating habits of children. The food industry spends billions of dollars on marketing fast food, sweetened cereals, and sugary soft drinks to young children. School-aged kids also have greater access to some of these foods through vending machines in schools and nearby fast-food restaurants. The result can set some children up for a lifetime of struggle with their weight.

We move less, too, since regular movement is no longer built into routines for most Americans. Jobs and leisure activities have become more sedentary and homes are filled with energy-saving devices. Physical activity has to be a conscious effort.[1]

Finally, there is some evidence to suggest that certain chemicals in our environment could have biological effects that change metabolism.[2]

Genetics and Evolution

While we don't *have* to eat all of this cheap, tasty, fattening food just because it's there, we're sort of programmed to do so. Since humans evolved in an environment where food availability was irregular—and where it took a lot of energy to get it—they took advantage of abundance when they could. Those who were able to put on a few extra pounds of stored fat had an advantage when times of famine rolled around and they could dip into fat stores for needed energy. Women also require a certain amount of fat in order to menstruate and reproduce. For early humans, it simply made good survival sense to eat a little extra when you could. And, our bodies haven't shed that hardwired push for more calories in the short time that our food environment has changed so dramatically.

Some people are also genetically wired to convert calories to fat more efficiently, which would once have been a distinct survival and reproductive advantage.[3] In contrast, those who can eat ice cream sundaes all day long without gaining an ounce wouldn't have stood a chance at survival in the Paleolithic age.

So far, more than four hundred genes that may contribute to obesity have been discovered. In addition to effects on metabolism, they affect appetite, satiety, how people react to food cues, and even brain circuitry regarding feelings of "reward" associated with eating. Some of these differences appear early in childhood.[4] For example, research shows that children who carry the FTO gene—also known as the obesity gene—have a preference for higher-calorie foods even though they may not eat more food overall. This suggests that those who nonchalantly pass up treats and high-calorie foods may be able to do so easily because of their genetic makeup, not because they exhibit exceptional self-control.[5]

It's this interplay between genetics and a dramatically unhealthy food environment, with maybe a few environmental toxins thrown into the mix that has made it easy for so many people to put on extra pounds. Other factors that are sometimes difficult to control can play a role, too. Sleep deprivation is associated with changes in hormones that control hunger and may cause increased hunger and weight gain.[6] Stress, which is often associated with depression and with poverty, can change metabolism in ways that promote weight gain.

Do Vegans Have a Weight-Loss Advantage?

Public health experts assess weight status using the body mass index (BMI), which measures body weight in relation to height. It doesn't consider how much muscle or fat you have—just how much you weigh. It also doesn't tell us anything about someone's health since it measures only size. So BMI is not useful for individuals, but it's used as a fast and inexpensive way to look for trends in populations.

On average, vegans have a lower BMI than either meat-eaters or vegetarians and they also have less body fat.[7–10] This doesn't mean that every vegan is thin, and in fact that's far from the truth. It also doesn't mean that adopting a vegan diet will automatically result in weight loss.

It's possible, however, that vegans are at lower risk for weight gain and that a vegan diet may have some advantages for weight loss management. Replacing animal foods with plant foods will automatically raise your fiber intake, for example, which could be important for weight loss.[11] Vegan diets are also typically somewhat lower in fat than diets built around animal foods, but it's not clear how much this matters. There is little evidence that higher-fat diets are the cause of obesity.[12] The lower glycemic index of vegan diets that are built around slow carbs may be more important since there is some (although very conflicting) evidence that diets with a high glycemic index promote obesity.[13,14]

Other possible explanations for benefits of eating more plant foods are pretty intriguing. For example, all people have colonies of bacteria living in their colon, but the type of bacteria varies depending on diet. Because of effects on metabolism, higher levels of the bacteria that tend to take up residence in vegetarian colons may be associated with lower weight.[15] Higher intake of fruits and vegetables might also help vegans avoid weight gain. These foods have bulk and volume because of their fiber and water content, which contributes to a feeling of fullness. Their rich phytochemical content could help with weight control, too. For example, the compound resveratrol, which is found in red grapes, grape juice, red wine, and peanuts, might increase activity of enzymes that induce fat breakdown.[16] Compounds in apricots, green tea, and chocolate have been linked to lower body weight and inhibition of fat formation.[17] Capsaicin, the chemical that gives red peppers their hotness, may increase energy expenditure.[18]

These are all new areas of research, and it's not likely that eating more phytochemicals will cause the pounds to start melting off. But, they may help to give vegans a little bit of an edge in preventing weight gain—and, these compounds also have a multitude of health benefits.

Low-Fat Vegan Diets and Weight

Some dieters have had success with vegan diets that stringently restrict, or even completely eliminate all higher-fat plant foods including oils, nuts, seeds, olives, and avocadoes. A gram of fat has twice the number of calories as a gram of carbohydrate or protein, so even without calorie counting, eating less fat can sometimes automatically reduce calorie intake. But, whether such low-fat intakes are practical and effective for the long term hasn't been shown. They work in part because they allow *only* lower-calorie foods and also because they limit variety. People who eat fewer types of foods tend to eat less food overall. There is no such thing as an "eat all you want and lose weight" diet unless food choices are very limited. Although a low-fat vegan approach is sometimes promoted as an alternative to "dieting," it is in fact, a fairly rigid, restricted approach to weight loss.

There is also evidence that including some higher fat foods in your diet can actually be beneficial for weight management. In the Nurses' Health Study, women who ate nuts the most frequently gained less weight over time compared to women who ate them less often.[19] Nuts seem to help promote a feeling of satiety, and they also might give metabolism a little boost.[20,21] It's also possible that we don't absorb all of the calories from nuts since they are often not completely digested.[22] It doesn't mean that you can snack on nuts all day long without gaining weight. But, there is no reason to cut these foods out of your diet completely.

Even diets that get a little extra fat from vegetable oils could have some advantages for weight management. In a study at Brown University in Rhode Island, researchers put women on test diets aimed at helping them shed about 5 percent of their weight. Study participants lost more weight when they ate a plant-based diet with the addition of 3 tablespoons of olive oil than when they ate a much lower-fat diet. All of the women had a chance to try both eating patterns, and most said they preferred the olive oil–enriched diet. They found that they were less hungry between meals with the higher fat intake and that their meals were more enjoyable.[23] In another study at Boston's Brigham and Women's Hospital, 101 subjects consumed either a 20 percent fat diet or a 35 percent fat diet for six months. The higher-fat diet was based on a Mediterranean-type plan with lots of fruits, vegetables, and whole grains, along with fat from nuts and olive oil. People in both groups lost weight, but only those eating the higher fat Mediterranean-style diet were able to keep the weight off for the long term.[20]

In contrast, some people claim to feel less hunger when they cut way back on fat intake. This could be because high-carbohydrate diets result in higher levels of leptin (a hormone produced by fat tissue) that signals satiety.[24] Protein is probably even better for satiety, though, since it can suppress hunger even when leptin levels are low.[25]

THE CHALLENGE OF LONG-TERM WEIGHT LOSS

One common belief is that most people regain the weight they lost because they return to the same eating habits that caused weight gain to begin with. While that may be true for some, it's evident now that maintaining a substantial weight loss takes far more work than once believed. Metabolism slows as you shed pounds, in part because fat loss is nearly always accompanied by reduced muscle mass. Anywhere from 14 to 31 percent of weight loss is comprised of lean tissue—muscle and bone—and the less muscle you have, the fewer calories you burn.[26] As your body gets lighter, moving it requires less energy, too, so that you'll burn fewer calories during exercise. For example, a woman who weighs 180 pounds will use about 190 calories in a half hour of brisk walking, while a 140-pound woman will need only 150 calories for the same exercise. As a result of these changes, women who have lost more than 10 percent of their body weight may need 300 to 400 calories less than a same-weight person who was never overweight.[27]

And it could be harder to trim those additional calories from the diet, since changes in hormone levels that occur with loss of body fat make it harder to eat less. As fat deposits decrease, so do levels of appetite-suppressing leptin.[28] At the same time, levels of the appetite-stimulating hormone ghrelin, which is produced by the stomach and pancreas, may increase with dieting.[29] It's all a part of your body's defense against starvation—which is how it perceives weight loss.

While the science shows that it is a challenge to maintain a weight loss, it doesn't mean that weight regain is inevitable. Some people lose substantial amounts of weight and keep it off for the long term. But it does appear that permanent weight loss requires some long-term diligence well beyond what someone who was never overweight needs to do in order to stay thin.[30] Among those who are a part of the National Weight Loss Registry, a database of 4,000 adults—mostly women—who have successfully maintained a weight loss of thirty pounds or more for at least a year, many have to pay meticulous attention to their food habits, often continuing to count calories in order to prevent weight regain. Particularly, those who were overweight since childhood need to work much harder to keep weight off and they experience more stress and depression.[31] Difficulty in maintaining weight loss may be an important public health concern since—as you'll see below—weight cycling may raise the risk for chronic disease. There are also questions about whether all overweight people *need* to lose weight. These issues and others have produced new perspectives and approaches regarding weight and health. They encourage a shift in focus away from dieting and toward health-enhancing behaviors as well as a more accepting and compassionate perspective on body size. Experts are exploring the benefits of small, realistic, and sustainable weight loss and the positive effects of compassionate self-acceptance and responsible self-care.

Should You Be on a Diet?

Being thin may lower risk for some chronic disease, but it doesn't guarantee it. As many as 20 percent of women whose weight falls in the target range for optimal health have risk factors for chronic diseases such as high blood pressure and elevated cholesterol. Nor does being overweight doom you to a life of health problems. We can't predict someone's health based on their weight alone. Researchers have coined the term "metabolically healthy obesity" or MHO to describe those who are above standards for "ideal" weight but don't appear to be at greater risk for chronic disease. In a study of more than 22,000 people in England, overweight people who didn't have risk factors like elevated cholesterol were no more likely to develop cardiovascular disease than slender people.[32]

Between 10 and 30 percent of obese people may be metabolically healthy and the percentages could be higher among women than men.[33,34] Unfortunately, some of those healthy people may increase their risk for chronic disease by going on a diet. When you lose weight, you shed both muscle and bone matter along with fat tissue. But, unless you're a body builder, weight gain is typically mostly fat.[35] If you're postmenopausal, that situation is especially bad since women typically lose muscle mass anyway as they age.

There is evidence that weight cycling also increases inflammation, which raises risk for chronic disease.[36,37] In fact, some of the increased risk in chronic disease associated with obesity may be a consequence not of being overweight but of weight cycling.[36,38,39] Weight cycling also often has damaging psychological effects that can impact quality of life and self-esteem—which in turn can interfere with good lifestyle choices. It's possible that some of the poor health attributed to obesity is the result of the stress that comes from discrimination and stigma.[40]

Some people lose considerable amounts of weight and keep those pounds off for the long term. It's not true of everyone, though. What does seem to be true is that many people are successful at maintaining weight losses of 4 to 5 percent of their initial weight for the long term. For a woman weighing 180 pounds, this represents a weight loss of around 7 to 9 pounds. It may be that at this smaller amount of weight loss, the body's fat-preserving defenses don't kick in.

While a small weight loss like this may not seem exciting, it can be significant from a health standpoint, resulting in lower blood pressure, lower cholesterol levels, reduced risk for diabetes, and improved insulin resistance.[41] (Although, whether it is the weight loss that produces those benefits or the adoption of healthier food and exercise habits isn't really known.)

Whether or not you should be striving for weight loss is a personal decision based on your own experience and goals. Maybe you put on some extra pounds following an injury, or after having a baby. Changes in lifestyle can also result in temporary weight loss or gain. For a healthy and balanced approach to shedding some of those pounds, use the Plant Plate in Chapter 2 as a guide. The sample menus on pages 36–38 will point you toward choices to meet different calorie levels.

But, if you have been weight cycling over the years and find it impossible to maintain a significant weight loss, then you know that striving to achieve a particular calorie intake doesn't present a long-term solution for you. Instead, consider shifting to an approach that optimizes health without a focus on the scale.

When you are eating a healthy vegan diet, consuming enough to satisfy physical hunger, and engaging in regular exercise, your body will settle at the weight that is normal for you. And embracing a health-promoting lifestyle can reduce risk factors for heart disease, hypertension, and diabetes at that normal weight.[42,43] In one study, for example, eating a diet that was rich in fruits, vegetables, and calcium and low in saturated fat caused blood pressure to drop in subjects even when their weight stayed stable.[43] This can be hard to embrace in a culture that isn't accepting of larger size bodies, but there are some wonderful online communities that can help you on this journey toward a more compassionate and realistic attitude toward your body and health. Check out the Health at Every Size (HAES) and Association for Size Diversity and Health, both listed on page 312. And be sure to take a look at JL's wonderful *Stop Chasing Skinny* blog for some inspiration to stop dieting and embrace foods that nourish both body and soul.

In the end, you are the person who must decide whether weight loss is important and realistic for you or whether the better choice is to move toward healthier food options and explore physical activities and movement that you enjoy without worrying about the numbers on the scale.

DITCH THE DIET: EAT AND MOVE FOR HEALTH AND ENJOYMENT

Whether your goal is to be healthier at your current weight or to put a stop to encroaching weight gain, an approach that is built around realistic principles of healthy, pleasurable eating and exercise is most likely the one that will bring success for the long term. It *might* also help you lose weight, but even if it doesn't, it will improve your health and reverse some of those psychologically damaging effects of chronic dieting. This is a realistic and wise approach because it concentrates on what you *can* change—your behavior and your health—not on achieving a weight that may or may not be reasonable for you. It's based on principles of intuitive eating, wise food choices to promote health and manage hunger, and compassionate self-care through exercise and stress management.

Intuitive Eating

Intuitive eating rejects the dieting mentality. Instead, it allows you to trust your body's hunger signals, eating when hungry and stopping when you are full. For women who regularly ignore those hunger and satiety signals, or who eat in response to other cues like stress or boredom, or who engage in binge eating, intuitive eating can lead to weight loss.[44] Even if it doesn't, intuitive eating produces meaningful improvements in health, body image, and self-esteem and also reduces symptoms of disordered eating.[42,44,45] Principles of intuitive eating include honoring your hunger, finding ways to resolve emotional issues without using food, respecting your body instead of being critical of it, and making food choices that are enjoyable. It means letting go of the belief that every choice needs to be perfect. At its core, intuitive eating means giving yourself unconditional permission to eat, eating for physical rather than emotional reasons, and relying on hunger and satiety cues.

It takes some practice to learn to recognize your body's signals regarding food intake, but it's a skill that can be learned simply by eating more mindfully—paying attention to the experience of eating. Principles of mindful and intuitive eating involve the following:[44]

- Pay attention to hunger and fullness cues rather than following a regimented diet plan. This means assessing your hunger—are you really physically hungry, or are you bored?—and allowing yourself to eat when you truly are hungry. And then paying attention to feelings of fullness so you know when to stop. It sounds simple, but many of us eat so unconsciously that practicing intuitive eating can be a real revelation. Give yourself a chance to assess hunger by slowing the pace of eating. Chew more slowly, take breaks to sip some water, and wait a few minutes to let hunger signals reach your brain before having a second helping.
- Eat away from distractions like the television or computer. You can't assess your hunger very well if you are focused on something else while you're eating.
- Engage the senses in order to appreciate and enjoy food. If you eat unconsciously, chances are you don't even taste your food. Pay attention to tastes and textures to enhance the pleasurable aspect of eating—something that gets lost for many chronic dieters.
- Be aware of the factors that drive you to eat "unmindfully," such as boredom or sadness. If you find yourself reaching for food when you aren't actually hungry, take a minute to assess your feelings. And be prepared to deal with them with a distraction other than food. Take a short walk, call or e-mail a friend, take a few minutes to work on your favorite hobby, get a little corner of the garden weeded, or give yourself a manicure. It can help to actually have a list of alternatives for those times when emotions draw you to mindlessly grab some food.

The intuitive eating approach doesn't forbid any foods. We vegans, of course, choose to eliminate certain foods from our diet for reasons that have nothing to do with weight loss. It's about eating more consciously and compassionately, and there is no reason why this can't fit with the intuitive eating paradigm. In fact, vegans see foods and food choices in a much larger—and I think, healthier—context. We recognize that our food choices have a positive impact on the world, whether they produce weight loss or not.

Eat Healthy Plant Foods with High Satiety Value

Intuitive eating encourages foods that you enjoy and that give you pleasure. But you still need to give some attention to food choices if you want to be healthy. Following the general guidelines in Chapter 2 will help you choose menus that meet nutrient needs—because that's something that *isn't* intuitive. You can also focus on the foods you enjoy that have greater satiety value, foods that do the best job of satisfying your hunger so that you won't feel compelled to overeat.

I encourage a generous protein intake since protein has greater satiety value than either fat or carbohydrates.[46] Higher protein intake may also increase energy expenditure and protect muscle mass during weight loss.[47,48] In fact, simply putting an emphasis on eating more protein and fiber—without giving any attention to calories—can even produce a small weight loss without a loss of muscle.[49]

I'm also in favor of choosing carbohydrates with a lower glycemic index (GI). The slower and more sustained rise in blood glucose following consumption of these foods may help you manage hunger. It doesn't mean you can't ever eat higher GI foods like white potatoes and chocolate cake. Whatever you do, don't fall into the trap of thinking that there are plant foods that you can never have. That's a fad diet way of thinking. If there are foods that trigger you to overeat—and eating intuitively doesn't help—then yes, it's a good idea to keep them at a distance. I don't have potato chips in my house because I can't eat just one (or ten). But I do enjoy them at parties and occasionally buy a small bag of chips for a snack. Only you can decide what works for you based on your experience.

As you work to incorporate practices of intuitive eating into your life, put an emphasis on these foods that have high satiety value:

- **Vegetables and fruits.** Packed with nutrition and with good-for-you phytochemicals, these foods are high in water and bulk that fills your stomach. Adding lots of them to meals is a great way to trick your eye—part of the satiety equation—by filling your plate with foods that contribute bulk without excess calories. Don't let this turn into a scenario, though, where you try to stave off hunger by munching on meals of "rabbit food." Without something a little more substantial, you won't be satisfied. But a huge salad with added beans, a tablespoon or two of sunflower seeds, and a drizzle of vinaigrette dressing provides both volume and satiety.

- **Slow carbs.** Carbohydrate-rich foods lend elements of comfort and satisfaction to meals. The ones that promote sustained levels of blood glucose, which may delay hunger, are sweet potatoes, pasta, oatmeal, barley, bread made from whole, unmilled grains (rather than from flour), and beans. Choose these most often.

- **Beans.** It's not too surprising that diets rich in beans have been found to help with weight loss.[50] No other food so perfectly packages fiber and protein—the dynamic duo for creating a feeling of fullness. Beans are also good for you regardless of any potential effects on hunger and weight. In overweight people, eating more legumes can improve blood pressure, blood cholesterol levels, and markers of inflammation.[51]

- **Soyfoods and seitan.** These foods represent an easy way for vegans to give diets a protein boost. One-half cup of extra-firm tofu or 1 cup of soy curls has nearly twice the amount of protein found in ½ cup of legumes, and seitan can have up to three times as much protein.

- **Healthy fats.** These foods can provide a sense of satisfaction and satiety that will prevent binging and overeating. Including nuts and even vegetable oils can actually help prevent weight gain in some women.

Take Care of Yourself: Rest, Relaxation, and Exercise

Chronic sleep deprivation and fatigue—not uncommon in busy women—could cause you to overeat. Sleep deprivation sometimes translates to increased hunger, possibly because of changes in levels of hormones that control hunger and satiety.[6,52,53] Likewise, stress may cause you to overeat, while missing cues that signal satiety. Depression may lead to overeating or sometimes to a lack of interest in self-care, which may mean you pay less attention to eating well. I talk more about tactics for dealing with stress and depression in Chapter 16. And it is so important to take steps to manage these problems for your overall health and certainly your happiness.

Exercise is a great way to make a dent in both stress and depression. It also energizes, helps you sleep better, and improves cognitive function. Exercise can enhance weight loss, but more important, it can prevent weight gain even in those who have a strong genetic risk for obesity.[54] Aerobic exercise like walking is great for burning calories and reducing stress. But weight training helps to protect muscle mass—especially important if you are losing weight, and as you move toward and beyond menopause. It's also just plain healthier to have plenty of muscle mass, which improves stamina and protects bone health. Again, as with healthy eating and managing stress and depression, there are so many advantages to exercise that have nothing to do with body weight.

Ideally, you'll find a physical activity that you enjoy, making exercise a pleasurable break in your day. If you're more like me—not especially enthused about any type of exercise or sports—and you find exercise to be a bit of a chore, you may need to give yourself a little push. Start small, and pay attention to the benefits. I don't especially enjoy lifting weights, but I love feeling strong. And I know that taking a break from work to walk for a few minutes really does improve my concentration and reduce stress.

If you don't like going to the gym, get a few exercise DVDs and work out at home. If you haven't exercised for a long time, start slowly and do something that feels comfortable. Maybe it's a walk around the block or maybe you'll start with lifting 3-pound weights while you're sitting in a chair. It doesn't matter; everybody has to start somewhere. And your goal doesn't have to be to run a marathon. It's enough to build some muscle, improve your cardiovascular health, sleep better, and feel better.

WHEN VEGANS ARE OVERWEIGHT

It's true that, on average, vegans have a lower BMI than people who eat meat. But for all the reasons I've talked about in this chapter, vegans can struggle with weight just like anyone else.

Some overweight vegans feel shy or embarrassed about talking to others about their vegan choices, believing that they aren't good role models for a vegan lifestyle. That's wrong for two reasons. First, because veganism is a set of choices built around an ethic of compassion, it has to be available to everyone. Race, religion, and political party don't matter. Nor does body size. It's hard to imagine that we can entice as many people as possible to a vegan lifestyle if we insist that all vegans have to be skinny.

Second, studies show that people are more open to a message when it comes from someone who is like them. This means that in vegan advocacy, there is a role for everyone.

Many, many women struggle with their weight. A vegan diet may help some women lose weight, but it's not a foolproof weight control program. However, without a doubt, eating more plant foods can improve your health at any weight. And, a vegan diet always delivers on its most important promises. It is *guaranteed* to make your diet more respectful and compassionate. Whether or not you can be thin, you can always choose to make the way you eat matter to yourself, to animals, and to the world.

VEGAN DIETS AND EATING DISORDERS

With rising rates of overweight and obesity among both children and adults, public health officials have launched The War on Obesity. In the media, however, it often feels more like a War on the Obese. Collateral damage is significant and it includes "weightist" prejudice, body dissatisfaction, and shame—as well as chronic dieting that can produce poor health outcomes. Along with media images that glorify ultrathin bodies and stigmatize overweight people, it might also promote eating disorders.

The two common eating disorders are anorexia nervosa, an exaggerated drive for thinness, intense fear of getting fat, and self-starvation; and bulimia nervosa, which is an overwhelming urge to eat followed by purging usually through vomiting. (I talk in Chapter 16 about orthorexia, a preoccupation with healthful eating that can become an unhealthy obsession. Some experts regard this as an emerging type of eating disorder.)

Although eating disorders are most common in teen girls and young women, they can occur at any age. In a survey of 1,000 women between the ages of six and seventy years, more than 60 percent said they were dissatisfied with their body and nearly half wanted to weigh less. Almost 5 percent of these women exhibited some behaviors typical of eating disorders.[55] Causes of eating disorders aren't well understood but experts now realize that they are the result of complex interaction among genetic factors, personality, and environment. Risk factors for eating disorders include perceived pressure to be thin, body dissatisfaction, and dietary restraint.

A true eating disorder is a serious mental illness that requires help from medical professionals. But, there is a continuum of restrained eating behaviors, some of which never progress to a condition that meets the clinical definition of an eating disorder. Intuitive eating can help with some of these disordered eating behaviors.[42,56] Some research has found that eating disorders are more common among vegetarian teens and young women. In the past, this raised concerns that vegetarians might be at risk for developing anorexia or bulimia. That's turned out to be untrue. First, in most cases, women develop the eating disorder before becoming vegetarian. Their vegetarian diet is a tool used to control food intake or mask the disorder.[57,58] In fact, in one study, girls who had tried and then abandoned a vegetarian diet were more likely to show signs of disordered eating than girls who stuck with a vegetarian diet.[59] For the ex-vegetarians, the diet was probably just one of many methods they dabbled in to control eating and weight.

In other studies, many of the girls with eating disorders weren't actually vegetarian even though they claimed that they were. Among girls and women who are truly vegetarian in practice, they don't appear to engage in disordered eating any more often than meateaters.[60] One of the most surprising findings is that girls and young women who adopt more strict types of vegetarian diets—like veganism—are less likely to have an eating disorder, compared to those who are semi-vegetarians.[61,62] This was the case among college women who filled out questionnaires about their eating habits, behaviors, and attitudes regarding food and diet, as well as the reasons behind their food choices. Women who ate more "flexitarian" or semi-vegetarian diets that included some meat had more restrained eating behavior than the vegetarians. They were also more concerned about the effect of their diet on weight control and less concerned about the effects on animal welfare.[61] This suggests that those who take a broader view of food choices and how they affect animals and the earth have healthier eating behaviors than those who limit animal foods strictly for reasons of weight control. It's another example of how a vegan ethic can help women develop perspective about food, diet, and body size.

FINDING YOUR WAY BEYOND THE SCALE

If yours is a history of weight cycling and years of struggle with your weight, it's time for a paradigm shift. Throw away the scale and turn toward habits that support your health, your self-esteem, and your happiness.

- Pay attention to hunger signals. Eat when you are hungry and stop when you are full. Eat more mindfully and practice principles of intuitive eating.
- Choose foods that protect health—slow carbs, healthy fats, legumes, and lots of fruits and vegetables. These are also the foods that promote satiety.
- Engage in regular exercise.
- Manage stress, deal with depression (see Chapter 16).
- Get adequate rest.
- Embrace the true consequences of your vegan diet—a way of eating and living that is a celebration of compassion and purpose.

CHAPTER TEN

HEALTHY AGING

The best diet in the world won't stop the clock, but your food choices, along with other lifestyle habits, can slow things down a little and help protect health throughout the decades—whether you change your diet for the better at age twenty or sixty.

You already know that diet and lifestyle affect risk for chronic diseases like cancer, heart disease, and osteoporosis, all of which are more common as women age. I'm going to talk more about those issues in the chapters ahead. In this chapter, I'll focus on dietary choices that affect the aging process itself, especially as it relates to cognitive function and skin health.

ANTIOXIDANTS AND THE AGING PROCESS

The process of aging—which starts as soon as we're born—is still a little bit of a mystery. Although scientists can see what happens to aging cells, they haven't yet uncovered exactly how or why the changes occur. One thing we do know is that aging is inevitable because the cells of the body can't live and reproduce forever. Stretches of DNA called telomeres sit at the end of chromosomes (which are strands of DNA) and these little tails get shorter each time the cell divides.

When the telomeres are gone, the cell has reached the end of its reproductive life. It becomes inactive, or it dies.

It seems that telomere length, other genetic factors, and oxidative stress all play roles in determining life span and all impact the process of aging. Accumulated oxidative damage from free radicals, which promotes mutations and cell damage, contributes to cell aging. A healthy diet may not be able to keep up completely with the damage wrought by free radicals—so far, no one has figured out how to live forever—but it does seem that eating lots of antioxidant-rich plant foods will provide a little bit of an edge when it comes to slowing the aging process. In older women living in Slovakia, for example, vegetarians had much lower levels of several markers of oxidative damage than nonvegetarians.[1]

HEALTHY BRAINS

Mild memory lapses are an annoying but common consequence of aging. You can't remember where you left your keys, or the name of the person you chatted with at a party last night. You might find that appointments and even important dates like birthdays slip your mind. It happens to everybody, but it happens with more frequency as we age. It's all perfectly normal and is due to chemical changes in the brain. This is different from dementia, which is a chronic progressive condition that can become severe enough to affect daily functioning.

Alzheimer's disease (AD) is the most common type of dementia. It's characterized by deposits of plaques in the brain that are the result of tissue degeneration, and also by changes within nerve cells. Another common disorder is multi-infarct dementia, which is caused by multiple small strokes in the brain. Dementia can also occur due to infections, chronic drug use, or severe depression. There is a clear genetic component to AD risk and for other types of dementia, but diet and lifestyle can offer some protection against these diseases.

Risk Factors for Dementia

There are no cognitive function studies involving older vegans, but what the research shows about diet and cognition suggests that eating more plants is beneficial. In one study, Seventh-day Adventists who ate meat had twice the risk of developing dementia as Adventist vegetarians.[2] People who eat a more Mediterranean-style diet—high in plant foods and good fats, low in animal foods and saturated fat—also tend to retain better brain function as they age.[3] It's not surprising given that underlying issues in dementia seem to be the same ones that raise risk for other chronic diseases. Both chronic inflammation and higher levels of advanced glycation end products (AGEs) are linked to risk for AD.[4-6] High cholesterol and insulin resistance are associated with accumulation of beta-amyloid, the hard deposit that is a pathological hallmark of AD.[7] Since people with low cholesterol tend to have healthier blood pressure readings, this could be one reason for their lower risk of dementia.[8-11] Even those who reduce their cholesterol through drug therapy are at lower risk for dementia.[12-13] Vegans tend to naturally have lower cholesterol levels and lower blood pressures.

The type of fat you eat may be important, too. In both the Nurses' Health Study and the Women's Health Initiative, women who ate the most monounsaturated fats like olive oil, canola oil, and nuts, had less age-related cognitive decline.[14,15] In contrast, older men and women living in Chicago were more likely to develop Alzheimer's Disease when their diets were high in saturated and trans fats.[16]

Since the long-chain omega-3 fat DHA is concentrated in some of the most active parts of the brain, it's also possible that higher intakes of these fats could protect brain function. The studies are a little conflicting at this point, but quite a few show that people with better DHA and EPA status have better cognitive function as they age.[17-19]

Oxidative stress might make the blood-brain barrier more permeable to proteins that lead to beta-amyloid accumulation.[20] So eating plenty of antioxidant-rich foods may be important for preventing the dementia seen with AD and could also prevent the cardiovascular problems that raise risk for dementia.[21] This is an easy one for vegans, of course, since whole plant foods are packed with antioxidants.

Another easy issue for vegans is vitamin B_{12}. Low intakes of this vitamin are associated with higher levels of homocysteine in the blood, which may be related to cognitive decline.[22,23] Again, it's important for all older adults to get vitamin B_{12} from supplements or fortified foods, which is the way vegans always get their B_{12}.

Finally, certain dietary minerals might affect cognition. In women especially, having iron levels that are too low or too high might speed up cognitive decline.[24] And while both copper and zinc are needed for brain function, excessive intakes of these nutrients might raise risk for dementia.[25] This is unlikely to be an issue for vegans, however, since absorption of these minerals is lower from plant foods. Whether or not aluminum plays a role in dementia is an ongoing issue of debate. To be on the safe side, you can reduce your exposure to this metal by choosing deodorant that doesn't include an antiperspirant, avoiding antacids that contain aluminum, and by choosing nonaluminum cookware.

Protecting Brain Health Goes Beyond Diet

Exercise doesn't just protect muscles and bones as you age; it can also improve cognitive function. It's possible that being physically active increases factors in the brain that are involved in neurological repair, and also reduces AGE formation in women.[26,27] And then there is the kind of exercise you do with your brain. Mentally stimulating activities slow cognitive decline, possibly by promoting more cell-to-cell connections in the brain.[20] Challenging your brain through crossword puzzles and other games, reading, learning a language, or learning to play a musical instrument are all activities that could help protect cognitive function. It's the challenge that makes a difference, so even using your nondominant hand to brush your teeth, move your computer mouse, or—most challenging of all—for writing can actually slow age-related changes in your brain.

Finally, people who suffer from depression have a higher risk of cognitive decline.[28-30] Scientists don't know why this is, but since depression is also associated with inflammation, which in turn is linked to cognitive decline, this could be part of the explanation. I talk more about the relationship of diet to depression in Chapter 16.

Soyfoods and Your Brain

Estrogen has a positive effect on cognitive function, so it seems like soy isoflavones could, too. But back in the year 2000, a study of Japanese men living in Hawaii found something quite unexpected. Men who ate the most tofu tended to have worse cognitive function as they aged.[31] So did their wives (although the researchers didn't measure the wives' soy consumption).

There were lots of limitations with this study, especially since it wasn't actually designed to look at cognitive function—it was a study on heart disease—and the assessment of soyfoods intake was limited and problematic.

Other research challenges these findings. For example, although tofu consumption was associated with worse cognitive function in older people living in Indonesia, a follow-up investigation didn't find any effect. And interestingly, Indonesians who ate more tempeh actually did better on tests of memory. In Hong Kong, isoflavone intake had no effect on cognition in older people.[32]

These three observational studies don't provide sufficient evidence for drawing a conclusion about isoflavones and cognition. We need clinical studies for that. So far, there have been as many as eight of these more robust kinds of studies. According to the North American Menopause Society, the findings suggest that eating soy can benefit cognitive function in women under the age of sixty-five, but, after that, it doesn't seem to have any effect. A more recent study, which lasted for three years and included more than 350 postmenopausal women, found a small benefit in visual memory (remembering pictures) among the women who consumed isoflavones, but no additional benefits.[33] Right now, the findings aren't strong enough to suggest that eating soy will protect your brain, but they are at least reassuring that it won't hurt your cognitive function.

Creatine and Cognitive Function

In Chapter 8, I talked about creatine, a compound involved in supplying energy to cells, as it relates to athletic performance. Because it's thought to reduce fatigue in weightlifting, athletes sometimes take supplements of creatine to improve their workouts.

There is no creatine in plant foods, but since both the liver and kidneys synthesize plenty of this compound, there is no indication that vegans are at a disadvantage. Recently, though, there has been some interest in creatine as a way of enhancing brain function, raising questions about whether vegans and vegetarians might benefit from a dietary source of this compound. Australian researchers measured the effects of creatine supplements in young vegans and vegetarians who took five grams of creatine per day for six weeks. At the end of the study, the subjects showed improvement in a number of tests of cognitive function.[34] Whether it would have had the same effect in omnivores is something we don't know. They already have some creatine in their diet, although they typically consume only about half the amount that was used in this study.

Another study did compare the effects of creatine on cognitive function between vegetarians and omnivores. In this group, all college-aged women, there were no differences in memory between the groups at the start of the study but, after five days, vegetarians who had taken creatine supplements did better on memory tests than vegetarians who didn't supplement. They also did better than meat-eaters who took creatine supplements. It may be that vegetarians are more sensitive to the benefits of creatine.[35] These studies tell us nothing, of course, about potential effects of creatine in protecting cognitive function in older women. Small doses—1 to 2 grams per day—seem to be harmless if this is something you would like to try, but the evidence isn't strong enough for me to recommend it.

TIPS FOR KEEPING YOUR BRAIN SHARP

- Eat a healthy diet—one that includes lots of slow carbs and healthy fats.
- Limit saturated fats and avoid trans fats.
- Eat lots of fruits and vegetables. Their rich content of antioxidants can reduce oxidative stress and they also help to keep blood pressure in check.
- Monitor your blood pressure. If it's high, watch salt intake and make sure you eat plenty of potassium-rich foods—fruits, vegetables, and legumes.
- Consider a supplement providing around 400 to 500 milligrams of the omega-3 fats DHA and EPA.
- Engage in daily exercise. You don't need to join the gym and buy lots of fancy equipment. Simply walking is great for body and mind. And don't drag your feet; people who walk more quickly may retain better cognitive function.
- Turn off the TV and exercise your brain with reading, crossword puzzles, or Sudoku.
- Pursue lifestyle practices that help you deal with stress and depression (see Chapter 16).

HEALTY SKIN THROUGH THE YEARS

It's your body's largest organ, weighing around 6 pounds and covering 18 to 20 square feet. Skin has a number of functions, but serving as a protective shield between you and the environment is its most important. Skin protects internal organs from trauma, ultraviolet radiation, temperature extremes, toxins, and bacteria.

The outermost layer of skin, the epidermis, prevents entry of foreign substances and also controls fluid losses. Beneath the epidermis, the dermis layer contains blood vessels, hair follicles (in some parts of the body), sweat glands, and nerves. It's held together by collagen, a protein that gives skin its strength, and it also contains the flexible protein elastin. The deepest layer of skin is the subcutaneous layer, which is a network of collagen and fat cells, helping to conserve heat and absorb shocks to reduce chances of injury.

Healthy Diet for Healthy Skin

The cells of your skin need the same good nutrition as the rest of your body. But certain nutrient shortfalls are likely to show up as skin problems in particular. Too little vitamin A, for example, can result in dry, scaly skin. Vegans get vitamin A from plant pigments—called carotenoids—found in dark green and deep orange vegetables. Because both zinc and vitamin C are needed for synthesis of collagen, they are especially important for healthy skin. The antioxidant activity of vitamin C might also help protect skin.[36] Vegans usually have diets that are rich in vitamin C, but zinc can fall short. Make sure your diet includes plenty of legumes and at least one or two servings of nuts or seeds to maximize zinc intake.

Avoiding fat-rich plant foods may take a toll on skin health. Both essential fatty acids—linoleic and alpha-linolenic acid (ALA)—are needed to keep skin healthy and vibrant. Everyone gets enough of the first, but some vegans could fall short in their intake of ALA, especially if they eat diets that are too low in fat. Low-fat intake might also interfere with absorption of important antioxidants and nutrients.

Aging Skin

The ravages of time that show up as crows' feet and laugh lines are among the inevitable and normal changes that occur as we age. Turnover of cells in the epidermis slows with the passage of time. In young adults, cells rejuvenate in about twenty-eight days. In older people it takes as long as 40 to 60 days.[37] The result is thinner skin that is also more susceptible to sunburn. In the dermis, decreased synthesis of collagen and elastin is a built-in consequence of aging that leads to wrinkles and loss of elasticity. A decline in tiny blood vessels reduces blood flow to skin in older people, too. And fewer oil-producing glands result in drier skin.

Many of the changes seen in skin are due to lower blood levels of hormones and also a reduction in hormone receptors in cells. Changes also occur in the muscles underlying the skin and in the way fat is distributed. In younger people, fat distribution is diffuse, while in older people, it tends to accumulate in pockets, which can lead to sagging. Many changes are due to genetics (you may find that people comment more and more on how much you look like your mother as you get older), and some are simply irrefutable signs of the passage of time along with the effects of gravity.

Because skin bumps right up against the rest of the world, environmental factors have a big effect on its health and the rate at which it ages. Stress, environment, and poor nutrition can all take a toll on aging skin. Things that cause premature aging can also raise risk for cancer, diabetes, and other chronic illnesses. So, eating in a way that protects skin from premature aging isn't all about vanity; it's about taking care of one of your body's important protective organs.

Dermatologists are in universal agreement about the most important factor in skin aging: sun exposure. Sun-induced skin aging, called photoaging, is a cumulative process that depends on the degree of sun exposure you experience over time. The pigmentation in your skin has a considerable effect, too, since light-skinned people are much more prone to sun damage and premature aging.

You'll need to weigh the negative consequences of sun exposure against its benefits for vitamin D production. The amount of sunshine needed to make vitamin D varies depending on where you live, your skin tone, and your age. Older people require more time in the sun to make vitamin D and they are also at higher risk for skin cancer. And, it's just hard to know exactly how much sun exposure is enough. Even people living in sunny parts of the world often don't synthesize enough vitamin D.[38–40] It's far better to take a vitamin D supplement and stick with good sunblock protection when you're in the sun. This is especially true for light-skinned people whose skin is far more susceptible to the damaging effects of sun exposure. UV radiation from sunlight is considered by major health organizations to be a carcinogen.

Good sunblock must protect against both UVA and UVB rays. UVB rays are the primary cause of sunburn and also play a key role in development of skin cancer. These are also the types of rays that produce vitamin D when skin is exposed to sunlight. SPF (sun protection factor) numbers are based on prevention of sunburn produced by UVB rays. But UVA rays have longer wavelengths that penetrate deeper into skin leading to oxidative stress, photoaging, and wrinkling. They also contribute to skin cancer. Tanning booths primarily emit UVA. It's important to look for sunblocks that protect against both UVA and UVB rays.

Protect Aging Skin with Antioxidants

Much of the sun's damage is due to oxidative stress, so it's not surprising that dietary antioxidants might offer some protection. In fact, even though people living in Greece get far more sun exposure than those living in Sweden, rates of melanoma are consistently lower in Mediterranean countries than in northern Europe. Part of the reason no doubt is differences in skin pigmentation, but their high fruit and vegetable intake could also offer protection for people living in southern Europe.[41]

Skin has its own antioxidant defense system, but it declines with aging, especially in sun-damaged skin.[42] Enhancing this built-in protection with an antioxidant-rich diet can help to keep skin as healthy as possible. When researchers compared diets of women in different countries to see how they might affect skin reactions to sun exposure, they found that the most protective diets were rich in vegetables, legumes, and olive oil.[43] Benefits of olive oil might seem a little surprising, but antioxidants in olive oil may protect against skin cancer and olive oil might affect the fat composition of skin in a way that is protective.[44–46]

Antioxidants in fruits and vegetables might aid in skin protection because they actually accumulate in the skin. Lycopene found in tomatoes is one of them, which may explain why consuming tomato paste can actually reduce sunburn damage.[47-48] The vitamin A precursor beta-carotene is another antioxidant that offers some protection against sunburn.[49] The protection from these antioxidant-rich foods is modest, so you can't just eat a carrot and then bake in the sun all day. No matter what you're eating, too much sun will damage your skin. But research does tell us that antioxidants work to reduce damaging effects of oxidation and that a diet rich in these compounds is likely to be very good for skin health.

In fact, a diet rich in beta-carotene from carrots, sweet potatoes, winter squash, and green leafy vegetables can give you a healthy glow. British scientists found that people with the highest intakes of fruits and vegetables and of beta-carotene had a more golden cast to their

Protecting Eye Health with Antioxidants

The higher antioxidant content of vegetarian and vegan diets may also protect against other aging processes. Cataracts, a clouding of the eye's lens, are a relatively common problem in older people in the United States. Since diets high in antioxidants appear to reduce risk for cataracts, it's not surprising that research shows that vegetarians, and especially vegans, are at reduced risk for cataracts.[55] There's also evidence that women who reduce their meat intake could be at lower risk for another age-related eye problem, macular degeneration.[56]

Two compounds in plant foods—lutein and zeaxanthin—are especially protective against age-related eye problems. They are actually pigments that accumulate in the eye and filter out harmful ultraviolet light. Spinach, broccoli, kale, and corn are good sources of both.

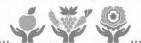

skin tone, regardless of ethnicity. Subjects liked the appearance of
the beta-carotene glow more than a tan.[50]

Finally, a diet rich in antioxidants from fruits and vegetables and
even from herbs and spices like cloves, allspice, cinnamon, sage, tar-
ragon, and rosemary can also reduce formation of AGEs, which are
especially damaging to collagen.[51–54]

Soyfoods for Your Skin

Because reduced estrogen production is associated with many of the
changes seen in aging skin, it's logical to wonder if soy isoflavones
could benefit skin health. The cosmetic industry has taken a particular interest in isoflavones, which have started to appear in a number of
skin creams. There is reason to think they work, too. An isoflavone-
enriched cream was found to enhance blood flow to the skin in postmenopausal women. That may be important since one effect of lower
estrogen levels is a reduction in small blood vessels in the skin.[57]

Soy isoflavones may also affect hyaluronic acid (HA), a compound
found within the matrix formed by collagen and that is responsible for
moisturizing the skin. In a study of postmenopausal women in São
Paulo, Brazil, a gel containing soy isoflavones was effective in raising
skin HA concentrations. After 24 weeks of using the gel on their face,
the concentration of HA in subjects' facial skin increased by about
two-and-a-half times.[58] Isoflavones may also work from inside to
protect skin. Postmenopausal women who consumed an isoflavone
supplement for six months experienced improved thickness of their
epidermis and improvements in collagen formation and blood vessels.[59] In another study, middle-aged women consumed 40 milligrams
of isoflavones—about the amount in 1½ servings of soyfoods—every
day for 12 weeks. They experienced improved skin elasticity and a decline in small wrinkles.[60] As I write this, some new research from
Dutch investigators that hasn't yet been published (but has been presented at medical conferences) shows that soy isoflavones are effective
in decreasing wrinkles and increasing collagen synthesis in postmenopausal women within less than four months.[61]

Plant-Based for Your Face

Although there is plenty of hype regarding skincare products, there is also quite a bit of research behind some of the ingredients. And some really do work to protect the health of your skin.

These are a few of the ingredients that are (or can be) derived from plants and that have demonstrated benefits when applied topically to your skin. One word of advice: some of these, the antioxidants in particular, are destroyed when exposed to air. As soon as you open the fancy jar of your new skin cream, many of its benefits will immediately dissipate. Opt for products that are packaged in tubes or bottles, which allows less surface exposure to the air.

Hyaluronic acid: This skin-identical ingredient—that is, it's a compound that is already in your skin—helps your skin retain moisture and may stimulate collagen synthesis.[62] Sodium hyaluronate is a non–animal derived version.

Alpha-hydroxy acids: These are exfoliants that remove the outer layer of built-up dead skin cells and can eliminate some wrinkling.[63] Although they can be derived from milk, most come from sugar or fruits. Look for products that contain 5 to 15 percent AHA.

Beta-hydroxy acids: The one used in skin preparations is salicylic acid, derived from a type of willow tree and also a key ingredient in aspirin. It's effective in treating acne.[64] Look for products that contain salicylic acid in 1 to 2 percent concentrations.

Vitamin C: Look for ascorbic acid or vitamin C on labels. It can protect skin from oxidative damage and may increase collagen production.[65]

Green tea: EGCG (epigallocatechin 3-gallate) from green tea can improve collagen synthesis and reduce damage from sun exposure.[66]

Soy isoflavones: These phytochemicals in soyfoods can improve blood flow to the skin, increase hyaluronic acid levels, and may benefit skin elasticity.[54,55]

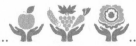

Eating for Healthy Skin

Time marches on and along with all that wisdom that you're accruing, you're going to collect a few wrinkles, too. The extent and timing is dependent somewhat on your genes, your skin tone, and how much sunbathing you did as a teen. It's never too late to take steps to protect the health of your skin, though. Granted, plant foods don't rival Botox or a face lift when it comes to reducing wrinkles. On the other hand, neither of those treatments will reduce your risk for skin cancer and other chronic diseases. To keep your skin healthy, and maybe even reverse some of the damage:

- Use a good sunscreen that provides protection from both UVA and UVB rays.
- Stay hydrated: drink enough water and limit intake of alcohol and caffeine, both of which are dehydrating.
- Make sure you get enough zinc.
- Get enough of the essential fatty acid ALA and choose healthy fats—especially extra-virgin olive oil—in general.
- Eat lots and lots of fruits and vegetables and make sure you're including plenty of the dark orange and green leafy vegetables that are rich in vitamin A.
- Include traditional soyfoods like tofu, tempeh, and soymilk in your diet if you like them. It's okay to eat veggie meats and cheeses occasionally if you enjoy them, but most don't contain the isoflavones that may protect skin health.

CHAPTER ELEVEN

PREVENTING BREAST CANCER

Every minute of the day, about 10 million of your cells are dividing, each passing along exact copies of its DNA. Given the astronomical number of cell divisions taking place over time, it's not too surprising that mistakes happen. Many factors, including diet, exposure to sunlight, and products of normal metabolism, can cause mutations, which are faulty copies of the cell's DNA that may lead to cancer.

These errors in DNA copying happen all of the time—hundreds of times a day—but, your body has numerous ways of repairing them so that most never go on to become a problem. The mutations become an issue only when the repair systems fail. Nor does a single mutation cause cancer. Instead, the abnormal cell that ignites the cancer process is a result of many different changes in cell function, usually taking place over decades.

Worldwide, the most common cancer in women is breast cancer. It's also the most studied of the cancers that are specific to women. Unfortunately, there is little available information about the relationship of diet to endometrial, ovarian, or cervical cancer. I'll talk about these other cancers, too, but most of this chapter deals with breast cancer.

Risk Factors for Breast Cancer

Between 5 and 10 percent of breast cancer cases are thought to be caused by inherited mutations in the breast cancer genes BRCA1 or BRCA2.[1] These mutations are found most often in Jewish women of Eastern European ancestry, although they are not exclusively confined to these women. Reproductive events also impact breast cancer risk. Early menarche—the time of a girl's first period—and late menopause extend lifelong exposure to estrogen, and this might increase risk for breast cancer.

Early pregnancy lowers risk, possibly because breast tissue is more sensitive to carcinogens between the time of the first period and first pregnancy—so shortening that time lowers lifelong risk.[2] Women who breastfeed have a lower breast cancer risk, too.

You can't change your genes, or the age at which you started your period, and you can't go back and reschedule the timing of your first child. There are plenty of things that affect cancer risk that you *can* control, though, and diet is one of them.

Breast cancer rates vary greatly around the world. You might think that this has something to do with genetics, but it actually seems to have more to do with where women live. Or more precisely *how* they live. When women move from a country or region where breast cancer rates are low to an area where women are at higher risk, breast cancer risk in their offspring begins to rise fairly quickly. So rates of breast cancer among Japanese-Americans, for example, are similar to those of non-Japanese women in the United States and are higher than those of women who stayed in Japan. This tells us that environment, lifestyle, and diet have a much greater effect on overall breast cancer risk than genetics.

The relationship of diet to breast cancer isn't entirely clear, but the evidence that certain plant foods reduce risk—and that some animal foods raise it—is considerable, despite the fact that there are some real challenges in uncovering links between diet and cancer.

RESEARCH ON DIET AND CANCER

It's difficult to study the effects of diet on cancer for a number of reasons. First, we lack good markers for most cancers, including breast cancer. It's easy to look at the effects of diet on conditions like heart disease because we can easily assess risk by measuring blood cholesterol and blood pressure. Aside from genetic tests for the BRCA1 and BRCA2 genes, there is no blood test for breast cancer risk, though. Certain factors like changes in breast density and also breast cell proliferation are related to risk—and some studies do look at these—but these are more difficult to measure and their relationship to breast cancer is less straightforward.

Second, there is evidence that diet might have varying effects depending on the type of tumor. Postmenopausal women are more likely to have ER+ (estrogen-receptor positive) tumors, whose growth is stimulated by estrogen—while younger women are more likely to have ER-tumors, which aren't affected by this hormone. One study found that higher fat intake raised cancer risk in postmenopausal women, but lowered it in premenopausal women. This might reflect the different types of tumors that pre- and postmenopausal women typically have.[3] Another type of tumor, called HER2-positive, is sensitive to a particular protein that stimulates breast cell growth. Interestingly, compounds in olive oil cause these tumor cells to die in cell culture studies but don't appear to have the same effect on other kinds of cancer cells.[4]

Finally, cancer develops over a long period of time so that a particular food, nutrient, or diet may contribute to the development of a tumor that doesn't become apparent for many decades. Compare that to heart disease where we can measure effects of different diets on cholesterol levels or blood pressure in a matter of weeks.

Animal studies can measure effects of diet much more directly and quickly by injecting animals with cancer cells and then looking at the effects of different dietary components and diets on tumor growth. These studies have limited value for us, though, since humans are different from other animals, and the diets fed to research animals don't reflect human diets very well.

As a result, we're lacking good clinical intervention studies that provide insight into the diet and breast cancer relationship. Instead, we need to rely on epidemiologic studies like the prospective studies I described in Chapter 4. And while these studies can uncover certain associations between diet and breast cancer, they don't establish cause and effect.

For all these reasons, there continue to be many questions around the link between diet and breast cancer. Even so, there is reason to think that basing diets on plant foods offers some protection.

BREAST CANCER IN VEGANS AND VEGETARIANS

Most of what we know about rates of cancer in vegetarians comes from just a handful of epidemiologic studies including the Adventist Health Study, the EPIC-Oxford study, and a few smaller studies in England. Although some of these found lower rates of breast cancer among vegetarians, none of the findings were statistically significant. That is, mathematically, there is a good chance that the findings were due to random chance. One exception is the Adventist Health Study-2, which found lower rates of cancer among vegan women. In this case, it's not clear whether the benefit came from their vegan diet or from other healthy habits.[5]

It's surprising, because so much of what we know about vegetarian and vegan eating habits suggest that these diets should lower risk for breast cancer. For example, vegetarian women consume more fiber, fruits, and vegetables, and less fat than women who eat meat. This may explain the lower blood estrogen levels seen in some vegetarian women as well as the fact that they begin menstruation later. Delayed menstruation could lower their overall lifetime exposure to estrogen, and possibly protect against breast cancer.[6–9]

So why don't studies show that vegetarians are less likely to develop breast cancer? There are several possible reasons. First, the evidence suggests—quite strongly in fact—that early life events have a big effect on breast cancer risk. Childhood dietary habits could be a much more important determinant of later breast cancer risk than habits adopted later in life. The studies that looked at breast cancer in vegetarians assessed only adult diets and, almost certainly, many of the women in these studies were not vegetarian before adulthood. Furthermore, even those who are lifelong vegetarians may have consumed more animal products such as milk, cheese, and eggs in childhood before alternatives were readily available.

Second, when it comes to research, *vegetarian* is a pretty fuzzy term. Many people who describe themselves as vegetarians actually consume some meat and/or fish.[10] Also, in the Adventist Health Study and EPIC-Oxford, many of the omnivore subjects ate a fairly healthy diet that was relatively low in meat. They had a lower risk for cancer compared to the general population. All of this tells us that diets weren't really that far apart for many of the meat-eaters and vegetarians in these studies.

None of this means, though, that vegan and vegetarian diets are not protective. When we start looking at studies on different plant and animal foods, we do see a pattern of protection for those eating plant-based diets. We may not have direct evidence for a protective effect of vegan diets—at least not yet—but there is a pretty good case to be made for eating more plants and less animal food.

PROTECTION FROM PLANT FOODS

Not too surprisingly, a standard American pattern of meat plus refined starches fails miserably at protecting against breast cancer compared to traditional patterns from other cultures. Women in the United States who adhere more closely to some of those traditional patterns from other parts of the world do much better in terms of breast cancer risk. In the Four-Corners Breast Cancer Study, among women living in the southwestern United States, those eating either a native Mexican diet or a more Mediterranean pattern were about half as likely to get breast cancer as women eating a more usual American diet.[11] Asian American women living in Los Angeles had a lower risk for breast cancer if they ate either a Mediterranean-type diet or a traditional Asian pattern with lots of vegetables and soy.[12] The common feature among traditional Mexican, Asian, and Mediterranean patterns is that they are all plant-based diets. Major health organizations including the National Cancer Institute (NCI) and the American Institute for Cancer Research (AICR) encourage adoption of plant-based diets to lower cancer risk.

Preventing Cancer

Phytochemicals in fruits and vegetables may affect cancer risk in a number of ways. Some are antioxidants, which means that they can prevent the oxidative damage that leads to mutations. Other compounds either enhance enzymes that detoxify carcinogens or inhibit enzymes that activate them.[13,14]

Most of these dietary compounds work to prevent development of cancer in its earliest stages, but some can affect later stages of the cancer process. For example, quercetin, a phytochemical found in citrus fruits, apples, onions, and red wine may inhibit an enzyme that digests tissue membranes and allows tumors to metastasize.[15] The isoflavones in soyfoods and compounds in green tea could also work at a later stage of cancer development by inhibiting angiogenesis, which is the formation of new blood vessels needed to supply nutrients and oxygen to tumors.

Although cooking can reduce both the nutrients and the phytochemicals in vegetables, it can also make some of them easier to absorb. For example, tomatoes are an excellent source of the carotenoid lycopene, but it's about four times better absorbed from tomato paste than from raw tomatoes. Adding a small amount of oil to cooked vegetables can also increase absorption of certain nutrients and phytochemicals.

The fiber content of plant foods also contributes to their protective effects. High-fiber diets are linked to lower blood estrogen levels, which are in turn linked to protection against some breast tumors.[16,17]

Table 11-1: Best of the Best: Some Phytochemical Stars

Phytochemical	Best Food Sources	How They Fight Cancer
Anthocyanins	Red, blue, and purple foods, especially berries	Antioxidants and also interfere with angiogenesis (growth of blood vessels to feed tumors), reduce cell proliferation, and induce cancer cell death (apoptosis)
Curcumin	Turmeric, a yellow-hued spice often used in curried dishes	Induces death of cancer cells, interferes with metastasis
EGCG (epigallocatechin-3-gallate)	Green tea	Antioxidant
Lycopene	Tomatoes are richest source. Also found in watermelon, grapefruit, guava, and papaya. It's absorbed best from cooked tomatoes.	Antioxidant
Resveratrol	Red grape seeds and skins, red wine, peanuts	Antioxidant, interferes with angiogenesis and metastasis
Sulforaphane	Broccoli, cabbage, Brussels sprouts, cauliflower, kale, collard greens, bok choy, and other members of the cabbage family	Interrupts cancer cell division and induces death of cancer cells. Enhances enzymes that detoxify carcinogens.
Quercetin	Apples, broccoli, green tea, onions, red wine	Antioxidant
Isoflavones	Soyfoods	Inhibit cancer cell growth, increase cell differentiation
Beta-carotene	Orange and yellow and green leafy vegetables	Antioxidant
Limonoids	Citrus fruits	Induce enzyme systems that detoxify carcinogens
Allicin	Onions and garlic	Destroy cancer cells

Soy Isoflavones and Breast Cancer

Some of the most interesting research on diet and breast cancer has focused on soy isoflavones. I talked about the relationship of isoflavones
to estrogen on pages 58–62 and the fact that these compounds act in
selective ways on estrogen receptors in breast and other tissue.

In 1990, the National Cancer Institute (NCI) began looking at the
relationship of soy intake to breast cancer risk. In fact, my husband,
who was a program director in the NCI's Diet and Cancer Branch in
the early 1990s, was largely instrumental in initiating this research
program, so it's an issue I've been close to for more than two decades. Since then, more than 1,300 scientific papers on soy and breast
cancer have been published.

Initial interest in soy and cancer stemmed from observations that
breast cancer rates were low in countries where soy is a usual part
of the diet. Because soyfoods contained isoflavones, which scientists
learned in the 1960s could have anti-estrogenic properties, this
seemed like an important part of the explanation. Surprisingly,
though, studies looking at this relationship have produced very
mixed results. There is little clinical evidence that soy consumption
in adulthood is protective against breast cancer.[18] In contrast, it appears that consuming soyfoods in childhood and/or the teen years
may reduce lifelong cancer risk by as much as 60 percent.[19] It seems
that compounds like isoflavones impact breast cells during breast development in ways that confer lifelong protection against breast cancer risk. Most girls in Asia grow up eating soyfoods, which may help
explain the lower rates of breast cancer in those countries.

Another emerging area of research that is especially interesting fo-
cuses on the relationship of soy intake to survival in women who
have had breast cancer. I'll talk more about this later in this chapter.

Fat and Cancer

Early cancer research suggested that diets high in fat might raise risk
for breast cancer. It's a theory that has weakened considerably how-

ever, over the past twenty years.[20,21] But even if the total amount of fat in your diet doesn't matter, the type of fat you eat might. And it's no surprise to know that the best fat comes from plants,[22] while both saturated and trans fats are believed to raise risk.[23,24]

Among fats, olive oil appears to have some unique benefits.[25–29] Of course, olive oil consumption tends to correlate with vegetable intake. That is, people who eat the most olive oil also eat the most vegetables. This makes it hard to tell whether it's olive oil or vegetables that are providing the protective effect. But extra-virgin olive oil also contains a number of compounds with demonstrated anticancer activity. One, called oleuropein, was found to inhibit growth in breast cancer cells and reduce expression of a cancer gene that codes for HER2-positive breast tumors.[30] This isn't to suggest that drowning foods in olive oil will lower your breast cancer risk. But when you do cook with added fats, extra-virgin olive oil is the best choice.

PREVENTING CANCER: WHAT TO AVOID
Animal Foods, Saturated Fat, and Breast Cancer

Not all studies show a relationship between meat intake and breast cancer,[31–33] but quite a few suggest that meat raises risk in both pre- and postmenopausal women.[32,34,35] In postmenopausal women in France, breast cancer risk rose by more than 50 percent for every 3½ ounces of meat consumed daily.[36]

Just like it's difficult to separate out what is protective in plant foods because so many beneficial compounds travel together, meat is rich in a variety of factors that may be cancer promoting. For example, meat-eaters have higher body stores of iron, which could raise risk for mutations. Cooking meat at high temperatures also causes mutagens to form.

In animal studies, very high doses of conjugated linoleic acid (CLA), which is a fat found in dairy foods, has shown some anticancer activity. But, as always, conclusions based on animal research are tenuous at best. The relationship of CLA to breast cancer is far less clear in humans.[37] For the most part, there is little information that links dairy intake to breast cancer one way or the other. One interesting finding is that dairy foods raise levels of insulin-like growth factor-1 (IGF-1), a hormone that stimulates cell division and, therefore, in theory, increases cancer risk.[38] Vegans have lower blood levels of IGF-1 than both meat-eaters and vegetarians, and women with lower levels of IGF-1 may be at lower risk for breast cancer.[39-41]

Alcohol and Breast Cancer

As little as a drink a day could increase breast cancer risk by as much as 10 percent according to a number of epidemiologic studies. Three drinks increase risk by 30 percent. One reason might be that alcohol acts as a solvent and could enhance penetration of carcinogens into cells. Also, products of alcohol metabolism in the body might be carcinogenic. Alcohol may also increase estrogen levels and estrogen receptors.

Despite the rather strong evidence for a link between alcohol and breast cancer, it's also true that women who eat Mediterranean-type diets, which typically include red wine, have a relatively low risk for breast cancer. Red wine is high in the cancer-protective phytochemical resveratrol.[42] In women who regularly drink alcohol, high intakes of the B vitamin folate, which is found in leafy green vegetables, orange juice, and legumes, seems to offer some protection.[43] It's possible that alcohol is less harmful for those of us eating diets abundant in fruits and vegetables, and especially rich in folate, which is typical of vegan diets. We just don't know, though, so it's a good idea to be moderate with your alcohol intake.

FOR WOMEN WHO HAVE HAD BREAST CANCER

If what you eat can raise or lower risk of getting cancer, it stands to reason that it can make a difference in prognosis for women who have had breast cancer. Probably the biggest area of interest has been in how soyfoods fit into the diets of breast cancer survivors.

Early research in animals raised some concerns. When mice were fed soy isoflavones and injected with estrogen-sensitive human breast cancer cells, the isoflavones stimulated tumor growth. These findings don't appear to be very relevant to humans, since we metabolize isoflavones differently than animals do. Furthermore, even in the mouse studies, there was no effect on tumor growth in animals who were fed whole soyfoods as opposed to purified isoflavones.

More important, as is often the case, the research in humans shows something completely different. It's not just that soy appears to be harmless for women with breast cancer; it may in fact be beneficial. The first indication of this came out of China, from the Shanghai Breast Cancer Survival Study. The study included more than 5,000 women who were diagnosed with breast cancer between the ages of twenty and seventy-five years. Those who consumed the most soyfoods—about two to three servings per day—were one-third less likely to have a recurrence of their disease.[44] Another study in China found that consuming soyfoods enhanced effectiveness of a breast cancer drug that works by inhibiting the body's production of estrogen.[45]

But these were studies in Asian women who presumably had been eating soy all of their lives. So might the findings actually be related to their early soy intake rather than what they ate after their diagnosis? That's certainly a possibility. But in two large studies in the United States that involved primarily Caucasian women—the Women's Healthy Eating and Living Study[46] and the Life after Cancer Epidemiology study[47]—women with breast cancer who consumed the highest amounts of isoflavones from soyfoods were much less likely to suffer a recurrence or to die from their disease. When the results from one of the Chinese studies and the two U.S. studies were combined, risk of recurrence was reduced by 25 percent in the high-soy consumers.[48] The benefits were similar in Chinese and non-Chinese women.

It's probably too soon to advise women to start eating soyfoods as a way to improve their prognosis after a breast cancer diagnosis. But we can at least say with confidence that soy is not harmful for women with breast cancer. The American Cancer Society and the American Institute for Cancer Research agree that women with breast cancer can safely consume soyfoods.

Although it's a little bit less compelling, there is also support for eating more plant foods in general. Reductions in saturated fat, and diets high in vitamin C, beta-carotene, vegetables, and fiber are all associated with improved survival in women who have had breast cancer.[49,50] Finally, women who exercise also have a better prognosis following a breast cancer diagnosis.[51,52]

ENDOMETRIAL, OVARIAN, AND CERVICAL CANCER

Unfortunately, we have much less information about female cancers other than breast cancer, in part because they are less common. Diets rich in vegetables may protect against both ovarian and cervical cancer, while dairy foods may raise risk for both.[53-55] Generally, the risk for these cancers is greatest in high-income countries and factors that cause women to become taller—like early sexual maturation—raise risk. These factors are clearly associated with a more Western-type diet.

Unlike other cancers that affect women, cervical cancer is far more common in poorer countries and occurs most often in Africa, Latin America, and India. It's also a cancer that affects younger women more often than older women. Virtually all cases of cervical cancer are associated with infection with a group of viruses called HPVs (human papilloma viruses), which are sexually transmitted. Not surprisingly, infection is higher in women who have a higher number of male sexual partners. However, most infected women don't develop cancer, and environmental factors definitely play a role in the development of cancer from HPV infection.

For the most part, there is little evidence of a role for diet in cervical cancer risk, especially in Western women, although a diet rich in folate might help prevent infection with HPV.[56] Regular screening through pap tests (pap smear) detects precancerous lesions on the cervix, which greatly reduces the risk of getting cervical cancer. Unfortunately, most women throughout the world don't have access to this simple and inexpensive test.

Contrary to popular belief, HPV can be sexually transmitted between women. Because evidence suggests that lesbian women are less likely to opt for cervical cancer screening through pap tests, some lesbian women might be at increased risk for this disease.[57]

NONREPRODUCTIVE CANCERS

What we know about vegan diets suggests protection from a host of cancers. In particular, levels and types of bacteria and enzymes in the colon differ significantly between vegetarians and meat-eaters in ways that confer protection for vegetarians.[58–60] Protection is probably due to the higher fiber content of plant-based diets. Vegans also tend to eat more fruits and vegetables and have a lower BMI on average, something that is linked to lower risk for several types of cancers, including colon cancer.[61,62]

In contrast, calcium appears to be protective against colon cancer and some vegans have low calcium intakes.

REDUCE YOUR CANCER RISK WITH A VEGAN DIET

Because of the limits and complexities of cancer research, it's difficult to define an anticancer diet with complete confidence. The evidence does point us in the direction of eating more plant foods and less animal food. Whether you're already vegan or you're headed in that direction, you may already be doing the most important thing to reduce your risk for cancer. Here are some ideas for making your vegan diet as cancer-protective as possible based on the current evidence.

- Eat lots and lots of fruits and vegetables. Truthfully, the evidence that these foods are protective has weakened a little over the years. But given what we know about their chemical makeup, it's pretty hard to believe that fruits and vegetables don't make a

difference. Because these foods vary so much in their phytochemical content, it's a good idea to eat a variety of them. Aim
for including lots of dark orange and leafy green veggies, along
with some from the cabbage family. Slice onions on your veggie
burger, spoon berries on top of your morning cereal, and sauté
a little garlic to stir into vegetable dishes. Stir orange wedges or
chopped apples into green salads. While some phytochemicals
are inactivated with cooking, others are better absorbed from
cooked foods, so aim for a mix of raw and cooked vegetables.
Cruciferous vegetables—the ones in the cabbage family—appear to be more protective when consumed raw. Try to snack
on raw cauliflower and broccoli, add shredded cabbage to salads, or try Apple Slaw with Goji Berry Dressing (page 256),
which includes uncooked kale.

- If you drink alcohol, choose red wine most of the time. Make
  sure your diet is rich in foods that provide lots of folate—leafy
  green vegetables, legumes, orange juice, and peanuts.

- Keep fat intake moderate. Choose healthy sources of fat like
  nuts, seeds, and avocado, and if you use added fats in your cooking, choose extra-virgin olive oil most of the time. Avoid trans
  fats; try to get them out of your diet completely by eliminating all
  foods with the words "partially hydrogenated oils" on the label.

- Make your diet as fiber-rich as possible by choosing whole
  grains most of the time. Most vegans really don't need to worry
  about fiber intake, though.

- Make exercise a priority.

- Encourage your daughter to eat soyfoods. Introducing soyfoods
  into your diet as an adult probably won't affect your breast cancer
  risk one way or the other. But girls who eat these foods in puberty
  or the teen years may have a lower lifetime risk for breast cancer,
  so make sure the ones in your family get to know these foods.
  And if you already eat them, by all means continue to do so.

CHAPTER TWELVE

EATING FOR A HEALTHY HEART

I n a survey by the Society for Women's Health Research, more than 50 percent of women said that the disease they fear most is cancer. Fewer than 10 percent called heart disease their top fear. Yet, heart disease is in fact the leading cause of death in women, killing more women than men. The good news is that the disease that kills more American women than any other is largely preventable.

HEART DISEASE STARTS WITH DAMAGE TO BLOOD VESSELS

Heart disease begins with damage to the endothelium, the layer of cells lining the interior of blood vessels. Smoking, high blood pressure, high blood cholesterol, chronic inflammation, and high blood glucose can all damage this lining.

Where arteries are damaged, cholesterol, fats, proteins, and calcium can enter the artery wall and begin to form a hard plaque within the endothelium. Atherosclerosis develops as arteries become rigid and narrowed by this plaque, making it more difficult for blood to flow through them. This raises blood pressure that, in turn, can cause more damage—sort of a vicious cycle. The plaque can also rupture, producing blood clots that can block blood flow.

If plaque forms in the arteries feeding the heart, diminished blood flow to that organ can cause shortness of breath and chest pain. If blood flow is severely diminished the result can be a heart attack, which causes severe damage to part of the heart. Decreased blood flow to the brain can cause a stroke, a sort of "brain attack."

RISK FACTORS FOR ATHEROSCLEROSIS

High LDL-Cholesterol and Low HDL-Cholesterol

Cholesterol is a waxy substance that is an important part of cell membranes and is used to synthesize many hormones including estrogen and testosterone. It's also the substrate for making vitamin D when skin is exposed to sunlight.

It's essential for life, but that doesn't mean that you need a dietary source of cholesterol. The liver makes all the cholesterol you need. Cholesterol travels through the blood in packages called lipoproteins. One type of lipoprotein, called LDL, picks up cholesterol in the liver and transports it to the cells of the rest of the body. When blood levels of LDL-cholesterol are higher than what the body needs, the excess can be deposited in the arteries, contributing to plaque formation. If the LDL becomes oxidized by free radicals, it becomes more dangerous to the artery walls. So, diets that raise blood levels of LDL-cholesterol and that promote oxidative damage promote heart disease.

In contrast, HDL packages are the "good cholesterol." HDLs act as scavengers, removing cholesterol from the arteries, and transporting it back to the liver to be destroyed. Higher HDL levels are protective against heart disease.

Studies of vegans show that their LDL-cholesterol levels are consistently lower than those of meat-eaters and usually lower than lacto-ovo vegetarians.[1-4] However, vegans also typically have somewhat lower levels of the good HDL-cholesterol, although levels are usually within the normal range.[4,5]

Table 12-1: How Vegans and Meat-Eaters Compare to Target Levels for Lipoproteins and Triglycerides			
	Optimal Levels (milligrams)	Average Vegan Levels*	Average Meat-Eater Levels*
LDL-cholesterol	<100 (or below 70 for those at very high risk for heart disease)	90.3	121
HDL-cholesterol	>60	52	55
Triglycerides	<150	86	107*

From http://www.veganhealth.org/articles/dxmarkers#totus. These average lipid levels were calculated from results of seventeen studies of western populations published between 1980 and 2003.

High Triglycerides

The fat stored in your body and the fat in foods is in the form of triglycerides, three fatty acids attached to a molecule of glycerol. Excess calories from any source promote formation of triglycerides in your body, which can be stored as fat. Experts debate the significance of high triglyceride levels in the blood and how much they matter for heart disease. They seem to be most dangerous when they occur along with other risk factors. Even if your LDL-cholesterol levels are in a good range, having high triglycerides along with low HDL levels may raise your risk for heart disease.

Hypertension

High blood pressure, or hypertension, damages the endothelial lining by putting constant pressure on it. A reading below 120/80 (mmHg) is considered "normal" blood pressure, but ideally, your blood pressure should be below 115/75. Hypertension is defined as a blood pressure above 140/90.

The effect of meat on blood pressure has been a topic of research for nearly one hundred years. In 1926 researchers reported that blood pressures of vegetarian college students rose markedly within two weeks when meat was added to their diets.[6] That relationship still holds true since vegans appear to have lower blood pressures in general and less hypertension than meat-eaters.[7] In the EPIC-Oxford study, meat-eaters were more than two and a half times as likely to have hypertension compared to vegans.[8]

Metabolic Syndrome

Although high LDL-cholesterol levels are an important risk factor for heart disease, having other risk factors—even in the absence of elevated LDLs—can be equally as dangerous. The metabolic syndrome refers to a cluster of conditions that doubles the risk for heart disease and raises risk for diabetes fivefold. People with metabolic syndrome have at least three of the following risk factors:

- Abdominal obesity or an "apple shape"
- High triglyceride level
- Low HDL-cholesterol level
- High blood pressure
- High blood glucose

Metabolic syndrome is more common in people who have a history of diabetes in their family, and it may also be more common in Asians and Hispanics. Lifestyle changes can be extremely effective in reversing symptoms of the metabolic syndrome, preventing diabetes and heart disease from occurring. Eating the healthy diet outlined in this chapter, along with exercise and a small weight loss—about 5 percent of your body weight—is very effective in reversing symptoms of metabolic syndrome.

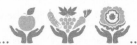

Abdominal Obesity

Most research shows that being overweight raises risk for heart disease. The jury is out, though, on whether it matters where the weight is carried. Generally, there is evidence that abdominal fat raises risk far more than fat that accumulates in the buttocks and thighs. Abdominal obesity is more likely to be associated with risk factors for heart disease like low HDL-cholesterol, high blood pressure, type-2 diabetes, and high triglycerides. However, overweight women who don't have these other risk factors may not be at elevated risk for heart disease.

Diabetes

People with diabetes are at greatly elevated risk for heart disease. Although there is a genetic component to diabetes, the most common type of diabetes, type-2, can often be prevented through diet and exercise. People with diabetes are likely to develop heart disease fifteen years earlier than people without diabetes.[9] I'll talk more about the role of diet in diabetes risk and management in Chapter 15.

Chronic Inflammation

This is the low-grade, chronic condition that occurs when the immune system goes into overdrive. Chronic inflammation is the silent condition I talked about in Chapter 3 that may raise risk for heart disease as well as diabetes, obesity, cancer, and possibly Alzheimer's disease. Smoking, stress, high blood glucose, and high blood cholesterol all promote inflammation. People eating plant-based diets have lower levels of inflammatory markers.

Beyond Diet

Smoking doubles heart disease risk, but the good news is that you can reverse the damage. Once you stop smoking, risk drops by one-third within two years. It continues to decline until by the end of ten

years, it's as though you had never smoked at all.[10] The effects of relaxation techniques like yoga or meditation on both inflammation
and blood pressure are rather impressive.[11] In older African American
people, regular practice of transcendental meditation cut their risk
for a heart attack or stroke by half. They were asked to meditate twice
a day for 20 minutes each time, but most averaged only about once a
day. That was enough to provide some benefits, although the subjects who met the twice-a-day goal had even better results.[12]

And of course, exercise is a crucial part of keeping the heart
healthy. Brisk walking for at least 3 hours per week or more vigorous
exercise for 1½ hours per week can lower your risk of heart disease
by 30 to 40 percent[13] Exercise improves the health of your heart, and
it also reduces inflammation.[14] Even gentle stretching exercises may
play a role in preventing heart disease since flexibility is linked to
healthier, more flexible arteries.[15]

HEART DISEASE IN WOMEN

Younger women have a little bit of built-in protection against heart
disease since estrogen lowers LDL-cholesterol and raises the good
HDL-cholesterol. But as estrogen production declines in
menopause, heart disease rates in women begin to increase until they
match—and then surpass—those of men. In fact, the total number of
deaths from cardiovascular disease has been greater for American
women than for men in the last 20 years.[16] And even though estrogen
therapy can improve some of the uncomfortable side-effects of
menopause, it may not reduce heart disease risk. In any event, because of the side-effects, hormone therapy is not recommended as a
way to reduce chronic disease risk.

Certain heart disease risk factors are even more dangerous for
women than for men. For example, while there is some debate about
HDL-cholesterol and heart disease, low levels seem to be more
harmful in women than in men.[17,18] Women also have smaller arteries, even compared to men of similar size.[19] This is probably due to

differences in sex hormones since hormone therapy affects artery size in both transgendered men and women.[20,21] These smaller arteries can mean less blood flow to the heart, so that even women who don't have significant plaque in their arteries can be at risk for heart disease. Their smaller arteries may also be part of the explanation for why women are at higher risk for rheumatoid arthritis and migraine headaches, something I'll talk about in Chapter 14.

Even though their higher estrogen levels help to reduce heart disease risk in younger women, actual risk factors can begin to develop well before menopause. Therefore, it's important for all women to live a heart-healthy lifestyle beginning when they are young. A diet based on plant foods is a good place to start.

PROTECTION FROM VEGAN AND VEGETARIAN DIETS

Their lower LDL-cholesterol levels, BMI, and rates of hypertension all help to protect vegans from heart disease.[22,23] Or at least we can assume that they do. Unfortunately, we don't have good information about actual rates of heart disease in vegans, since studies often group vegans and other vegetarians together. And surprisingly, when we look at the rates of heart disease in those vegan/vegetarian groups, the findings aren't especially impressive, especially for women. In the Adventist Health Study, vegetarian men had lower risk than nonvegetarians, but there was no difference between vegetarian and nonvegetarian women.[24] In another analysis that pooled findings from five studies, a vegetarian diet was protective for both sexes, but somewhat less so for women.[25] And in the EPIC-Oxford study, there was no difference in heart disease rates between vegetarians and meat-eaters at all.[26]

Again, one reason for this might be that the nonvegetarians in these studies had such healthy lifestyles that they weren't all that different from the vegetarians. Since vegans were mixed in with the lacto-ovo vegetarians—and dairy foods and eggs are high in saturated fat and cholesterol—it's also possible that any protective effect of vegan diets was lost in these studies.

It's also not true that every single vegan or vegetarian diet is as heart-healthy as it could be. Some vegans may make food choices that cancel out some of the benefits of a plant-based diet. If you're on the cookies and potato chip vegan diet, you probably aren't expecting much in the way of health benefits. But even vegans eating healthy fiber-rich meals built around whole grains, legumes, fruits, and vegetables can fall short of the optimal pattern for protecting heart health. For example, vegans may be at risk if they don't consume adequate vitamin B_{12}. Low vitamin B_{12} levels are associated with elevated blood levels of the amino acid homocysteine, which is linked to damage to endothelial cells and increased risk for heart disease.[27] Studies of vegans who don't supplement with vitamin B_{12} show that their levels of homocysteine are consistently high.[28,29] These higher levels are seen even in vegans whose B_{12} status is good enough to prevent overt deficiency symptoms, but still not high enough to be considered optimal.

The types of fats and carbohydrates in your diet can affect risk for heart disease, too. By looking at the research on different eating patterns, and the effects of different foods, we can pull together guidelines for a vegan diet that is likely to be protective for almost anyone. One place to start is in cultures where people have a lower risk for heart disease.

Lessons from Crete and Asia

Beginning in the 1950s, Dr. Ancel Keys from the University of Minnesota studied fifteen different populations in Italy, Greece, Yugoslavia, the Netherlands, Finland, Japan, and the United States. His findings were published as the now-famous Seven Countries Study.[30] Although heart disease rates rose as average fat intake increased among these populations, there was one surprising exception. The people with the highest fat intake of all—those living on the Greek Island of Crete—had the lowest rates of heart disease. One big problem with the Seven Countries Study for our purposes is that it looked only at men. It was also an ecological study, the weakest type of epidemiologic study.

But subsequent research has revealed that the food pattern that was a part of peasant cultures around the Mediterranean Sea—despite being high in total fat—includes numerous protective factors against chronic diseases like heart disease and cancer.[31-33] There is evidence that this style of eating improves the health of the endothelial lining,[34] and we know now that it does indeed reduce heart disease risk in women.[35]

On the other side of the world, heart disease was also low in Asian countries where diets are traditionally modest in animal foods and rich in vegetables. As mentioned throughout this book, Asians consume something else that isn't common in Mediterranean diets: soyfoods. You'll see later in this chapter that this might be part of the explanation for the lower rates of heart disease in that part of the world.

A vegan diet that incorporates protective factors from these cultural styles of eating brings together—literally—the best of all worlds.

EATING TO REDUCE HEART DISEASE RISK

Choose Healthy Fats

The Seven Countries Study brings to light one of the most important findings about diet and heart disease. That is, the *type* of fat you eat is far more important than the amount. Saturated fat, the kind that is abundant in red meats, whole milk, cheese, and eggs, raises blood cholesterol levels and promotes atherosclerosis. But the polyunsaturated and monounsaturated fats that predominate in plant foods, and that are important components of the Mediterranean diet, don't.

Although very low-fat vegetarian diets have been successful in reducing risk for heart disease, these studies have included a number of dietary changes, making it difficult to determine which factors are most important. In a study published in 1990, for example, Dr. Dean Ornish showed that a comprehensive plan that included a lacto-ovo vegetarian diet could actually reduce (not just prevent further accumulation) the amount of plaque in arteries.[36] He put subjects on a diet that was low in total and saturated fat, and very limited in animal foods. The participants also ate plenty of fruits and vegetables, exercised, and engaged in stress management practices like meditation. And they lost more weight than subjects in the control group.

Which of those many differences was or were responsible for the benefits? We can only make educated guesses about that. It's very likely that the weight loss, low saturated fat intake, higher intake of antioxidant-rich plant foods, and use of stress-management techniques all contributed to the positive outcome. Research shows that each of these factors is protective. But because fat from plant foods is also protective, it's not at all likely that eating less of this type of fat was the reason for the benefits seen in this study.

While this study shows that vegetarian diets can be part of a powerful program to heal people who have heart disease, it doesn't make the case for avoiding higher-fat plant foods like nuts, seeds, vegetable oils, avocado, and soyfoods. These are all foods that can be a part of a heart-healthy diet, and there is abundant research—some of it on women—to back this up. For example, among nearly 49,000 women in the Women's Health Initiative Dietary Modification Trial, the amount of dietary fat consumed was unrelated to heart attacks or strokes.[37] And while eating more red meat and trans fats was linked to higher heart disease risk in the Nurses' Health Study, higher intakes of poly- and monounsaturated fats were protective.[38,39]

There is a downside to eating too little fat, too. Very low-fat diets cause both the bad LDL and the good HDL-cholesterol levels to drop. In one intervention study, where subjects consumed very low-fat vegan diets—just 10 percent of total calories came from fat—LDL-cholesterol levels decreased, but HDL levels dropped to the same extent. Consequently, there was no difference at study end in the ratio of bad to good cholesterol, which is a standard measure of heart disease risk. At the same time, triglyceride levels went up.[40] In contrast, including monounsaturated fats in a heart-healthy diet improves the ratio of LDL- to HDL-cholesterol.[41]

Very low-fat diets might also affect LDL-cholesterol particles in unfavorable ways. High carbohydrate and low fat intakes produce LDL particles that are very small and dense, which makes them more likely to contribute to atherosclerosis. In people who eat more plant fats, LDL particles are larger and more buoyant, a type that is less harmful.[42]

Very low-fat intakes are achieved by eliminating foods that have demonstrated heart-healthy effects. Nuts are strongly associated with protection against heart disease. And many experts believe that olive oil consumption is responsible for some of the health benefits of the Mediterranean diet pattern. It's rich in antioxidants and is a unique source of a phytochemical called oleocanthal. This is the compound that gives extra-virgin olive oil its characteristic peppery bite to the back of the throat. It's an antioxidant that also reduces inflammation. In postmenopausal Italian women, higher olive oil intake was associated with lower risk for heart disease.[43] A higher intake of extra-virgin olive oil may improve antioxidant status and reduce oxidation of LDL-cholesterol.[44,45] Generally, eating more healthy unsaturated fats helps to reduce inflammation, too.[46,47]

What About Dietary Cholesterol?

The amount of cholesterol in your diet isn't the most important determinant of blood cholesterol levels, since production of cholesterol in the liver decreases when dietary cholesterol intake increases. This doesn't mean that dietary cholesterol doesn't matter. Diets very high in cholesterol can overcome this feedback system. Also, some people are more sensitive to the effects of dietary cholesterol than others. While small amounts of cholesterol in the diet are not harmful, eating too much of it can raise heart disease risk. It's not something you need to worry about as a vegan, though, because plants are always free of cholesterol.

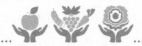

In contrast, single meals that are extremely high in fat—like the type you might find at a fast-food restaurant—can damage arteries.[48] The key here is to find the happy medium that comes from including a few servings of nuts and a couple teaspoons of vegetable oils in a diet that is built around low-fat grains, fruits, vegetables, and legumes, while avoiding the saturated fats and trans fats (more about these below) that are found most often in animal products and processed foods.

Plant Sources of Saturated Fat

The biggest sources of saturated fats in American diets are meat, chicken, cheese, butter, eggs, and milk. But even plant foods contain small amounts of saturated fat. And a few plant foods are actually very high in it. The most common saturated fat-rich plant foods are tropical oils—those made from coconut, palm, and cocoa beans. But here is where things get a little bit complicated, because saturated fat isn't just one type of fat; it's a group of fats with different effects on cholesterol levels.

There is a particular mystique surrounding coconut oil, which is often believed to have special curative and health promoting powers, despite its high content of saturated fat. In fact, studies do show that the fats in coconut oil have antimicrobial properties. And, the predominant fat in coconut oil—called lauric acid—is a saturated fat that raises the good HDL-cholesterol. However, other saturated fats in coconut oil can raise LDL-cholesterol. So the overall impact of coconut oil on heart disease risk isn't clear.

In countries where people eat plant-based diets that include these tropical oils as their primary source of fat, heart disease rates are typically low. This suggests that there is room for these fats in vegan diets. Because they are solid at room temperature and have pleasant aromas and flavors, they can be fun and useful in some vegan recipes. Until we know more about their true effects on chronic disease, don't make these the predominant fats in your diet. If you are at high risk for heart disease and are using a vegan diet to help lower that risk, it's a good idea to avoid these fats for the most part.

Avoid Trans Fats

While some animal foods naturally provide small amounts of trans fats, they are mostly the result of processing. These are the fats that are produced when vegetable oils are hydrogenated. They are definitely off the heart-healthy menu since they raise LDL-cholesterol, lower HDL-cholesterol, and promote inflammation.[49] Even small intakes are associated with increased risk for heart disease and diabetes. Just a 2 percent increase in calories from trans fats is associated with a 23 percent increase in incidence of coronary heart disease.[50]

Consider a Source of Long-Chain Omega-3 Fats

DHA and EPA are the long-chain omega-3 fats found in fatty fish and fish oil supplements. Although we can synthesize them from the essential omega-3 fat ALA (which is found in flaxseeds, chia seeds, walnuts, and canola oil), you may remember from Chapter 2 that this synthesis may not be efficient enough to produce adequate amounts of DHA and EPA.

Initial interest in the possible benefits of DHA and EPA came from observations that Eskimos, who have very high intakes of these fats, have low rates of heart disease. DHA and EPA are associated with lower triglyceride levels, reduced inflammation, improved endothelial function, and reduced tendency to form blood clots. They may help to modulate blood pressure as well.

While there is every reason to believe that they are good for your heart, studies looking at their benefits are conflicting. It remains unclear whether those of us who already eat a heart-healthy vegan diet would benefit further from supplements of DHA and EPA. I suggest a small dose of these fats—200–300 milligrams combined, two to three times per week—for vegans. Many health organizations recommend higher amounts—closer to 500 milligrams daily.

Choose Healthy Carbs

Saturated and trans fats aren't the only dietary threats to heart health. Replacing harmful fats with refined and highly processed starches and sugars doesn't translate to much improvement for heart health. In fact, the evidence suggests that it doesn't do any good at all.[51] Eating more white bread, mashed potatoes, and sugary low-fat desserts instead of animal fats will lower your LDL-cholesterol, but it also lowers the protective HDL-cholesterol and it raises triglyceride levels.

It's not clear whether all high-carbohydrate diets raise triglyceride levels, or just those that contain high amounts of processed, refined carbohydrates. In the Women's Health Initiative, higher carb intakes didn't raise triglyceride levels as long as the carbohydrate-rich foods were unrefined and high in fiber.[52] In fact, you have to eat carbohydrate-rich foods if you want to have a fiber-rich diet. Whole-grain fiber in particular can lower risk for heart disease in women by as much as 25 percent.[53,54] Replacing some carbohydrate-rich foods with healthy fats can be one way to lower triglyceride levels, but as long as you are choosing fiber-rich foods with a low glycemic index—the slow carbs I talked about in Chapter 3—there is no reason to avoid carbohydrate-rich foods.

Reduce Sodium

Since salt is very much an acquired taste, you can retrain your taste buds to enjoy less salty food. It takes some time, but when people eat lower salt diets to reduce their sodium intake, the foods that they once enjoyed begin to taste excessively salty.

Diets high in sodium have been linked to higher blood pressure and increased risk of heart disease and stroke. Because of this, government guidelines suggest that people should consume no more than 2,300 milligrams of sodium per day—the amount in about 1 teaspoon of table salt. These guidelines recommend an even lower intake of no more than 1,500 milligrams per day for those at the highest risk for stroke: older people, those with hypertension, and African Americans.

(African Americans are twice as likely to suffer a stroke as Caucasians, a difference that may be due in part to genetic factors.)

Getting sodium intake down to less than 1,500 milligrams per day is a challenge, and not all experts agree that it's warranted. Some studies have failed to find any relationship between sodium intake and risk for dying from heart disease or stroke.[55] Some people are also more sensitive to the effects of sodium than others, which means that limiting salt is not beneficial for everyone.

The easiest way to reduce sodium intake is to limit your use of processed foods since veggie meats and cheeses can pile on the sodium. It doesn't mean you can't have these foods, but they should play a supporting role in vegan diets. Being generous in your cooking

Table 12-2: Sodium Content of Selected Vegan Foods	
Food	Sodium Content, Milligrams
Tofurky beer brat, 1 sausage	620
Table salt, ¼ teaspoon (about fifteen shakes of an average five-hole salt shaker)	590
Tamari, 1 teaspoon	310
Miso, 1 teaspoon	225
Boca Burger	280
Daiya vegan cheese, ¼ cup	250
Amy's Vegan Chocolate Cake, 1 slice	210
Chickpeas, canned, ½ cup	177
Whole wheat bread, 1 slice	170
Chickpeas, canned, rinsed, ½ cup	161
Ketchup, 1 tablespoon	160
Celery, 1 medium stalk	32
Chickpeas, cooked without salt, ½ cup	6
Brown rice, ½ cup cooked without salt	5
Plum tomato, 1 medium	3
Apple, medium	2
Tofu, ½ cup	0
Balsamic vinegar, 1 tablespoon	0
Olive oil, 1 teaspoon	0

with herbs and spices and taking advantage of umami-rich ingredients (see Chapter 1) can be useful in weaning yourself from more
salty foods. It's fine to use salt in cooking, and iodized salt can be an
important source of iodine in vegan diets.

Protective Plant Foods

Getting animal foods out of your diet goes a long way toward protecting your heart. But, it's not just the lower saturated fat and cholesterol content of vegan diets that makes them so beneficial. Plant
foods have their own advantages, and some of them are powerhouses
of heart-healthy compounds.

Beans

One of the biggest advantages to vegan diets is that beans typically replace meat. It's a replacement that automatically sends saturated fat
and cholesterol intake plummeting, while increasing fiber intake. Not
surprisingly, women who eat more beans have lower risk for both
heart disease and type-2 diabetes.[56,57] Consuming beans just four
times per week—and most vegans eat them every day—can lower risk
for heart disease by more than 20 percent.[58]

It's possible that the fiber in beans lowers cholesterol by binding it
in the intestines, or it might inhibit synthesis of cholesterol in the
liver. The soluble fiber in beans increases LDL cholesterol particle
size making it less damaging.[59] Finally, the phytochemicals in beans
might have a role in reducing heart disease, too.

Soyfoods

Because they are rich in protein and so versatile, soyfoods often
stand in for meat in Asian dishes and they are natural replacements
for meat in vegan meals. The fact that they are lower in saturated fat
(and free of cholesterol) than the meat and dairy products they replace means that they can automatically make your diet more heart-
healthy. But both the protein and the isoflavones in soyfoods give
them some unique benefits.

Soy protein has a direct cholesterol-lowering effect so that simply adding these foods to your diet—even if they don't replace foods high in saturated fat—can lower LDL-cholesterol.[60] It's a modest effect, but even the small reductions seen in LDL-cholesterol levels from eating soy protein can have a significant impact on heart health over time. Incorporating soyfoods into a diet that includes other heart-healthy factors can produce a significant effect on LDL-cholesterol, lowering it by as much as 30 percent.[61]

Soy isoflavones also impact heart health. They improve the health of the endothelial lining of the arteries and may increase LDL particle size.[62,63] The combination of these effects could be very powerful in reducing disease risk. For example, in the Shanghai Women's Health Study, higher soyfoods intake was associated with an 86 percent reduction in the risk of having a heart attack in postmenopausal women.[64] And in another study of postmenopausal women, isoflavone-rich soy protein was linked to a marked reduction in thickening of the carotid arteries (the arteries that go to the brain) over time.[65]

Nuts

Nuts are definite proof that heart-healthy diets can include higher-fat foods. Research consistently confirms that they are wonderful little packages of beneficial compounds. Because they are high in healthy fats, they reduce LDL-cholesterol, especially the small, dense LDL that is so harmful to arteries.[66] The protein in nuts is especially high in one particular amino acid called arginine, which promotes production of a compound that keeps arteries flexible.[67] They're also high in antioxidants and fiber and may reduce inflammation.[68]

In both the Nurses' Health Study and the Iowa Women's Health Study, women who ate the most nuts had the lowest risk for heart disease.[69,70] If you aren't allergic to nuts, they should be considered an essential part of a diet for protection of heart health. Enjoy a serving or two of nuts—a serving is a quarter cup or about an ounce—as daily snacks or use small amounts of nuts added to grain dishes or in oatmeal or salad.

Fruits and Vegetables

Fruits and vegetables provide the mineral potassium, which helps to keep blood pressure at healthy levels.[71] Eating lots of these foods might also reduce inflammation and insulin resistance and improve endothelial function.[72] Since oxidative damage to LDL-cholesterol makes it more harmful to arteries and more likely to contribute to plaque formation, the antioxidants in fruits and vegetables could be a protective factor, too.

A HEART-HEALTHY DIET FOR VEGAN WOMEN

Going vegan is among the best things you can do for heart health. To make your vegan diet as protective as possible, follow these guidelines

- Choose healthy fats. Get most of your dietary fat from nuts, seeds, olives, avocado, soyfoods, and vegetable oils. Avoid meals

Diet and Alcohol

Red wine—like red grape juice—is particularly rich in phytochemicals that protect against oxidation and improve the health of the endothelium. But there is evidence that other alcoholic beverages, including beer, have similar effects.[73] Moderate alcohol intake—one drink per day—is also consistently shown to raise HDL-cholesterol levels. In postmenopausal women, it's also been linked to small decreases in triglycerides and LDL-cholesterol.[74] But you'll need to weigh this against the potential increase in breast cancer risk that comes with alcohol consumption. If you drink alcohol, aim for no more than one serving per day. If you don't drink, don't start since there are plenty of other ways to lower heart disease risk.

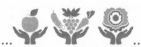

that are excessively high in fat, but ultra–low fat eating isn't necessary for heart health and may not be advisable.

- Make sure you meet needs for vitamin B_{12}. The easiest way to do so is to take a daily supplement providing 25 micrograms.
- Follow the guidelines on pages 43–44 for choosing slow carbs.
- Get trans fats out of your diet.
- Consider a supplement of the long-chain omega-3 fats DHA and EPA.
- If you have high blood pressure, reduce your sodium intake and monitor it to see if this helps.
- Eat lots and lots of fruits and vegetables to keep your potassium intake high.
- Eat at least a cup of cooked beans every day.
- Include one or two servings of traditional soyfoods in your diet every day.
- Include a serving of nuts in your daily menu.
- If you drink, choose red wine most of the time.
- Need a treat? Try dark chocolate, which is a good source of antioxidants and is associated with lower blood pressure and better artery flexibility.[75]

MediterrAsian Meals for a Healthy Heart

Food patterns from Asian countries and the Mediterranean region share certain healthful features—namely lots of vegetables, protein from legumes, and very little in the way of animal protein and fat. Each of these patterns offers its own unique heart-healthy elements, too. Soyfoods play a big role in Asian meals and extra-virgin olive oil is the primary fat used in Italy, Spain and Greece. Here are a few heart-healthy menus that bring the best of these regions to your plate—a sort of MediterrAsian approach to eating.

Sample MediterrAsian Menus

DAY ONE

Breakfast

Miso soup with tofu and vegetables and noodles (Dissolve 2 tablespoons miso in 1 cup of water, add chunks of tofu and veggies, and simmer for a minute or two. Or, for something a little different, try **Creamy Kale Miso Soup (page 268)**

Snack

Fruit smoothie

Lunch

Salad with greens, raw vegetables, orange segments, walnuts, almonds, edamame (green soybeans), and dressing of extra-virgin olive oil and balsamic vinegar

Whole wheat couscous (add chopped dried fruit and mint)

Snack

Whole wheat pita with hummus

Dinner

White beans seasoned with garlic, sundried tomatoes, and lemon juice

Sauteed Vegetables

Red wine

DAY TWO

Breakfast

Whole-grain toast with almond butter

Fresh figs or grapes

Green tea

Lunch

Socca Pizza (page 291)

Snack

Instant lentil soup cup

Dinner

Stir-fried vegetables with tofu or tempeh over brown rice

DAY THREE

Breakfast

Rolled oats with chopped walnuts, raisins, and soymilk

Snack

Fruit salad with almond milk yogurt

Lunch

Vegetable soup with navy beans

Snack

Apple slices spread with peanut butter

Dinner

Adzuki Bean Potato Salad (page 258)

CHAPTER THIRTEEN

STRONG BONES FOR LIFE

Strong bones without milk? Most people can't imagine it. But for most of human history, milk wasn't on the menu. It wasn't until animals were domesticated some 10,000 years ago that dairy products began to appear in human diets. And even then, they were common only in certain parts of the world since most humans couldn't (and can't) digest milk very well.

We're born with the ability to synthesize the enzyme lact*ase*, needed to digest the sugar in milk, called lact*ose*. Human breast milk is rich in this milk sugar, as is cow's milk, so the ability to produce lactase is crucial for survival. But, by early childhood, levels of lactase decline by 75 to 90 percent.[1] This is a part of normal human development and it makes it difficult to consume dairy foods.

In northern Europe, a mutation occurring around 8,000 BCE resulted in continued production of lactase and the ability to comfortably consume dairy foods throughout life. Even today, milk-drinking is far more common among people of northern European ancestry than it is in parts of the world like Asia. So in the scheme of things, the idea that milk is an important source of calcium for anyone but infants is pretty new, and it's relevant to only a small group of the world's population. Our early ancestors still got plenty of calcium without dairy foods, by foraging for calcium-rich leafy greens.

THE LIFE CYCLE OF YOUR SKELETON

Bones are so hard and solid that it's easy to think of them as inert. But your skeleton is actually dynamic and constantly in flux. It releases bone matter to the blood and then takes up nutrients to rebuild. That's because, in addition to providing the body with structure and mobility, the skeleton is a storage facility for calcium and other compounds that are needed for biological processes.

Calcium contributes to bone strength and is also required in other parts of the body for a variety of functions. It's needed for muscle contraction, dilation and relaxation of blood vessels, nerve transmission, and blood clotting. Because it's so vital to processes that support life, blood levels of calcium are maintained within a very tight range. Bones supply calcium to the blood when it's needed and then take up new calcium—supplied by the diet—to rebuild. You can't ascertain your calcium status—whether you're getting enough of this nutrient—by measuring amounts in the blood, because those levels are always pretty much constant.

Throughout childhood and the teen years, bones rebuild faster than they break down allowing them to become heavier and longer. The process continues even after adult height is reached for another decade or so as bones get heavier. By the early thirties, bone accumulation maxes out. Bones are as heavy and dense as they are ever going to be. This is called peak bone mass, and it's a major factor that determines risk of getting osteoporosis.

Then somewhere around the midforties, hormonal changes cause bone loss to speed up. This is a normal part of aging, but if it occurs at too rapid a pace, the result can be excessive bone loss or osteoporosis. In women, the drop in estrogen production that signals menopause is largely responsible for increased bone loss over the next decade. This stepped-up bone loss, along with the fact that women's bones are less dense than men's to begin with, means that women are at greater risk for osteoporosis and fractures than men.

Continuing to get adequate calcium is important throughout life, but a lifestyle that slows bone loss matters, too. Vegans sometimes fall short of meeting calcium needs—an issue that needs attention. On the other hand, plant foods are rich in a host of other nutrients that play a significant role in protecting bone health.

Protein, Calcium, and Bones: Unraveling the Relationship

Long-time vegans may have heard that the real reason for osteoporosis is excess dietary protein, not insufficient calcium. And when I first started looking at the research on vegan calcium needs twenty-five years ago, it seemed like that was the most obvious thing in the world. Unfortunately, it's not so obvious any longer. In fact, this theory has been pretty much turned on its head.

Some of the early misunderstanding about protein and bones came from studies comparing hip fracture rates around the world. This is a quick and easy way to look at bone health and its association with diet. One study found that rates of hip fractures were highest in countries where people ate the most animal protein. A possible explanation for this goes back to research conducted nearly one hundred years ago. Studies from the early 1900s found that feeding high-protein diets to subjects caused excess calcium to show up in the urine. It seemed that somehow protein was leaching calcium from the bone.

One explanation has focused on the effect of protein on blood acidity. High protein intake, especially when it comes from animal foods and grains, causes blood pH to drop—that is, blood becomes more acidic. Since many of the metabolic reactions that support life can't occur in that environment, the body needs ways to quickly counter the formation of acid-producing compounds. One of these processes involves release of compounds, including calcium, from bones. Once calcium is leached from bones into the blood, some of it ends up being excreted in the urine.

Not surprisingly, evidence suggests that vegan diets—since they don't contain any animal protein—are less acid-forming.[2] It would *seem* to follow that vegans have lower calcium needs.

But while this all seems to come together to suggest an advantage for vegans regarding bone health, it's a theory that is now widely challenged.

Is Protein Bad to the Bone?

Interestingly, while older people in Japan and Hong Kong are less likely to break their hips, they actually have higher rates of spinal fractures than older people in Western countries.[3] If their low protein intake protected them from hip fractures, it seems like this would have the same protection in other parts of the skeleton. The fact that it doesn't tells us that something else is going on.

The worldwide comparisons of hip fracture rates and protein intake are ecological studies, and you may remember from Chapter 4 that this type of study produces more questions than answers. It's because ecological studies ignore a host of potentially confounding variables. For example, exercise protects bone health, and people in countries with lower protein intakes tend to be more physically active. So is it their low protein intake or their more active lifestyle that is protective? Ecological studies can't answer that question.

In some countries, older people are also less likely to fall on hard cement—either because they leave the home only on the arm of a younger family member or because there is no cement on which to fall. Ethnicity also plays a big role in bone health. People of African descent have a higher peak bone mass, putting them at lower lifelong risk for osteoporosis. And hip structure in Asians is slightly different in a way that may protect against breakage.[4]

When we start looking at all of these issues, it becomes clear that there are many factors affecting hip fractures rates throughout the world. A focus on protein alone doesn't tell us too much of anything. In addition, newer research shows that protein-rich diets enhance calcium absorption by the body. This greater influx of calcium into the blood may compensate for any calcium losses that occur when blood becomes more acidic. When we look at studies within similar populations—as opposed to those that compare different populations around the world—it turns out that there is no clear pattern linking increased protein intake to bone turnover, calcium loss, and fracture rates.[5-8]

In fact, some studies show that eating more protein protects bone health.[9-12] It's not really that surprising; in addition to its effect on calcium absorption, protein is an integral part of bones. It also supports muscles, which are important for overall health of the skeleton.

NUTRIENTS FOR STRONG BONES

The more we study bone health, the more it becomes clear that maintaining healthy bones throughout life depends on the interaction of numerous dietary and lifestyle factors. In addition to calcium and protein, healthy bones need adequate vitamin D, vitamin K, magnesium, potassium, and even vitamin C. There are a few challenges here for vegans, but mostly advantages.

Calcium: Many women, whether or not they drink milk, fall short of meeting calcium recommendations. In vegans, there is evidence that calcium shortfalls take a toll on bone health. In the EPIC-Oxford study, vegans were more likely to suffer broken bones than nonvegans, but it was only because they had low calcium intakes. Vegans with higher calcium intakes were at no greater risk.[13] The best sources of calcium for vegans are collard and turnip greens, kale, bok choy, calcium-set tofu, fortified plant milks and juices, figs, tahini, and blackstrap molasses. As you'll see below, the other nutrients in calcium-rich plant foods make them especially good choices for protecting bone health.

Vitamin D: There is evidence that vitamin D might protect against a wide range of chronic illnesses, including fibromyalgia, cancer, hypertension, and rheumatoid arthritis. But its most important function is in boosting calcium absorption in the intestines and reducing its excretion from the kidneys in order to provide adequate calcium for bones. While osteoporosis results from loss of bone content, a vitamin D deficiency can lead to osteomalacia, which is a defect in bone building.

If our early human ancestors had depended on food for vitamin D, our species would have been in trouble, because there are very few natural sources of this nutrient. A few high-fat fish provide it and so do eggs from chickens who are fed a vitamin D-rich diet. As a result, throughout all of human history, most people were not getting vitamin D from their diet. The main source of vitamin D has always been what we synthesize ourselves when skin is exposed to sunlight. When humans started to move farther from the equator and also began to spend more time indoors, they had more trouble making enough vitamin D. As a result, it was added to cow's milk, which became an important source of this nutrient for many people. Today, many foods, including plant milks, are fortified with vitamin D.

Exposing arms and legs to the sun three times a week for 10 to 30 minutes during midday on a day when sunburn is possible, and without using sunscreen, should produce enough vitamin D in light-skinned young women. The darker your skin and the older you are, the more exposure you need. And it's important to weigh this exposure against skin cancer risk. For this reason, a daily dose of 600 to 1,000 IUs of vitamin D can be a good idea for most women. Most supplements of vitamin D come from animals, but vegan vitamin D—called vitamin D2 or ergocalciferol—is available.

Protein: After decades of criticism for its alleged bone-damaging effects, protein is back on the list of bone-protective nutrients. Most vegan women have no trouble meeting the RDA for protein. But some, especially those who eat low-calorie diets or who don't include legumes in their menus, can fall short. The minimum servings in the

Plant Plate on page 30 provide around 50 grams of protein and about 1,500 calories. If your calorie needs are higher than this, you probably need more protein as well, since both protein and calorie needs are tied to body weight. (Multiply your healthy body weight by 0.4 to find out how many grams of protein you need.) Keep in mind that all legumes, grains, nuts, seeds, and vegetables provide protein, so as you increase your calorie intake from healthy foods, you'll automatically increase your protein intake.

Vitamin K: Vitamin K plays an essential role in the activation of a protein needed for healthy bones. In the Nurses' Health Study, women with the lowest vitamin K intake were most likely to experience a hip fracture.[14] And low vitamin K intake was linked to poorer bone mineral density.[15] Leafy green vegetables are the best sources of this vitamin. Soy, canola oil, and olive oil provide some vitamin K, too. Fat enhances absorption of vitamin K so giving your kale a quick sauté in one of these oils will go even further in helping you meet needs.

Vitamin C: Eating lots of vitamin C–rich fruits and vegetables will do double duty for your bones since vitamin C is needed for synthesis of connective tissue in bones and these foods also help to prevent blood from becoming acidic. In older people, vitamin C helps prevent bone loss.[16] Vegetarians and vegans typically have high vitamin C intakes.

Potassium: Potassium-rich foods help to balance out acid-causing dietary factors and may reduce calcium loss from bones.[17] One reason why vegans have less acidic urine might be because the main sources of protein in their diet—legumes—are also rich in potassium. It's difficult to meet potassium needs if you aren't eating a diet that's rich in fruits, vegetables, and legumes. Most Americans fall woefully short in meeting the RDA for this nutrient. Truthfully, so do many vegans and vegetarians, but their intakes are at least typically much higher than those of people who eat meat. Best sources of potassium

are legumes, avocado, beet greens, spinach, Swiss chard, sweet potatoes, tomato juice, bananas, and orange juice.

Magnesium: Magnesium deficiency raises risk for osteoporosis in
women,[18] and older people with higher magnesium intakes have
better bone health.[19] Vegetarian diets are typically higher in magnesium than omnivore diets—in fact, many omnivore women don't
meet the RDA for magnesium—and vegans may have the highest
intakes of all.[20] It's not surprising since the best sources of this
nutrient are whole grains, legumes, nuts, seeds, and leafy green
vegetables.

Isoflavones: Since estrogen protects bone health, there has been lots
of interest in the possible effects of soy isoflavones on bones. Epidemiologic studies of women in Shanghai[21] and Singapore,[22] and also
of American Seventh-Day Adventists, have linked soy consumption
to better bone health.[23]

But in order to see a true cause and effect, again, we have to look
at clinical studies. Since 1998, there have been more than twenty-five
of these, and the findings are conflicting. Most of the recent ones
show no protective effects of isoflavone supplements. It may be that,
as with breast cancer, it is lifelong intake that matters, since the
women in the studies in Shanghai and Singapore were presumably
eating soyfoods throughout childhood. Alternatively, it's possible
that eating traditional soyfoods is more beneficial than getting
isoflavones from the soy supplements and extracts used in clinical
studies. But so far, neither of those theories seems to explain the differences in these findings.

For now, we don't have strong evidence that soy isoflavones protect
bone health. If you remember the discussion about isoflavones in
Chapter 5, this isn't necessarily surprising. Isoflavones aren't the same
as estrogen, so they can't be expected to act like estrogen in all tissues.

SUPER FOODS FOR STRONG BONES

When we look at the nutrients that play a big role in protecting bone health, it's pretty clear that many vegan foods are advantageous. Emphasizing these foods in your diet will help you plan menus that keep your bones strong well into later years.

Leafy greens: Long before people started milking cows, they were getting plenty of calcium by foraging for leafy greens. Of the cultivated greens available to us today, collard greens, kale, turnip greens, and bok choy are the best sources of this nutrient. Other greens—spinach, Swiss chard, and beet greens—aren't good sources of calcium because their calcium is bound to compounds (especially oxalate) that inhibit its absorption. However, they are among the best sources of potassium and magnesium, two minerals that are important for bone health. All greens also supply vitamin K and vitamin C, two other nutrients needed for healthy bones. Eating a variety of leafy greens, and eating lots of them, is a good way to protect bone health.

Soyfoods: While research on bone-protective effects of soy isoflavones has been disappointing, these foods still have a role to play in protecting bone health. They're among the richest sources of plant protein and some, like calcium-set tofu and fortified soymilk, are good sources of well-absorbed calcium. Whole soybeans and tempeh are also good sources of potassium and magnesium.

Beans: In addition to providing protein, beans are among the best sources of potassium and magnesium. The fact that vegans and vegetarians often replace meat in meals with beans is part of the reason for their higher intakes of these two minerals. Most beans also make a small contribution to calcium intake.

	Calcium-rich	Protein-rich	Vitamin K-rich	Vitamin C-rich	Potassium-rich	Magnesium-rich
BEANS						
Black beans	✓	✓			✓	✓
Great northern beans	✓	✓			✓	✓
Navy beans	✓	✓			✓	✓
SOYFOODS						
Tofu, firm	✓	✓			✓	✓
Tofu, soft	✓	✓				✓
Soybeans	✓	✓			✓	✓
Tempeh	✓	✓			✓	✓
Calcium-fortified soymilk	✓	✓				✓
NUTS/SEEDS						
Almond butter	✓	✓			✓	✓
Tahini	✓	✓				✓
VEGETABLES						
Acorn squash					✓	✓
Bok choy	✓			✓	✓	✓
Broccoli			✓	✓	✓	✓
Cabbage			✓	✓	✓	✓
Collard greens	✓	✓	✓	✓		✓
Kale	✓		✓	✓		✓
Spinach	-			✓	✓	✓
Swiss chard				✓	✓	✓
Calcium-fortified tomato juice	✓			✓	✓	✓
Turnip greens	✓		✓	✓		✓

Table 13-1: Super Foods for Bone Health

— *continues* —

Table 13-1: Super Foods for Bone Health — *continued* —						
	Calcium-rich	Protein-rich	Vitamin K-rich	Vitamin C-rich	Potassium-rich	Magnesium-rich
FRUIT						
Figs	✓				✓	✓
Calcium-fortified orange juice	✓			✓	✓	✓
OTHER FOODS						
Calcium-Fortified hemp, rice, almond milk	✓					

BONE THIEVES: SMOKING, SODIUM, AND ALCOHOL

Moderate drinking is linked to better bone density, but too much alcohol leads to both poorer bone health and risk of fracture. This is another instance where it is important to keep alcohol in check.[24]

Women who smoke also tend to break more bones and to lose bone mass more rapidly.[25] Smoking may impair calcium absorption, and it might bring on an earlier menopause, which raises risk for osteoporosis.[26]

Finally, diets high in sodium promote loss of calcium in the urine in women regardless of their calcium intake.[27] It doesn't mean you have to go salt-free. It's fine to lightly salt your food, and iodized salt can be a good way to meet iodine needs. But use a light hand with the salt shaker and keep processed foods to a minimum in order to keep sodium intake from going too high.

STRONG WOMEN HAVE STRONG BONES

If you're carrying around a few more pounds than you would like, you can take some satisfaction in knowing that this may protect the health of your bones. Slender women are more likely to break bones.[28] Weight loss also takes a toll on bones and raises risk for osteoporosis, although exercise can counter these effects.[29] Exercise and adequate weight protect bones by placing stress and impact on them, two things that keep the skeleton strong. Being sedentary is by far the worst thing you can do for bone health.

Exercise that creates impact like jogging or high-impact aerobics can be especially beneficial. But the muscle mass that comes with strength training can also increase bone mass. Stronger muscles plus the improved balance and agility that come with many types of exercise, also make it less likely that you'll fall.

If you already have osteoporosis, avoid high-impact activities or exercise that increases your risk of falling. If you're restricted in the types of exercise you can do, even low-impact movements like water aerobics can improve muscle strength.

A Vegan Prescription for Bone Health

- Make sure your diet is rich in protein by including at least three servings of legumes in menus every day.
- Eat plenty of calcium-rich foods. Aim for 3 cups per day of foods that provide calcium—leafy greens (collard greens, turnip greens, kale, and bok choy), fortified plant milks and juices, calcium-set tofu, soybeans, tempeh, and figs. Almond butter and sesame tahini are other good calcium sources.
- Get adequate sun exposure or take a supplement providing at least 600 IUs of vitamin D.
- Pack your menus with fruits and vegetables.
- Eat lots of leafy greens—all different kinds—for their calcium, vitamin K, magnesium, and potassium.
- Exercise every day and include strength-training in your regimen. If you are limited in the type of exercise you can do, talk to a physical therapist to find a plan that fits your needs.
- Cut back on sodium by avoiding processed foods and limiting added salt in the foods you prepare yourself.
- Keep alcohol intake moderate.
- Stop or cut back on smoking.

CHAPTER FOURTEEN

FIGHTING PAIN WITH PLANT FOODS

Few things can challenge your quality of life as much as chronic pain. It saps your energy, hampers concentration, and can make it difficult to perform even the simplest household tasks. The most common causes of chronic pain—rheumatoid arthritis, osteoarthritis, fibromyalgia, and migraine headaches—affect women more often than men. One reason may be the smaller arteries in women. I talked in Chapter 12 about how this can raise heart disease risk. It can also contribute to rheumatoid arthritis and migraine headaches. Both inflammation and insulin resistance may also lie at the heart of some of these diseases. So it's not surprising that there is a potential for diet to make a difference in the management of pain.

RHEUMATOID ARTHRITIS

Rheumatoid arthritis (RA) is an autoimmune disease in which the immune system attacks the joints and their surrounding tissues, causing inflammation, pain, and stiffness. Affecting three times more women than men, it's also associated with a higher risk for cardiovascular disease.

In Europe, rates of rheumatoid arthritis increase as you travel from south to north. One reason could be differences in diets since Mediterranean-type diets have been used with some success to treat pain in people with RA.[1,2]

As many as 150 different studies—many focusing on vegetarian diets—have looked at the effects of diet on RA, but many of them have such serious shortcomings that it's been difficult to learn much from their results. One group of Finnish researchers has had some success in reducing symptoms of RA with a raw foods vegan diet. Besides being high in antioxidants, which may be beneficial, a raw foods diet might produce helpful changes in intestinal bacteria.[3-6] This increase in "friendly" bacteria might reduce inflammation-inducing compounds in the bloodstream.[3] Another theory is that RA is linked to a pathogen called *Proteus mirabilis* that is also involved in urinary tract infections. One group of experts recommends antibacterial medications along with a vegetarian diet as a way to counter the effects of these microbes. It's a theory that hasn't yet been validated, however.[7]

Since certain foods are thought to trigger inflammation in people with RA, elimination diets are another approach to dealing with symptoms.[8] Common problem foods are removed from the diet for a period of time, and then slowly added back one at a time to assess their effects on symptoms. A vegan diet is a good first step toward this approach since milk and meat are believed to be common RA triggers.[9] Among plant foods, the possible culprits are corn, wheat, oats, rye, coffee, and citrus fruits, so these should also be removed on an elimination diet.

The problem with studies using elimination diets is that it's often not possible to pinpoint the actual foods that make a difference. For example, one study found that a gluten-free vegan diet was useful in treating people with RA. But was it the absence of some particular animal food or the lack of gluten that made a difference? There is no way to know without gradually adding back individual foods one at a time.[10] That's hard to do in studies, but you can do it on your own.

Start with a vegan diet that eliminates all sources of gluten (see the list on page 200), along with coffee and citrus fruits. Give it about four weeks to see if there is any improvement in your RA symptoms. If you don't feel better, then these foods are probably not triggers for you. If you do feel better, you can try to add the foods back one at a time—one food every four days or so—to see how you react. If your symptoms worsen after adding back a food, eliminate it again for a few days and then try another challenge. Since this is a subjective test, you'll want to give foods a thorough testing. You don't want to eliminate a food from your diet permanently unless it is a genuine trigger. If you find that wheat triggers symptoms, it doesn't necessarily mean that you can't consume other sources of gluten. You may be just fine with gluten in general but still have problems with wheat or rye. Since you'll probably end up testing a number of foods, it can help to keep a food log or journal.

Regardless of their direct effects on symptoms of RA, vegan diets that are low in saturated and trans fats, and rich in slow carbohydrates, vegetables, and healthy fats are an ideal choice for anyone who has this disease since it's a way of eating that reduces inflammation. Because of their anti-inflammatory properties, DHA and EPA supplements may also help. Another type of fat called gamma-linolenic acid, which is found in borage and evening primrose oils, was effective in patients in an arthritis clinic.[11] Although it hasn't been thoroughly tested, it's worth a try.

Also, because RA is so much more common in women than men, there is interest in understanding the role that hormones may have on this disease. Women taking birth control pills may be at lower risk[12] although whether having taken oral contraceptives at one time lowers lifetime risk is a topic of considerable debate.[13] Isoflavones and other compounds in soyfoods might play a protective role, too, but there is only very preliminary research on this.[14,15]

Gluten-Free Diets

Gluten is a type of protein found in wheat. People with celiac disease have an abnormal immune reaction to certain compounds that are produced when gluten is digested. Those same compounds are found in other grains such as barley and rye. A gluten-free diet—which is the standard treatment for celiac disease—is one that eliminates all grains that produce these immune reactions. Whether a gluten-free diet can also help other kinds of conditions isn't known. But if you want to try one as part of an elimination diet to reduce symptoms of rheumatoid arthritis, you'll need to avoid these grains and grain products.

Barley	Rye
Barley malt/extract	Seitan
Bran	Semolina
Bulgur	Spelt
Couscous	Triticale
Kamut	Udon
Panko	Wheat
Pasta	Wheat germ

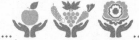

Finally, in both the Nurses' Health Study and the Iowa Women's Health Study, women who smoked were more likely to develop RA.[16,17] So we can add this to the long list of reasons why, if you smoke, you should start taking steps to quit.

Fighting Pain from Rheumatoid Arthritis

Despite a large number of studies on RA and diet, the findings remain sketchy. The research does point toward some promising approaches, however, and maybe some of what has helped others will be beneficial for you. Here are some things you might try.

- Eat a healthy vegan diet aimed at reducing inflammation—that is, lots of slow carbs and antioxidant-rich foods.
- Add more raw foods to your diet. Replace some of the cooked grains and beans in your diet with sprouted versions of these foods. Eat raw, unroasted nuts instead of roasted nuts. Eat plenty of raw fruits and vegetables.
- Take a supplement providing about 400 to 500 milligrams of DHA/EPA.
- Increase your vegetable intake to make sure your diet is especially rich in antioxidants.
- Take supplements of evening primrose or borage oil providing about 1,400 milligrams (1.4 grams) of gamma-linolenic acid. (Don't take this if you are pregnant, though, since it's associated with miscarriages. As with any supplements, check with your health-care provider. There can be contraindications with some medications and some supplements.)
- Try eliminating foods that are common triggers—corn, wheat, oats, rye, coffee, and citrus—and then slowly add them back one at a time to see if it affects your symptoms.

OSTEOARTHRITIS

Osteoarthritis (OA) occurs when cartilage, the tissue that cushions bones at the joints, breaks down, allowing bones to rub together. The result is pain, swelling, and stiffness. It's a common consequence of the wear and tear on joints that comes with age. Among older people, it's more common in women than in men.

Exercise and weight loss (in those who are overweight) are mainstays of both prevention and treatment. This is another instance where even small amounts of weight loss can bring some relief.

It's possible that a diet that promotes inflammation makes symptoms of OA worse, which would suggest that a vegan diet is helpful. And since oxidative stress can promote cartilage damage, the higher antioxidant content of plant foods might be beneficial in preventing

OA or slowing its progression.[18] Even a relatively moderate intake of the antioxidant nutrient vitamin C—around 120 to 200 milligrams per day—can reduce OA progression.[19] You could get this much vitamin C in your diet by consuming an orange plus one cup of gently cooked broccoli, peppers, or Brussels sprouts.

A number of supplements are also being studied for possible benefits in managing OA. Among the most promising are ASUs (avocado/soybean unsaponifiables), which are extracts of avocado or soybean oils. These supplements, taken in doses of 300 milligrams per day, could slow the progression of OA and/or relieve symptoms.[20-22]

One of the best studied supplements is glucosamine which is either made from crustacean shells or produced synthetically. There are a couple of different forms of this supplement and one, glucosamine sulfate, seems to be the most effective at reducing pain and slowing progression of OA.[23-25] In contrast, chondroitin, a (nonvegan) supplement usually derived from cartilage tissue of cows, doesn't seem to have any advantage over glucosamine or provide any additional benefits.[26]

Managing Osteoarthritis

Aside from the benefits of weight loss for overweight women, we have very little information about the type of diet that might prevent or control OA. Here are some things you might try.

- Eat an antioxidant-rich diet and make sure you are getting plenty of vitamin C. Vegans usually have high intakes of this nutrient.
- Consider supplements of ASUs and/or glucosamine sulfate.
- Although there isn't much research on it, some people have found relief from acupuncture.
- Exercise that takes weight off your joints—like swimming or water aerobics—can be soothing and beneficial. Regular exercise in general is important for both the prevention and management of osteoarthritis.

FIBROMYALGIA

Fibromyalgia wasn't even recognized as a distinct disease until 1992. It's a condition that causes widespread and chronic muscle pain along with fatigue, and it's thought to be due to abnormalities in the way the nervous system processes pain. Some people with fibromyalgia also suffer from memory and concentration problems, commonly referred to as "fibro fog." About 1 to 2 percent of the American population has fibromyalgia and it is much more common in women.

Only a handful of studies have looked at effects of diet on fibromyalgia, and they have generally been poorly designed or have failed to report enough data to guide us in making recommendations. When a vegetarian diet was compared to drug therapy, those consuming the vegetarian diet experienced some reduction in pain, but it wasn't nearly as effective as drug treatment. In fact, it wasn't impressive enough for any of the subjects to stick with the diet after the study was over.[27] In two other studies, subjects who followed raw foods vegan diets saw improvement in their symptoms, but the findings from these studies were fairly limited and it wasn't clear whether subjects felt better because of the diet or because they lost weight. Again, none chose to continue with the diet, which might suggest that the benefits weren't sufficiently motivating.[3,28] In a third study of a raw vegan diet, there was no control group and many of the subjects didn't even meet diagnostic criteria for fibromyalgia.[29]

This isn't to say that vegan diets aren't helpful; it's just that the current evidence isn't strong enough for us to know. However, the most common food triggers for fibromyalgia symptoms are animal foods: fish and dairy. So it's not surprising that some women say their symptoms improve when they adopt a vegan diet. Other triggers include caffeine, food coloring, and chocolate. Certain food additives, aspartame and monosodium glutamate, may make fibromyalgia worse, too. I talk more about that on page 206.

Diet Plan for Reducing Symptoms of Fibromyalgia

With so little known about the relationship of diet to fibromyalgia, you'll need to be a little bit of your own researcher, looking for foods and other factors that trigger symptoms. Here are some things you can try.

- Avoid monosodium glutamate.
- Avoid foods and drinks sweetened with aspartame.
- Cut caffeine and chocolate out of your diet and see if this affects symptoms.
- Manage stress and get enough sleep.

MIGRAINE HEADACHES

Women are three times more likely than men to suffer from migraines, which are due to abnormal blood vessel function. These headaches occur most often in younger people, those between the ages of ten and thirty. There is a strong genetic predisposition to migraines, but lifestyle, environment, and dietary factors can all act as triggers, bringing on a migraine headache.

Triggers seem to be most important during times when you are most vulnerable to a migraine anyway—during the week before your period, or when you're tired or stressed. One of the most important triggers is skipping meals, which is strongly related to risk of getting a migraine, especially in women.[30] Letting yourself get dehydrated can also bring on a headache. So, for some women, preventing migraines can be as simple as eating regular meals and drinking plenty of water.

The effects of individual foods vary quite a bit from person to person, so you might find it useful to keep a food diary to watch for migraine triggers. Keep in mind that a trigger can cause a migraine even 24 hours after you consume it. Vegan diets automatically eliminate some of the most common migraine triggers like cured meats and cheeses. Other foods that can often act as triggers are alcohol, citrus fruits, and icy cold foods like ice water or ice cream. Chocolate can bring on a migraine, but in women, carob can be even more harmful.[31] As with fibromyalgia, both aspartame and monosodium glutamate (MSG) can cause migraines in some women.

Drinking more than three cups of regular coffee per day may cause you to have more migraines. On the other hand, as most migraine sufferers know, quickly drinking a cup or two of coffee when you feel a migraine coming on can be very effective at stopping it in its tracks.

Some research shows that magnesium deficiency is a common underlying problem of migraine headaches. Most vegans meet needs for this nutrient with ease, but you might want to take a look at the table on pages 317–320 to make sure you eat plenty of magnesium-rich foods. Researchers from the New York Headache Center suggest that the supplements listed below could be helpful in preventing migraines.[32] Don't take all of them, but rather try them one at a time, starting at the top of the list. And be sure to talk to your health-care provider first to get advice about whether these supplements are right for you, especially if you're taking other medications. Some of these amounts are well above the RDA and should be taken with care.

- Magnesium: 400 milligrams daily
- *Petasites Hybridus* (an herb, commonly called butterbur): 75 milligrams twice daily for a month and then 50 milligrams twice daily
- Feverfew (an herb): 100 milligrams daily
- Coenzyme Q10: 300 milligrams daily
- Riboflavin (a B-vitamin): 400 milligrams daily
- Alpha lipoic acid: 600 milligrams daily

Diet Plan for Preventing Migraine Headaches
- Eat regular meals; don't skip meals or let your blood sugar get too low.
- Drink plenty of cool (but not icy) water.
- Eat plenty of magnesium-rich foods. The best sources are wheat bran, almonds, spinach, cashews, soybeans, wheat germ,

shredded wheat cereal, oatmeal, peanuts, peanut butter, potatoes, black-eyed peas, pinto beans, brown rice.

- Avoid monosodium glutamate (MSG) and aspartame.
- Avoid icy foods.
- Track your food intake and compare to headache frequency,
  with particular attention to effects of alcohol, citrus fruits,
  chocolate, and carob.
- Try one of the supplements of nutrients or herbs listed above.

MONOSODIUM GLUTAMATE AND ASPARTAME

Two amino acids—glutamate and aspartate—might be related to both fibromyalgia and migraine headaches. Glutamate is found in MSG or monosodium glutamate, the common ingredient in Chinese restaurant food, and aspartate is part of
the sugar substitute aspartame. These are both "excitatory neurotransmitters,"
and they could adversely affect the nervous system in fibromyalgia. For example, higher levels of glutamate in spinal fluid correlate to pain levels in people
with fibromyalgia. Infection and stress can make the blood-brain barrier more
permeable to glutamate, and many people with fibromyalgia report that their
symptoms are worsened by stress.[33] Glutamate is also linked to migraines, and
about 80 percent of people with fibromyalgia have migraines.[34] Ingredients that
contain MSG include hydrolyzed vegetable protein, autolyzed yeast, sodium
caseinate, yeast extract, hydrolyzed oat flour, texturized protein, and calcium
caseinate. Some veggie meats may contain one or more of these ingredients,
so be sure to read labels carefully. Despite suspicions about glutamate and aspartate in fibromyalgia, there isn't much good research on them. But some
people do see a reduction in their symptoms when they eliminate aspartame
and MSG from their diet. The relationship with MSG is interesting since, despite the fact that it is a very common ingredient in cooking throughout China,
rates of fibromyalgia are extremely low there.[35] It's possible that some populations have genetic protection from this disease, and so, not having fibromyalgia, they don't need to worry about trigger foods and food components.

You might remember that in Chapter 1, I talked about the importance of seeking out foods that are rich in umami as a way to enhance your vegan diet. Umami-
rich foods are high in glutamate. Whether these foods—like umeboshi plum
sauce, nutritional yeast, sundried tomatoes, and ketchup—act as triggers for fibromyalgia symptoms or migraine headaches isn't known. There is no research on
this and they are generally lower in free glutamate than MSG. Eliminating these
foods as a test to see if it improves your symptoms is certainly worth a try, though.

CHAPTER FIFTEEN

CONTROLLING DIABETES

Hundreds of years ago, physicians recognized a mysterious and fatal wasting disease in people who also produced excessive amounts of urine. Their urine was especially attractive to ants. In the middle of the seventeenth century, British physician Thomas Willis bravely sampled the urine of one his patients and noted that it was "wondrous sweet." The disease came to be called diabetes mellitus, which translates to "honey siphon" reflecting the characteristic sugar-laden urine of the disease.

Diabetes is a problem of inadequate or ineffective insulin. I talked in Chapter 3 about how cells require insulin in order to absorb glucose—their main fuel—from the blood. When insulin can't do its job, glucose builds up in the bloodstream. The only way the body can get rid of it is to excrete it in the urine. That's why early signs of diabetes are frequent trips to the bathroom and excessive thirst. At the same time, although cells are bathed in a sea of glucose, they're starving because they can't absorb it. Hunger and sometimes weight loss are other early signs of diabetes.

TWO TYPES OF DIABETES

Type 1 diabetes is an autoimmune disease in which the body's own immune system attacks cells in the pancreas that secrete insulin. Its cause isn't well understood. Children who are breastfed appear to be at a much lower risk for developing type-1 diabetes, and there is evidence that early consumption of cow's milk could raise risk, although there are also studies that refute this link.[1-4]

Only a small percentage of people with diabetes have this type, which usually has a sudden onset and tends to occur in younger people. In type-1 diabetes the pancreas fails to secrete insulin or it produces very little of it. People with type-1 diabetes always require daily insulin delivered either by injection or pump. Before the discovery of insulin in the 1920s, type-1 diabetes was a death sentence.

The far more common kind of diabetes is **type-2 diabetes,** which is a disease of insulin resistance rather than insufficient insulin production. That is, while enough insulin is produced, cells are insensitive to its effects. At some point, the overworked pancreas—which keeps pumping out more and more insulin in response to high glucose levels—may lose its capacity to produce insulin. Sometimes insulin injections are helpful in the control of type 2 diabetes, and it can also be managed with oral medications that make cells more sensitive to insulin. Like those with type-1 diabetes, people with insulin resistance and type-2 diabetes are at higher risk for nerve damage and heart disease.

Type-2 diabetes is caused by some combination of genetics and lifestyle. It's only been recently recognized that chronic inflammation is an underlying cause of type-2 diabetes, but there were actually hints about this connection more than a hundred years ago. In the late 1800s, physicians recognized that giving patients high doses of sodium salicylate (a close cousin to aspirin) could lower blood glucose in people with "mild" diabetes, which was most likely type 2-diabetes.[5]

Gestational diabetes develops in pregnancy and then disappears after the baby is born. Women who have had gestational diabetes are at higher risk of developing type-2 diabetes. Optimal lifestyle choices, including exercise and healthy diet, can prevent that from happening.

The recommendations in this chapter can be helpful for women with either type-1 or type-2 diabetes. However, most of the research and findings I'll talk about are from studies on people with type-2 diabetes. If you have type-1 diabetes, you'll want to work with your health-care provider when making dietary changes and also keep close tabs on your blood glucose levels. This is true as well for women with type-2 diabetes who are using insulin or other medications that affect blood glucose levels. In people taking certain medications, diet changes that improve insulin sensitivity (a measure of how cells respond to insulin) can produce hypoglycemia, or low blood sugar. If you haven't already, make sure you talk with your health-care provider or dietitian about what to do in the case of hypoglycemia.

DIET TO PREVENT TYPE-2 DIABETES

Most people will have prediabetes before they develop type-2 diabetes. At this stage, blood glucose levels are higher than normal due to insulin resistance, but not yet high enough to be diagnosed as diabetes.

High calorie intake and excess body fat, especially around your middle, raise risk for prediabetes. However, the insulin resistance that underscores prediabetes can itself cause weight gain and it isn't entirely clear which comes first—the weight or the insulin resistance. Regardless, weight loss—even when it's modest—can be very effective in preventing the progression of insulin resistance and prediabetes to diabetes.[6] This is one of those areas where losing just 5 percent of body weight can have an important benefit, by decreasing insulin resistance and improving blood glucose measures.[7]

Being vegan appears to be protective, too. In the Adventist Health Study-2, vegans were less than half as likely as meat-eaters to have diabetes and their lower body weight was only part of the explanation.[8] Studies in women show that getting protein and fat from plant foods lowers risk for diabetes.[9-11] Nuts, legumes, and whole grains also seem to help prevent this disease.[9,12-14] One reason might be that many of these plant foods are rich in the mineral magnesium, which lowers risk for diabetes.[15] Conversely, women who consume more red and processed meats have a higher risk.[16,17] Trans fats, which promote inflammation, also raise risk for diabetes.[11]

Carbohydrates and Fats in Diets to Control Diabetes

Although lifestyle changes can often prevent prediabetes from progressing to diabetes, there is some debate about whether it is possible to "cure" type-2 diabetes once it occurs. What is clear, however, is that diabetes can be very well controlled to the point where the signs that you had/have diabetes aren't measurable. That is, you can get blood glucose under control, reverse insulin resistance, improve your cholesterol levels, and reduce or even eliminate medications.

If you use insulin to manage your diabetes, you've already been taught how to keep tabs on your blood glucose levels after meals. For long-term assessment of blood glucose status, a test called HbA1c (glycosylated hemoglobin) is used. The HbA1c test measures how much glucose enters red blood cells and attaches to hemoglobin, the component that delivers oxygen to cells. Since red blood cells have a life span of only three to four months, their glucose content reflects how well blood glucose is controlled over that time period.

A common misconception is that the best way to manage blood glucose levels is to restrict carbohydrates. In fact, slow carbs—the ones that cause a slow and steady release of glucose to the bloodstream—are effective in controlling blood glucose levels and improving insulin sensitivity.[18] Emphasizing whole grains and other fiber-rich foods can improve insulin sensitivity in people with normal or impaired glucose status even when they are overweight.[19] This isn't a newfangled idea, either. Nearly thirty-five years ago, researchers showed that when men with diabetes followed a diet that was very high in fiber-rich carbohydrates, more than half of them were able to stop taking insulin. And the change happened in about just two weeks.[20] More recently, a vegan diet that was low in fat and very high in slow carbs was used successfully to control blood glucose levels and help people reduce or eliminate their diabetes medications.[21]

It's also not necessary to eliminate all higher-fat foods to control diabetes and its risk factors. In fact, there are some good reasons to include healthy plant fats in your diet. Even when blood glucose levels are well controlled, many people with diabetes have high triglyceride levels and low HDL-cholesterol (the good cholesterol). They often have higher levels of small, dense LDL-cholesterol particles, the type that is especially harmful.[22] Replacing some of the carbohydrate in your diet with healthful sources of fat can lower triglycerides, raise HDL cholesterol levels, and produce LDL-cholesterol particles that are more buoyant, and therefore less likely to contribute to heart disease. Blood glucose may sometimes be more easily controlled with higher intakes of monounsaturated fats (nuts, avocado, canola, and olive oils) and more Mediterranean-style diets.[23–26]

Diets that strictly forbid all higher-fat foods including nuts and seeds are also likely to be too low in omega-3 fats. Consuming too little alpha-linolenic acid (ALA), the essential omega-3 fatty acid, is especially harmful for people with diabetes since their bodies are less efficient at converting ALA to the long-chain omega-3 fats DHA and EPA.

This isn't to suggest a free-for-all with fat. Diets with excessive amounts of fat can worsen insulin sensitivity in women.[27] Even though this appears to be due mostly to saturated fats and isn't seen with more usual fat intakes,[28,29] it's still a good idea to keep your fat intake on the moderate side—around 20 to 25 percent of calories—with most of it coming from nuts, seeds, avocados, soyfoods, and small amounts of healthy oils. Capping your fat intake at this level also encourages a more varied food intake, which is good overall for nutrient status and health.

VEGAN DIETS: BENEFITS FOR PEOPLE WITH DIABETES

Menus built around plant foods bring a host of benefits for control of diabetes. Since people with diabetes have a higher risk for heart disease, the low saturated fat content of vegan diets is extremely beneficial.

Certain plant foods, like nuts that have anti-inflammatory properties, can also be powerful tools in diabetes management.[30,31]

Poor blood glucose control is associated with low antioxidant status, and also with formation of AGEs (advanced glycation end products). (See page 46.) People with diabetes produce high amounts of these compounds, which may contribute to the blood vessel damage that occurs in poorly controlled diabetes.[32–34] Keeping blood glucose under control and feeding your body with plenty of antioxidants—which are abundant in fruits and vegetables—can help prevent the formation of AGEs.[35]

Even herbs and spices are excellent sources of compounds that improve the control of diabetes and reduce risk for complications. Cinnamon has a 1,000-plus year history of use in the treatment of what the Chinese called "thirsty disease," which was no doubt diabetes. Among modern Chinese people with type-2 diabetes, taking extracts of cinnamon was found to improve blood glucose levels and diabetic control.[36]

I mentioned above that magnesium-rich diets seem to lower risk for developing diabetes. For those who have diabetes, it can help make cells more sensitive to insulin. Magnesium supplements are sometimes recommended for that reason, but chances are that you won't need to take one. In one study showing magnesium to be protective, high intakes were about 400 milligrams per day. Vegan women typically have intakes that are at least that high, and often quite a bit higher.[37,38]

Supplements for Vegans with Diabetes

One nutrient that may need a little extra attention in your diet is chromium. This mineral enhances the activity of insulin and is important in blood glucose control. Although many foods provide chromium, most have only small amounts and some people might fall short. Broccoli is an excellent source of chromium and so is grape juice (and some red wines). Whole grains (but not processed grains) also contribute chromium to the diet. You should be able to meet chromium needs by eating a variety of whole plant foods, but it's also possible that a small supplement would be beneficial. The RDA for women is 20 to 25 micrograms.

A popular supplement used to improve treatment of diabetes is alpha-lipoic acid. This is a naturally occurring compound that is involved in energy production, acts as an antioxidant, and may improve insulin sensitivity.[39] It's not considered essential in the diet since humans synthesize it, but if you want to increase your intake of alpha-lipoic acid, supplements are the only way to do so. The benefits of taking them aren't clear, but if you are struggling to manage blood glucose levels, it's something to consider.

Finally, supplements of gamma linolenic acid (GLA) may also be useful for people with diabetes who experience nerve damage, a potential complication of poorly controlled diabetes. Sources of this fat include borage, blackcurrant, hempseed, and evening primrose oils.[40,41] As always, check with your health-care provider before you start taking supplements.

MANAGING DIABETES: GUIDELINES FOR VEGANS

The American Diabetes Association has recommended a diet that provides about 60 to 70 percent of calories from a mix of carbohydrates and monounsaturated fats, but there is no ideal ratio of carbohydrates, fat, and protein in the diet—or at least, it isn't known. It's really a matter of what works best for you. You may need to experiment to find the ideal diet that you enjoy and that supports good control of blood glucose. Here are some guidelines for making the best choices for managing diabetes.

- Choose slow carbs, using the tips on pages 43–44 to guide you. Although it's fine to include some refined carbohydrate treats in your diet, aim to limit them.
- Choose healthy higher-fat foods like nuts, seeds, avocado, olives, soyfoods, olive oil, and canola oil. If you tend to eat a

low-fat diet, and you find your triglycerides creeping up, you'll want to replace some of the carbohydrates in your diet with foods that provide some fat.

- Make sure you meet needs for the essential omega-3 fat ALA (alpha-linolenic acid) by following the guidelines on pages 22–24. People with diabetes should also take supplements providing at least 300 milligrams per day of DHA and EPA from algae. If you suffer from nerve pain, talk to your health-care provider about adding a supplement of GLA (gamma linolenic acid) from borage, evening primrose, or blackcurrant oil to your diet. The amount shown to reduce neuropathy (nerve pain) is found in about 2 grams of borage oil, 3 grams of blackcurrant oil, or 5 grams of evening primrose oil.

- Avoid trans fats. They can worsen insulin resistance and promote inflammation. Avoid any food with "partially hydrogenated oil" on the label.

- Limiting saturated fat and cholesterol is especially important for people with diabetes. You don't need to worry about it, though. Your vegan diet is cholesterol-free and, unless you're eating lots of coconut and palm oil, it's also low in saturated fat.

- Protein needs are higher for people with poor glucose control and also for those eating low-calorie diets.[22] Vegans have an advantage since plant proteins may help to preserve kidney function in people with diabetes.[42]

- Eat a diet rich in fruits and vegetables. The antioxidant content of these foods can help prevent formation of AGEs and reduce your risk of complications from diabetes.

- Spice up your diet. Cinnamon appears to be a powerful spice for normalizing blood glucose levels. If you like its flavor, adding cinnamon to dishes is a pretty easy dietary habit to adopt. Cinnamon is wonderful in oatmeal, of course, but you can also add it to savory dishes like **Cinnamon-Ginger Seitan** (page 299) or **Cinnamon Tofu** (page 297).

- Use acidic ingredients like lemon and lime juice, tomatoes, and vinegar in dressing and marinades. They slow absorption of carbohydrates and can also reduce formation of AGEs from baked and broiled dishes.
- Eat a diet rich in magnesium. It's easy to do so when you're emphasizing whole plant foods in your menus. You can get 400 milligrams of magnesium—an amount that has been associated with improved control of diabetes—by eating ½ cup of tofu, 1 cup of beans, ½ cup of cooked spinach, and a cup of brown rice.
- If you drink alcohol, limit intake to one drink per day. Interestingly, moderate alcohol consumption improves insulin sensitivity and lowers risk for type-2 diabetes.[43,44] If you don't drink, this isn't sufficient reason to start doing so; there are plenty of other ways to improve insulin sensitivity. If you take insulin, be sure to avoid drinking alcohol on an empty stomach, which may cause hypoglycemia.
- If you're having trouble keeping blood glucose levels controlled, talk to your health-care provider about supplements of chromium and alpha-lipoic acid.
- Be certain to get exercise. Women with diabetes can improve insulin sensitivity by exercise alone, even without weight loss.[22]
- If you take insulin or other glucose-lowering drugs, you'll want to continue checking blood glucose levels. As your control of these levels improves, you may need to cut back on medication to avoid hypoglycemia.

Using the Plant Plate to Manage Calories

There are plenty of phone apps and websites that will help you track calories if you find that helpful in controlling your diabetes. You can also use the Plant Plate (page 30) to guide you toward a specific calorie intake that supports weight loss or maintenance. These guidelines aren't meant to be a prescription, but rather will help you see how choices from the Plant Plate—with an emphasis on the foods I talked about above—stack up against calorie needs.

Table 15-1 shows food choices at different calorie levels for a diet that gets about 25 percent of calories from fat, 15 percent from protein, and 60 percent from carbohydrates. Oils are included here not because they are necessary but because many people find it easier to plan appealing meals when you can use a little bit of vegetable oil. A serving is just 1 teaspoon of vegetable oil, which is often enough to enhance texture and flavor of salads or sautéed vegetables. If you don't use vegetables oils in your food preparation, you can replace 2 teaspoons of oil with 1 tablespoon of nut butter or 2 tablespoons of chopped nuts (either of these equals one-half serving of nuts.) Or, if you prefer a lower fat diet, something a little closer to 20 percent of your calories, replace those 2 teaspoons of oil with one serving of either whole grains or legumes. I also separated out soyfoods from other legumes to encourage one serving of soy per day. This is an easy way to increase the protein content of your diet but it's not absolutely necessary. If you don't like soyfoods, just replace them with another serving of legumes.

Table 15-1 Food Choices for Diets to Control Diabetes			
	1,500 Calories	**1,800 Calories**	**2,100 Calories**
Whole grains/ starches	5	5	6
Non-soy legumes	3	4	4
Soyfoods	1	1	2
Nuts and seeds	1	1½	1½
Vegetables	5	5	5
Fruits	3	3	3
Oils	2	2	3

CHAPTER SIXTEEN

FEELING GOOD: MANAGING STRESS AND DEPRESSION

Depression, anxiety, and stress—almost everyone experiences them at one time or another. Sometimes you just feel down in the dumps for no particular reason. Or you suffer a bout of depression due to loss or disappointment. It's the same with anxiety. You feel anxious or stressed in certain situations, but when the situation is resolved, the stress goes away. Those are the normal ups and downs of life. It's when these conditions are chronic that they become problematic.

Diet and lifestyle changes can help with all types of depression and stress. In this chapter I'm going to look at how diet may impact the more chronic types but will also talk about how certain supplements and lifestyle choices can prevent and manage more everyday kinds of sadness, stress, and anxiety. The tips on pages 223–225 can help whether you've been diagnosed with depression or just find yourself occasionally needing a little bit of a lift.

Women are more likely to suffer from depression and anxiety than men. Before puberty, rates of depression are roughly equal between boys and girls. Once the teen years hit, young women become twice as likely to suffer from depression and it's a difference that lasts throughout the life span.[1] This suggests a hormonal link since women are most vulnerable to depression during puberty, at certain times of the menstrual cycle, right after pregnancy, and around the time of menopause.[2-4] Women may also respond differently to stress than men and in ways that raise risk for stress-related depression.[5]

Magnetic resonance imaging (MRI) shows that the brains of depressed people actually look different. In women with depression, one part of the brain—the hippocampus—was found to be 9 to 13 percent smaller than in women who weren't depressed.[6] Chronic stress, which is related to depression, might be part of the explanation since it suppresses production of new nerve cells in the hippocampus.[7] This could be one reason why chronic depression raises risk for dementia later in life.[8]

Depression doesn't just make you feel bad; it also takes a toll on overall health by raising risk for heart disease and diabetes.[9] So managing even mild depression can have far-reaching benefits on your overall health.[10]

Is Depression Another Chronic Disease Related to Inflammation?

Stress and depression in women have both been linked to markers of inflammation.[11,12] This suggests that there is something about stress and depression that *causes* inflammation, and there is evidence that this is true. For example, stressors like negative social interactions and chronic relationship problems both increase inflammation.[13] In contrast, people who have good social support have lower blood levels of inflammatory markers.[14]

But it's also possible that the cause-and-effect relationship goes the other way. That is, the same inflammation that promotes diseases like diabetes and heart disease might be a causative factor in depression. Even mildly elevated levels of inflammatory markers are associated with the development of depression over time.[15,16] And, interestingly, anti-inflammatory medicine—like aspirin—enhances the effects of antidepressant drugs.[17] Lifestyle habits that are effective in reducing symptoms of depression, anxiety, and stress include exercise, meditation, and adequate rest, all of which happen to also reduce inflammation.[18-20]

This might mean that a diet that reduces inflammation could be helpful in dealing with depression, anxiety, and stress. It's not to say that adopting a healthy diet is a cure for mood disorders. For one thing, some people with depression don't show signs of chronic inflammation, and plenty of people with evidence of inflammation aren't depressed.[21] Even so, eating more healthfully is, at the very least, a way to take care of yourself with the potential to also reduce some symptoms of depression and anxiety.

SUPPLEMENTS

Falling short on certain nutrients can be a cause of depression and could make existing depression worse. Vitamins D and B_{12} are especially important in protecting emotional health, and the long-chain omega-3 fats (DHA abd EPA) may be, too.

In the Iowa Women's Health Study, women with lower dietary intakes of vitamin D were more likely to be depressed.[22] Other research agrees with this and shows that low blood levels of vitamin D, due to either inadequate intake or lack of sunlight, are significantly associated with depression.[23] For everyone—omnivores included—the only sources of vitamin D are supplements, fortified foods, and sun exposure. (Actually, there are a few animal sources of vitamin D, but it is very unlikely that omnivores can eat enough of them to meet needs.) If you aren't certain that you're getting adequate vitamin D from sunshine—which is not always easy—make sure you're taking a supplement.

Inadequate intakes of the B vitamins folate, B_6, and vitamin B_{12} can cause high blood levels of the amino acid homocysteine, which has been linked to depression.[24,25] Vitamin B_6 is also needed for the synthesis of certain neurotransmitters, including serotonin. Low serotonin levels are implicated in depression. Vegans tend to get plenty of

Low Cholesterol and Depression

Several studies have linked very low blood cholesterol levels with an increased risk for depression, particularly in men.[32,33] It's a confusing observation that could have any number of explanations that have nothing to do with diet. Since low cholesterol levels protect against heart disease, and depression raises risk for heart disease, it doesn't really seem like low cholesterol and depression go together very well. But it's possible that certain genetic predispositions might cause low blood cholesterol while also raising risk for mood disorders.[34] Drugs used to treat high cholesterol may also have transient negative effects on mood and depression.[35]

In women, it is low levels of HDL-cholesterol—the good cholesterol—that seem most likely to raise risk for depression.[36] This might be because HDL-cholesterol has anti-inflammatory properties.[37,38] But this is another issue where cause and effect isn't so clear. It might be that lower HDL levels are the result, not the cause, of depression. At least in men, the pro-inflammatory hormones associated with depression can cause HDL levels to drop.[38] It's reasonable to think the same thing might happen in women.

Regardless of the reasons, it's important to adopt a lifestyle that promotes healthy HDL cholesterol levels. This means getting enough exercise and including some higher-fat foods in your menus.

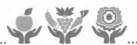

folate, which is abundant in beans and leafy green vegetables. It's also easy to meet needs for vitamin B_6 from plant foods; bananas, avocado, orange juice, potatoes, leafy green vegetables, and soyfoods are all great sources. The only sources of vitamin B_{12} for vegans, however, are supplements and fortified foods. This nutrient is needed for nerve cell function, and inadequate intake can cause a wide range of neurological problems including cognitive decline and depression.[26,27] Always make sure you're getting enough. The easiest way is to take a daily supplement providing around 25 micrograms of vitamin B_{12}.

The role of the long-chain omega-3 fats DHA and EPA in fighting depression isn't well understood. One statistical analysis of twelve studies found little benefit of omega-3 supplements.[28] Two others found that these fats were helpful in reducing depression.[29,30] They were also beneficial for medical students suffering from anxiety. The students' symptoms declined by about 20 percent when they took supplements of the omega-3s.[31] Even though the findings are conflicting, there are enough suggestions of a benefit that I think it's well worth trying a supplement of these fatty acids if you suffer from depression or anxiety.

VEGAN DIETS AND SEROTONIN

Tryptophan is an essential amino acid that is needed to make the neurotransmitter serotonin, and low levels of serotonin are linked to depression. One theory is that diets higher in tryptophan might help relieve depression—or at least that getting too little of this amino acid could make depression worse.

While it's true that meat is higher in tryptophan than plants, a well-balanced vegan diet is almost guaranteed to provide more than enough of this amino acid. Tryptophan requirements for vegan women are generally between 300 and 400 milligrams per day. If you're building menus around the Plant Plate (page 30)—consuming at least three servings per day of legumes (which includes beans, soyfoods, and peanut butter) along with a few servings of grains and plenty of vegetables—you won't have any trouble meeting those requirements. Table 16–1 shows tryptophan content of selected vegan foods.

A cup of soymilk or ½ cup of black beans has about the same amount of tryptophan as 1 cup of cow's milk—a food often touted for being high in tryptophan and (erroneously) regarded as useful

Table 16-1: Tryptophan Content of Plant Foods	
Food	Milligrams of Tryptophan (Women require 300 to 400)
Tofu, ½ cup	155
Oatmeal, ½ cup cooked	118
Soymilk, 1 cup	105
Beans, ½ cup cooked	70 to 90
Baked potato	80
Peanut butter, 2 tablespoons	80
Quinoa, ½ cup cooked	50
Walnuts, 1 ounce	50
Whole wheat bread, 1 slice	30
Brown rice, ½ cup cooked	20
Broccoli, ½ cup cooked	25
Kale, ½ cup cooked	15
Spinach, 1 cup raw	12

against insomnia. Foods like legumes also provide carbohydrates, which are needed for tryptophan to get into the brain.

And, compared to some omnivores and lacto-ovo vegetarians, vegans may even have the edge when it comes to converting tryptophan to serotonin. According to research in both adolescents and adults, depression is more common among people with lactose intolerance, the inability to digest the sugar that occurs naturally in milk. The theory is that undigested lactose in the intestines interferes with tryptophan metabolism, leading to low serotonin levels. So people with mild undiagnosed lactose intolerance who still consume some dairy foods could actually be at higher risk for depression.[39,40]

In people with low serotonin levels, eating more tryptophan-rich foods doesn't appear to raise those levels. It probably requires supplements to do that.[41] At this time, the evidence isn't strong enough to support pharmacological doses of tryptophan for treating depression.

If it's something you want to try, be sure to talk with your health-care provider first, especially if you are taking medication for depression.

There are other potential ways to give your serotonin levels a boost. Exposure to bright light may be helpful, even in people who don't suffer from seasonal affective disorder (SAD), a type of depression that occurs only during winter months.[42] If it's an option for you, even sitting near a brightly lit window can make a difference.

Exercise is also linked to improvements in serotonin levels, and, as I'll talk about below, it combats depression in other ways as well.[43]

COPING WITH STRESS, ANXIETY, AND DEPRESSION

If you suffer from depression that interferes with daily tasks and causes a feeling of hopelessness, there are effective treatments including medications, counseling, and cognitive therapy. If you need to take advantage of those options, you should definitely do so. Don't feel that you need to do it all on your own or "pull yourself up by your bootstraps." Depression is a disease, and sometimes it requires medical treatment.

But like most chronic diseases, lifestyle choices can help. In some cases, these choices are all that is needed to manage mild depression, stress, and anxiety. In others, they can be beneficial in augmenting other treatments.

- Try to get daily exposure to outdoor light. Move your work space close to a window if you have that option. If you can't get outside during the day, consider a light therapy box.
- Be sure to get adequate sleep since sleep deprivation increases markers of inflammation and may also worsen depression.[20]
- Exercise can be a powerful antidote to depression. In addition to its effects on serotonin levels, it can also reduce the inflammation that may contribute to depression.[19] Most research has looked at aerobic exercise, but strength training appears to be

beneficial, too. Exercising in the gym is great, but if you have the chance to get outdoors and take a walk, even briefly, that can help. And even better, if you can stroll in the woods (or on the beach or through a park), all the better. Most of us intuitively understand the restorative power of being in nature, and the science backs this up.[44] The Japanese call it *shinrin-yoku* or "forest bathing." In Japan, the "Therapeutic Effects of Forests Project" is looking at the benefits of spending time outdoors in nature on mental health.[45]

- Boost your endorphin levels. These neurotransmitters help to reduce pain and also promote a feeling of well-being. They are another beneficial by-product of exercise and are responsible for the "runner's high" that some athletes experience.[46] Laughter can increase endorphin levels, too. Spicy foods like jalapeño peppers can give a short little burst of endorphins.[47] So when you're feeling blue, some vigorous exercise, a funny movie, or a spicy snack may help you feel better.

- Some women find that certain daily practices make a big difference in how they feel. Talking to a friend, spending time in meditation or prayer, or simply writing in a journal are all good ways to decrease symptoms of depression.

- Some research suggests that a more Mediterranean-style diet—rich in plant foods and healthy fats—is associated with a lower incidence of depression in women.[48] Choosing more slow carbs can also help to combat inflammation.

- Make sure you are getting adequate vitamin B_{12}.

- Include plenty of vitamin B_6-rich foods in your diet. Some good choices are avocado, white and sweet potatoes, spinach, tomato juice, sea vegetables, bananas, oranges, soybeans, and soymilk.

- Consider a supplement of the long-chain omega-3 fats DHA and EPA. In Chapter 2, I suggested getting around 200 to 300 milligrams of these two fats combined several times a week. If you are dealing with depression, you may want to try a higher intake of around 400–500 milligrams per day.

- If you don't have adequate sun exposure throughout the year, take a vitamin D supplement providing 600 to 1,000 IUs per day.

DON'T LET YOUR DIET BE A SOURCE OF STRESS

When the first government food guide was developed in 1916, nutritionists put the focus on what they called "protective foods," those that provided plenty of calcium, vitamin A, and vitamin C. As long as people were meeting nutrient needs, there was little concern about other parts of the diet. One early nutrition expert suggested that you could "eat what you want after you eat what you should."[49]

That was reasonable advice in the days when grocery stores weren't packed with Doritos, Twinkies, and miles of soft drinks, and when there wasn't a fast-food restaurant on every corner. Once you had met nutrient needs, you couldn't really do yourself all that much harm by eating "what you wanted."

Today, if we want to be healthy, we definitely need to use a little bit of restraint. But, it's important to keep that restraint from morphing into restrained eating. Demonizing whole categories of plant foods, like fats, cooked foods, and gently processed foods, can progress toward an unhealthy attitude regarding dietary choices. Researchers have coined the term *orthorexia* (Latin for "correct eating") to describe an unhealthy preoccupation with eating healthy foods. People with orthorexia become fearful of eating *anything* that doesn't fit strict definitions of acceptable foods. They might believe that their food choices can guarantee good health and feel extremely stressed and guilty if they eat any food that doesn't fit their own guidelines for optimal eating.

Some popular approaches to vegan diets encourage that type of attitude toward food, but most vegans bring a healthier perspective to their food choices. And that's fortunate—because the truth is that you are likely to fall short of perfection no matter how hard you try to eat well. Nutrition is ever-evolving, and we learn new things about how to eat healthfully every day.

Striving to eat a healthy diet, based on the best available evidence, *is* important. But it is how you eat *most of the time* that matters. Minor deviations from your usual healthy diet are unlikely to have much impact on overall health. Build your food choices around the Plant Plate (but, don't stress if you aren't eating the "right" number of servings every day) and around healthy fats and slow carbs. Strive to get enough calcium and be sure to take supplements of vitamin D and vitamin B_{12}. Listen for hunger and satiety signals and take pleasure in the food you eat.

WHEN BEING A VEGAN IS STRESSFUL

Going vegetarian might in and of itself be an instant mood elevator. At least that was the experience of one group of omnivores who dropped meat, fish, and poultry from their menus for two weeks. They reported improved mood (according to their scores on a series of written tests) compared to subjects in the study who continued to eat meat or who traded in meat for fish.[50] In contrast, research in a group of young Australian women found that vegetarians were more likely to experience depression.[51] The researchers didn't have any explanation for this, and there is no reason to believe that being vegan or vegetarian raises risk for mood disorders or depression. Instead, one possibility is that people who choose to be vegetarian are more sensitive in general.

According to a study in Italy, many vegetarians and vegans may simply be hardwired for compassion.[52] The researchers recruited sixty subjects—twenty omnivores, nineteen vegetarians, and twenty-one vegans—and conducted a series of written tests aimed at measuring empathy. The results revealed that the vegetarians and vegans were significantly more empathetic.

Using brain scans, the researchers then showed that the "empathy related" areas of the brain were more active among the vegetarians and vegans as they viewed images depicting both human and animal suffering. In addition, when they viewed images of animal suffering, the vegetarians and vegans experienced activity in empathy-related areas of their brains that weren't affected by the images of human suffering.

Although this study is preliminary and hasn't been confirmed by other research, it wouldn't be especially surprising to learn that those of us who bring compassion into our dietary choices may somehow be different from the rest of the population—and in a good way.

But is there a downside to being part of the compassionate crowd? Vegans tend to be much more aware of the suffering of animals. If we are also more sensitive to that suffering, it can produce feelings of despair or depression about the state of the world and treatment of animals. We also live in a world where many—or really most—people don't feel the way we do. Most of us are forced to dine with friends, family members, and colleagues who are eating meat. It's often uncomfortable, but we're expected to grin and bear it.

Without a doubt, these are issues that can bring on feelings of loneliness, sadness, and isolation. But by embracing the reasons for being vegan, appreciating both short- and long-term successes, and seeking out support systems, you can find ways to counter feelings of hopelessness and adopt a more positive outlook.

- Accentuate the positive. Good things happen for animals and for veganism every day. Focus on the victories: the animals who get rescued, and the people and groups who are making a difference. You might worry that this will make you complacent regarding your own choices or your commitment to veganism. But I think most of us find that these stories of success keep us motivated and dedicated to continuing the work of changing the world for animals.
- Keep perspective by taking the long view. Paraphrasing a nineteenth-century abolitionist, the Reverend Martin Luther King famously told his followers that "The arc of history is long, but it bends toward justice." It's true that the results of our vegan choices may not be realized as quickly as we'd like. Sometimes progress is slow, but by embracing an ethic of justice, living it, and modeling it, you are part of the momentum toward a more fair and just world.
- Find your community. Whether it is where you live or over the internet, get support from others who share your goals and understand your feelings. Certainly the internet can be a double-edged sword, and some gathering places are more toxic than nurturing. But there are groups and blogs that are welcoming and nonjudgmental and that don't allow hurtful comments about your vegan choices, your perspective on diet, or about

body size and appearance. You'll find the discussions and articles at www.VeganForHer.com a great place to get support and encouragement.

- See your nonvegan communities as opportunity. You may often find yourself the only vegan among family or at work, your place of worship, or in your knitting or book group. That can be a little lonely, but it also is a wonderful opportunity. Not every setting is conducive to talking about your vegan choices, but you can always do a little nonconfrontational outreach by sharing food or showing off your latest vegan fashions.

- Get active for animals. Even if you don't think of yourself as an activist, there are all kinds of ways to make a difference for animals and to move veganism forward. There are choices for introverts and extroverts, for those who love to talk about veganism to others and those who don't. If you're looking for ideas on how to be more involved for animals, and also want some fun tips for taking veganism beyond your plate, turn the page for some ideas from JL.

CHAPTER SEVENTEEN

VEGANISM BEYOND THE PLATE

By JL Fields

Are you scratching your head? Veganism beyond the plate? Veganism *is* more than just food, right? Well, yes.

You may have picked up this book because you're curious about the health benefits of a plant-based diet or are concerned about the environment. Perhaps you are already on the path to a totally animal-free diet or you have just started out with one vegan meal a day. Whatever your path, there is a key part of veganism that I want to talk about here: the animals. As Ginny reminded us in the introduction to this book, veganism—as defined by Donald Watson in 1944—is "a way of living that seeks to exclude, as far as possible and practicable, all forms of exploitation of, and cruelty to, animals for food, clothing and any other purpose." My veganism, which began after I turned forty, grew from a connection with a goat in Africa (more on that in the recipe section), and, once I started on this journey, there was no turning back. While some people may call this a fad diet, it is not so for me. Once I learned more about animal food production, animal testing, and animals in entertainment, my veganism shifted from dietary to ethical. That was a seismic shift for me, personally, and frankly it has made it easier for me to adhere to a plant-based diet. It's not about me; it's about the animals. That is my personal experience; whatever your reasons for picking up this book, I hope the information in this chapter, which stems from my own journey as a relatively new vegan, will help you take your own veganism beyond the plate.

THE CLOSET

As a vegan lifestyle coach and educator, I work with clients on eating a plant-based diet, naturally, but I also work with them on taking veganism beyond the plate. We usually start with the closet, which is exactly where I started, because, let's face it, we have some serious products of cruelty stored on our shelves and hangers.

I am a shoe and handbag junkie. When I went vegan almost everything in my closet was leather. How could I possibly get rid of all of my shoes and bags? What would I wear? I would go broke replacing everything! But a funny thing happened. I started to feel uncomfortable when I espoused my veganism while wearing my favorite pair of pointy toe patent-leather boots. I got some really great advice from fellow vegans: do what you can, learn to do better, and consider this a process. I started slow, with one pair of vegan boots, which I ended up wearing every single day. The next season, spring, I picked up a new pair of shoes. Over time, my shoe and boot collection—as well as handbags—grew enough so that I was ready to get rid of the animal products in my closet. I didn't want to waste the items, however, so I gave some items to friends and donated the rest. I actually considered it a bit of vegan activism because I always told the recipient why I was giving them away.

It's not just about leather, though. It's about silk, wool, down, and fur. Fortunately, fur was never a part of my fashion sense, but I was once again surprised by the amount of down and silk I had in my closet. Wool was a real heartbreaker, as a knitter, but once I thought about the sheep holistically, not just as a being that was sheared but about what would happen to that sheep once she was spent, well, I couldn't do it. I started knitting with plant fibers, like bamboo, soy, and cotton. I had several coats with down—as well as a comforter and a few pillows—that I also thought couldn't be that bad. I mean ducks and geese weren't killed for their feathers right? Well, there's death and there's cruelty and when I learned that feathers are plucked in bunches, with bare hands, leaving the birds bloodied, I had to move on.

There are so many cruelty-free alternatives to wearing animal skin, including natural options such as cotton, linen, and hemp and man-made materials such as polyester, acrylic, and nylon. Synthetic leather, known as "pleather," is everywhere these days (and so much more affordable than leather!), as well as breathable microfiber. While going through vegan lifestyle coaching certification with the Main Street Vegan Academy I toured Vaute Couture, a company that was launched specifically to offer a fashionable, vegan coat that was ultrawarm. Frankly, I started making it a challenge—how to find the most stylish, compassionate clothing. I will never forget walking into my hair salon, carrying a GUNAS tote bag, and two different women walked up to me to ask me about my bag. "It's made by GUNAS, a vegan company, no animals were harmed in the making of this bag!" I loved that little moment of activism (they both wrote down the GUNAS website address).

Here are some great resources for cruelty-free wearables that look as good as they are compassionate:

Shoes and Handbags
Big Buddha
Chinese Laundry
Compassion Couture
GUNAS
Madden Girl
Matt & Nat
Novacas

Payless
Susan Nicole
Target
Vegan Cuts
Zappos (use the "vegan" filter)

Non-Down Coats
Merrell
Vaute Couture

Yarn
Elann
Michael's
PurlSoho
Yarnmarket.com (search by fiber)

HEALTH AND BEAUTY

While I jumped on the closet pretty quickly, it took me a while to connect my veganism to the products I used on my body. I actually got a wake-up call from my own blog readers. A friend gave me samples of a new shampoo by L'Oréal, which were labeled as, and being marketed as, vegan. I was excited and shared it with my blog readers. Someone immediately asked how I could consider it vegan, since L'Oreal still tests its products on animals. "How vegan am I?" I wondered. I actually took that question back to my readers and while responses reflected two extremes, most of us landed in the middle. We do the best we can. For me, that means that once I learn something, it's hard to ignore it. I therefore became obsessed with finding products that were "bunny-friendly." I wanted plant-based ingredients that did not harm animals in the process. I started using the smartphone apps Be Nice to Bunnies and Cruelty-Free while shopping. I also started sampling products from Vegan Cuts, an online deal site and market that features only vegan products. Once you know where to look it's actually quite easy to find compassionate skin and body care. Here's a tip: look for logos on packaging that indicate "vegan," a leaping bunny image or the PETA bunny ears. Also watch for palm oil on the ingredient list of soaps. Its production is responsible for considerable loss of rain forests and results in suffering for animals who live there, especially orangutans. Look for soaps that use coconut oil instead, like the inexpensive Kirk's Castile soap.

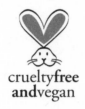

JL's Top Sources for Cruelty-Free Personal Care Products
Abba
Aubrey
Earth Sourced by Paula's Choice
Hurraw! Lip Balm
Kiss My Face
MuLondon
Red Apple (vegan and gluten-free makeup)
So Balanced
Tom's of Maine

HOUSEHOLD PRODUCTS

I used to think that vegan household products would be the hardest items to locate. Then it dawned on me—just turn to my local health food market, when all else fails. When I lived in New York I could find kitchen and cleaning supplies in an aisle at Mrs. Green's Natural Market. Now, in Colorado, I find them at Mountain Mama's Natural Market. The good news is that you can find them in your supermarkets, Target, and Wal-Mart, too. Dr. Bronner's, Method, Mrs. Meyer's, and

Seventh Generation make up my dishwasher and dish soap, hand soap, and my bathroom and multipurpose cleaning supplies.

You can find extensive resources to build a compassionate closet, health and beauty routine, and household supplies: PETA (http://www .peta.org/living), Girlie Girl Army (http://www.girliegirlarmy.com), Total Image Consultants (http://totalimageconsultants.com/), and The Discerning Brute (http://www.thediscerningbrute.com), to name a few. I encourage you to visit all four sites to learn more about the impact of fashion, health and beauty products, and home furnishings on animals and find alternatives to help you live more compassionately.

One More Thing—Care to Be a Change Agent for Animals?

I am going to confess that I am an activist at heart—and it's probably one of the many reasons Ginny and I were drawn to one another. In college I conducted antiracism trainings on campus. In my twenties, in postgraduate school, I worked at a gay, lesbian, bisexual, and transgendered community-based organization for six years. Immediately after that I spent the next eight years working professionally to end violence against women and girls.

If I care about a cause I do something about it. In this case I started my vegan activism with a food blog. I write as a woman who made big changes, like going vegan, postforty. I develop and share recipes to demonstrate how easy and accessible vegan food and cooking is. But I wanted to go further.

Animal sanctuaries have a special place in my heart. Visiting farm animal sanctuaries turns the notion of meat into what meat really is— an animal. These animals have names and personalities and unique, often tragic, stories and circumstances that brought them to a sanctuary. When you meet them, and look into their eyes, you can't help but think of the millions of animals who did not get so lucky. Sanctuaries need volunteers—to feed the animals, scoop poop, take visitors on tours. That is activism. Most sanctuaries are nonprofits and they need financial resources. Write a check, attend a fund-raiser, pass out fliers on the street corner, join a board of directors—it's all activism!

When I'm not in the kitchen creating recipes or blogging about my latest "oops" moment in my vegan journey, I'm actually earning a living. I am a nonprofit and education consultant and one of my clients is PETA. I am a writer and I started a vegan online column for the *Journal News*, in Westchester County, NY. I found ways to merge my profession with my passion. I am also a volunteer; I serve on the board of directors for Our Hen House, a multimedia hive with a mission to effectively mainstream the movement to end the exploitation of animals.

Ginny also finds ways to volunteer beyond the work she does in vegan nutrition. She serves on the board of directors of her local spay/neuter organization and volunteers at her animal shelter.

Every single one of us can help end animal suffering. You don't have to go underground to get a video or start your own farmed animal sanctuary or even sit on the board of directors for an organization. Change for animals comes from all kinds of big and little actions. What do you already know how to do? What are your skills and hobbies? How can you match them with a like-minded organization?

- Hold a vegan bake sale at your children's school.
- Design a brochure for a vegan campus campaign.
- Volunteer at your local animal shelter.
- Rescue a cat, dog, ferret, guinea pig, or rabbit.
- Offer your professional services pro bono to an animal rights nonprofit organization.
- Hand out leaflets on vegan diets at local events or on college campuses.
- Write letters to the editor about animal issues.
- Start a blog to share your vegan recipes with your friends and family.

We all, in our own special way, can be a change agent for animals.

Sometimes I still feel overwhelmed. I realize I cannot live 100 percent vegan. When I am overcome with those feelings I look at a quote hanging over my desk from activist Colleen Patrick Goudreau: "Don't do nothing because you can't do everything. Do something. Anything." My vegan journey is not about perfection. Try as I may to do everything "right," I have made my mistakes—whether eating a veggie burger at a restaurant and learning later it was made with cheese or buying a pair of shoes and discovering a tiny strip of suede on the toe. Do I just give up when I make mistakes? Nope. I learn from them. I ask better questions and through the process I become better informed. I keep going because it really is a journey. A joyful journey.

PART FOUR
Recipes

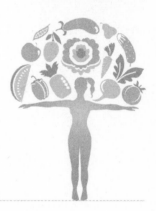

LIST OF RECIPES

RECIPES

By JL Fields

Most of my life I was a comfort-food cook. I grew up in the rural Midwest where we plopped a pot roast in the crockpot with onions, potatoes, carrots, salt, and pepper, and dinner was served. Shortly after getting married I discovered that my husband loved to cook. Thank goodness. I stopped.

A few years into the marriage, I was in Kenya for work. We were in a small village in the Rift Valley. There was a celebration held for an auspicious occasion and my colleagues and I were guests of honor. Early in the day an elder from the community brought a goat to the site of the celebration—a true demonstration of generosity. The goat was presented and subsequently killed, butchered, and cooked throughout the day. That evening we were offered the goat for dinner. I told myself that to refuse it would be an affront. Essentially I met a goat, shook his hand, then I ate him. I became a vegetarian the next day. I phoned my husband with the news—he needed to figure out how to press tofu before I got back to the States.

For eight years my omnivore husband made most of my vegetarian meals. One January I began working with a nutrition counselor to eat healthier. She had me follow a whole foods meal plan for two weeks. During those fourteen days I consumed no dairy and just one hard-boiled egg. Hey, I was practically vegan! I decided to give a plant-based diet a try. About a year into my vegan lifestyle I learned about farm animal sanctuaries. I found the website for Woodstock Farm Animal Sanctuary, clicked through the animal links and was mesmerized by a video of a goat named Clover. I immediately hit the donation button and began sponsoring Clover on a monthly basis. I went vegetarian because of a goat, I went vegan for my health, and I remain vegan for my health, for a goat, for all animals.

In the Kitchen

I wanted to get this vegan thing right so I decided it was time to learn to cook. First I turned to vegan cookbooks such as *Veganomicon, Vive le Vegan! Color Me Vegan, The 30-Minute Vegan, Christina Cooks,* and *Great Vegetarian Cooking Under Pressure.* Then I was ready to create, dive in, and explore. I signed up for public education courses at culinary institutes—such as Natural Gourmet Institute and the Christine Pirello School of Integrative Health and, though not classically trained, I got it. I got how to turn a plant into something delicious, to turn a grain into the star of a multifaceted meal.

Like you, I am pretty busy and though I now love to cook, I don't want to spend every waking hour in the kitchen. I've found that you can make tasty, healthy meals in no time—sometimes with some advance planning. The recipes are based on the nutrition advice you've been reading throughout this book—these recipes show you how to take all that theory and put it into delicious practice in your own kitchen.

Eat for Life

As you adopt a plant-based way of eating, you'll find what works best for your lifestyle and kitchen. Myself, I am a typical beans, greens, and grains vegan—those three foods play a central role in every meal. I also try to have something raw each time I dine. For instance, I love eating bowl meals: I'll start with a hot grain in a bowl—brown rice, quinoa, farro, or pearled barley—before adding cooked beans and then topping it off with a raw green, such as arugula.

You'll discover what works best for you—maybe you'll find that green smoothies are great for breakfast, or you'd rather have toast with mashed avocado. I've found that eating a lot of large salads as meals with a hearty nut-based dressing is a terrific way to get greens and protein. You'll find a lot of salad recipes, as well as creamy dressings that can accompany your favorite veggies or be used as dips or spreads.

As noted throughout the book, fat certainly isn't an enemy—and you'll find lots of good fats in these recipes. Most of the recipes call for extra-virgin olive oil (I use cold-pressed); however you will see avocado oil in several. You can use extra-virgin olive oil in place of avocado oil but I do love that avocado oil has a high smoke point (particularly when refined) and is high in monounsaturated fat. I find that the rich, creamy—I'll even say buttery—flavor adds a little something special to cooking and baking.

My recipes are easy to prepare, healthy, and satisfying—but by no means are they set in stone. Christina Pirello taught me the art of intuitive cooking—to cook with seasonal foods, to use a variety of cooking (and raw) preparation methods, and to trust your instincts— and I encourage you to do the same. You may want to substitute quinoa for millet or almonds for cashews. Feel free to experiment— there is so much variety and flexibility in a vegan diet that you can truly make it your own.

REAL-WORLD COOKING TIPS

To put it bluntly, I am not a fancy cook. But I do make flavorful, healthy dishes that I am sure you will enjoy. Most of my recipes can be made in no time (though sometimes I'll spend a few hours in the kitchen on Sundays to make big batches of meals so that I do not have to cook during the week). You'll find plenty of time-savers in these recipes; when I'm in the kitchen, I use shortcuts, namely a pressure cooker, a rice cooker, and a few other appliances. If you don't have these appliances, not to worry: you can still make the recipes but, pardon me for a moment, while I try to convince you to consider using a few.

The Pressure Cooker

This nifty appliance helps you make beans and grains in minutes. Sure you can buy canned beans or instant rice, but once you realize how quickly you can prepare home-cooked beans and grains, I don't think you'll want to. How fast?

- Quinoa: 1 minute
- Bulgur: 5 minutes
- Pearled barley: 18 minutes
- Brown lentils: 8 minutes
- Black-eyed peas: 10 minutes
- Adzuki beans: 14 to 20 minutes
- Navy beans: 16 to 20 minutes
- Red kidney beans: 20 minutes

You can also save money: One 15-ounce can of beans is about 1½ cups that, if organic, can cost $2 or more. A 16-ounce package of dry, organic beans, which will cost between $3 and $3.50, will make 7½ cups of cooked beans. Your home-cooked 1½ cups of beans costs .64 cents; you save nearly $1.30.

The pressure cooker is great for one-pot meals: stews, soups, and more. For an easy, healthy, filling dinner, I will heat onions and garlic in a little olive oil in the pressure cooker and then mix and match vegetables and beans. Another quick and filling meal is based around cubed or small potatoes, which cook up in 6 minutes in the pressure cooker. I cook the potatoes with packaged seitan or tofu, carrots and celery, maybe a diced tomato or two, and enough vegetable broth to cover everything. Six minutes under pressure and I am enjoying a hearty stew with a raw salad or sautéed greens.

For those of you with pressure cookers, you're in luck! Many of these recipes offer pressure cooker instructions. For those who I have yet to convert, those same recipes offer stove top instructions.

The Rice Cooker

While a rice cooker may not speed up your cooking process, it will absolutely make it easier. Electric rice cookers on the market today have a variety of settings (white, sushi, brown, porridge), and some can even be set for an auto start. I prepare oatmeal in the rice cooker in the evening, set the auto start for about 30 minutes before I plan to get up, and awaken to the smell of a home-cooked, hot breakfast! Oatmeal? That's right! In addition to rice you can make oats and other grains, as well as beans and vegetables. I see my rice cooker as a fast crockpot—toss the ingredients into the rice cooker and open it when it's done.

Other Kitchen Tools

I have made a point to provide recipes in this book that do not require a high-speed blender. I do think a standard blender is a great tool for vegans because you can make smoothies, as well as dips, dressing, hot and cold soups, and sauces (you can use an immersion blender for the last two). I find that a food processor can work just as well and you'll note that I use blenders and food processors interchangeably in the recipes.

Otherwise, you don't need anything special for these recipes. I use standard skillets, saucepans, and baking dishes.

Vegan Pantry Staples

You may find some ingredients in these recipes that are new to you; here is a list, along with some of my pantry staples:

Adzuki beans: Also spelled azuki or aduki, these tiny red beans are popular in Asian cooking.

Black salt: Also called kala namak, this salt is mined from the Himalayan region. And it's actually pink in color, not black. It has an aroma and flavor that is remarkably similar to hard-boiled eggs.

Bragg Liquid Aminos: A condiment. I use Bragg Liquid Aminos as an alternative way to salt vegetables and salads and often use it when recipes call for soy sauce.

Chia, hemp, and flaxseeds: Tiny seeds that can absorb liquid and help thicken dishes. All three are good sources of the omega-3 fat ALA.

Coconut aminos: This gluten-free source of aminos is a raw alternative to Bragg Liquid Aminos.

Garbanzo flour: Made from dried chickpeas, you'll also see this called *besan*.

Goji berries: Orange-red berries that are native to China. They are rich in vitamin A and antioxidants. Great in oatmeal, cookies, smoothies, and salad dressings.

Marmite: A thick, yeast-based spread. It's a very salty condiment so a little goes a long way. This is an umami-rich food.

Miso: This salty, fermented soybean paste captures the essence of Japanese cooking. It comes in different colors—white, red, and yellow—and some are somewhat more sweet than others. It's used extensively in vegan broths, soups, and sauces.

Nutritional yeast: A flaked or powdered condiment, this yeast is grown on a nutrient-rich medium. It gives foods a cheesy flavor. Look for Red Star brand Vegetarian Support Formula, because that's the type that provides vitamin B_{12}.

Plant milks: You'll find milk made from rice, almonds, soybeans, hempseed, and coconut in the refrigerated section of stores and also packaged aseptically. These are usually interchangeable in recipes. Look for brands that are fortified with calcium and vitamin D. (Note: don't confuse coconut milk sold as a beverage with coconut milk sold in cans. The latter is used in cooking, especially for curried dishes. It's much higher in fat and calories than the type sold as a beverage.)

Sea vegetables: Often referred to as seaweed, since they grow wild in the ocean. These vegetables, which include nori, kombu, dulse, arame, and kelp, play a big role in Japanese cooking. They are usually sold dried and then can be added to soups or used to make vegetarian sushi. All add umami to dishes.

Soy curls: They are made by Butler Foods from textured whole soybeans. Soy curls need to be rehydrated before cooking. Find them at local natural food stores or online at VeganEssentials.

Sriracha hot sauce: Not just any hot sauce, this is the bottle with a rooster that you have probably seen on the table at your favorite Chinese restaurant. It is my hot sauce of choice.

Syrup: I often use agave, maple, date, or brown rice syrup as an alternative to sugar.

Tempeh: An ancient food from Indonesia, this cake of fermented soybeans has a tender and chewy texture and a savory flavor sometimes described as "yeasty" or "mushroomlike." Tempeh can be made from soybeans only or soybeans in combination with grains.

Tofu: Made in the same way that cheese is made from cow's milk, tofu is produced by adding a curdling agent to soymilk. Throughout Asia tofu is made fresh daily from soybeans in small shops and sold on the street by vendors. If you are stir-frying chunks of tofu with veggies to serve over rice, choose firm tofu. Soft tofu is perfect to mash or puree as a filling for sandwiches or lasagna. And the tofu that is traditional to Japanese cooking, silken tofu, is a soft, custard-like food that can be blended or pureed for sauces, smoothies, or desserts. It makes a great replacement for the cream in creamed soup recipes. Frozen tofu takes on a chewy, spongy texture that makes it a useful meat substitute. Freeze it right in the unopened package. Then defrost, squeeze out the liquid and chop or shred it. Several recipes call for pressed and drained tofu. You can do this by using a tofu press or simply be wrapping the tofu in fresh or paper towels, placing in a bowl, and setting a pan or heavy cookbook on the tofu to press out the liquid.

TVP (texturized vegetable protein): This fun soyfood is easy to use—you simply rehydrate the dry TVP granules with water or vegetable broth, and they absorb the flavors in your dish. The texture is perfect for making vegan "meatballs" or burgers or as "meat" in chili.

Umeboshi: Japanese pickled plums used as a condiment.

Ume Plum Vinegar: The pickling brine from umeboshi. Both are high in umami.

Vegan margarine/vegan "butter": There are a number of vegan butters on the market, but the vegan world was rocked when Bryanna Clark Grogan developed a homemade vegan "butter" recipe (http://vegan.com/recipes/bryanna-clark-grogan/bryannas-vegan-butter/). I make it and find the recipe simple, delicious, and compassionate to all animals.

Vegan mayonnaise: Eggless mayonnaise products include Vegenaise (Follow Your Heart), Nayonaise (Nasoya), and Mindful Mayo (Earth Balance). All are great vegan alternatives to egg-based mayonnaise.

Vital wheat gluten: Wheat protein, used in bread baking to add extra gluten, which helps whole-grain bread loaves to rise well (and it makes a nice crust). It's also the key ingredient in making quick seitan recipes.

Whole grains: I cook with a variety of these foods including brown rice and barley, as well as grains that may be new to you, such as quinoa, farro, amaranth, millet, and kasha. Look for them in the bulk food section of natural food stores.

GET COOKING!

As you go through the recipes remember that I am not a chef. I am just like you. I want to prepare healthy, nutritious, and delicious vegan foods as quickly and easily as possible. The recipes I provide support Ginny's sound nutritional advice for women across the life span. I hope you find the recipes as accessible as I intend them to be.

BREAKFAST

"ICE CREAM" FOR BREAKFAST

This is a quick and filling breakfast that also makes for a great dessert. If mangoes aren't to your liking, any frozen fruit will do.

½ cup cashews
½ cup frozen mango chunks (or your favorite fruit from the frozen food aisle)
Half a frozen banana, cut into chunks
¼ cup uncooked, rolled oats

Place all ingredients in a food processor (use the S blade).
Pulse, scraping down the side of the bowl as necessary, to an ice cream consistency.

YIELD: 2 SERVINGS

COCONUT-MANGO-AVOCADO SMOOTHIE

Kick-start your day with this rich, healthy smoothie or enjoy it anytime as a hearty snack. The avocado adds a lush creaminess and the hemp seeds provide omega-3 fats. For an alternative to mango try papaya, peach, cantaloupe, or banana.

2 cups coconut water (fresh, from 2 young Thai coconuts, or bottled)
2 tablespoons hemp seeds
½ cup frozen mango
Half an avocado
1 medjool date
½ cup ice

    Blend all ingredients.

YIELD: 2 SERVINGS

SILKY STRAWBERRY SMOOTHIE

Get your isoflavones here! Tofu not only adds protein, it gives this smoothie a great creaminess. No strawberries on hand? Try other berries or stone fruits. Add spinach or kale to make a green smoothie!

½ cup silken tofu
1 cup fresh strawberries
1 banana
1 cup ice
1 teaspoon agave syrup (optional)

    Blend all ingredients.

YIELD: 2 SERVINGS

OAT-AMARANTH-CARROT PORRIDGE

I studied macrobiotic cooking in an intensive program with Christina Pirello and discovered the joy of less "conventional" breakfast meals, ranging from miso soup to braised root vegetables to this hearty porridge. Porridge is so easy to make in your rice cooker; stove top instructions are provided, as well.

2 tablespoons vegan butter
¼ cup yellow onion, diced
2 carrots, diced
2½ cups water
1 cup amaranth
1 cup rolled oats
1 teaspoon iodized sea salt
½ teaspoon cinnamon

RICE COOKER INSTRUCTIONS:

Add all ingredients to your rice cooker and select the porridge cycle.

Serve with a dab of vegan butter and a sprinkle of cinnamon and sea salt to taste.

STOVE TOP INSTRUCTIONS:

Sauté the vegan butter, onion, and carrots in a large saucepan for 3 to 5 minutes.

Add water and amaranth.

Bring to a boil.

Reduce to simmer for 10 minutes.

Add the rolled oats and bring back to a gentle boil.

Reduce heat and simmer for 10 to 15 minutes.

Stir in salt and cinnamon before serving.

YIELD: 4 SERVINGS

CREAMY VEGETABLE
BREAKFAST CASSEROLE

With its wealth of veggies, this dish does double duty as comfort food that is also good for you—providing lots of calcium from the kale and tofu. It is also great to serve for brunch.

1 tablespoon extra-virgin olive oil
1 small yellow onion, diced
3 cloves of garlic, minced
3 stalks of celery, diced
3 carrots, diced
1 small green pepper, diced
4 cups of kale, torn into small pieces
¼ teaspoon thyme
¼ teaspoon saffron threads
¼ teaspoon dried sweet basil
Salt
1 package extra-firm tofu
¼ cup almond milk
Ground black pepper (optional)
1 cup shredded vegan cheddar cheese
1 cup quartered cherry tomatoes

Preheat the oven to 375°F. Lightly grease a baking dish with olive oil.

Sauté the first eleven ingredients in a large skillet for about 8 minutes.

Blend the tofu, almond milk, and pepper to a thick, creamy consistency (about 20 seconds in a high-speed blender).

In a large bowl mix the blended tofu and cooked veggies. Fold in the cheddar cheese and ¾ cup of the quartered cherry tomatoes and pour into a casserole dish.

Spread the remaining cherry tomatoes over the top. Add ground black pepper, if desired.

Bake for 35 to 40 minutes.

YIELD: 8 SERVINGS

SALADS, SIDES, AND DIPS

CHOPPED SALAD WITH CREAMY CHIPOTLE DRESSING

This salad has it all: greens, beans, and rich, smoky dressing. For the corn, I steam two ears of fresh corn, run them under cold water, then cut off the kernels. Canned or frozen and thawed corn will also work.

For the salad:

3 cups chopped romaine lettuce
1 cup red kidney beans (home-cooked or canned), rinsed and drained

1 cup corn
1 cup diced cucumber
2 pinches salt
Ground black pepper

For the dressing:
¼ cup cashews (raw, unsalted)
¼ teaspoon ground chipotle powder
2 tablespoons red wine vinegar
¼ cup water

Toss all salad ingredients in a large mixing bowl.
Blend all dressing ingredients in a blender or food processor.
Pour the dressing on the salad, toss, and serve with fresh ground pepper.

YIELD: 1 ENTREE SALAD OR 2 SIDE SALADS

 # CUCUMBER AND QUINOA SALAD

Many of us grew up eating sliced cucumbers and onions as a dinner side dish on hot summer evenings. This recipe is a twist on that old favorite. The addition of quinoa—a gluten-free, protein-rich whole grain—turns a familiar small vegetable side salad into a hearty and delicious vegetarian entree! Serve as side dish or over raw greens for a hearty salad entree.

For the salad:
1½ cups quinoa, rinsed and drained
2¼ cups water
½ teaspoon salt
1½–2 cups, cut into half-moons, bunching and cipollini onions
2 cups diced cucumber (I like to leave the peels on)
1 tablespoon chopped fresh dill

For the dressing:

⅓ cup white wine vinegar

2 tablespoons extra-virgin olive oil

1 ½ teaspoons vegan sugar (I use Florida Crystals pure
   cane sugar)

Iodized sea salt and ground black pepper

   Bring quinoa, water, and salt to a boil in a saucepan, cover
the pan, reduce the heat, and simmer for 15 minutes. When the
quinoa is finished cooking, fluff it with a fork. Transfer it to a large
mixing bowl and set it aside.

   Dry-sauté the onions with a pinch of salt over medium heat (or
use extra-virgin olive oil pan spray) until they are golden around
the edges.

   For the dressing, whisk the vinegar, oil, and sugar with a fork
in a small bowl.

   To assemble, add cucumber, onions, and dill to the quinoa
and lightly toss in the large mixing bowl. Drizzle the dressing
over the quinoa and toss gently. Salt and pepper to taste.

   Chill in the refrigerator for at least two hours before serving,
but this salad is even better the next day so plan ahead to chill
overnight! Garnish with dill and serve.

YIELD: 6 SIDE SERVINGS OR 3 TO 4 ENTREE SERVINGS

 # NUTTY QUINOA AND CHERRY SALAD

I made this dish for Christmas. The nonvegan guests enjoyed it as
a side dish and it served as my entree. You can use a variety of
dried fruits (try cranberries). You can easily turn this into an even
heartier salad by adding black beans.

1 cup dried cherries

1 cup quinoa, rinsed and drained

2 cups water

A pinch of salt

1 teaspoon extra-virgin olive oil
¼ cup fresh lemon juice (about 1½ lemons)
½ cup chopped pecans
Sea salt

Rehydrate the cherries by soaking them in water for 30 minutes. Rinse and drain.

Bring the quinoa, water, and salt to a boil in a saucepan, cover the pan, reduce the heat, and simmer for 15 minutes. When the quinoa is finished cooking, fluff it with a fork. Let it cool and refrigerate it for at least two hours.

Mix the quinoa with the olive oil and lemon juice. Toss with the cherries and pecans and add salt to desired taste.

YIELD: 8 SIDE SERVINGS OR 4 ENTREE SERVINGS

APPLE SLAW WITH GOJI BERRY DRESSING

The blend of goji berries with apples and carrots makes a distinct slaw that's sure to impress.

For the salad:
1 large apple, cored and quartered (no need to peel)
2 large carrots
1 large stalk of celery
3 curly kale leaves (with stems)

For the dressing:
1 tablespoon avocado oil (or extra-virgin olive oil)
2 tablespoons apple cider vinegar
1 teaspoon whole-grain mustard
¼ cup water
1 clove garlic

¼ cup dried goji berries (or other dried, unsulfured fruit, such
  as raisins, currants, cranberries, or mulberries)
Ground black pepper

  Shred the apple, carrots, celery, and kale in a food processor
(use the slicing blade) or on a mandoline slicer.
  Transfer the shredded apple mixture to a large bowl.
  Blend all dressing ingredients in a blender or food processor.
  Pour the dressing over the shredded apple mixture and toss.
  Store in an airtight container and refrigerate for at least 30
minutes.

YIELD: 4 SERVINGS

VEGAN SEVEN LAYER SALAD

Many of us grew up with the thick, multilayered salad full of meat
and dairy. Here is a vegan version that is both hearty and light—
the best kind of comfort food.

1 5-ounce package vegan bacon
2½ cups chopped iceberg lettuce
¼ cup diced red onion
½ cup chopped celery
2 cups frozen peas, thawed (lightly salted, optional)
¾–1 cup vegan mayonnaise (enough to cover the salad)
Shredded vegan cheese (enough to sprinkle over the top of
  the salad)
Ground black pepper (optional)

  Prepare the vegan bacon according to package instructions,
crumble, and set aside.
  Layer lettuce, onions, celery, and peas, in this order, in a large
bowl (a glass bowl offers a great presentation).

Spread vegan mayonnaise over the peas, just enough to cover them.

Add a layer of shredded vegan cheese and add pepper to taste.

When ready to serve, add the final layer, the crumbled vegan bacon.

YIELD: 6 TO 8 SERVINGS

Note: Even though a seven layer salad looks cool, I tend to toss it together before serving.

ADZUKI BEAN POTATO SALAD

This dish is rich with umami foods, including kombu, ume plum vinegar, and potatoes. This stick-to-your-ribs meal just might please everyone in your multivore household.

1 medium red potato
2 carrots
2 scallions
2½ cups adzuki beans (home-cooked or canned)
1 teaspoon white miso
2 tablespoons vegan mayonnaise
¼ cup diced green pepper
2 tablespoons fresh lime juice

Steam the potato (no need to peel) in a microwave and dice once cool. If preparing on the stove top, dice first, then steam in a pan of water using a steamer insert, for 20 minutes.

Shred the carrots and scallions in a food processor or chop by hand.

Mix all the ingredients in a large bowl and refrigerate for at least two hours before serving.

YIELD: 4 TO 6 SERVINGS

CREAMY STRAWBERRY
SALAD DRESSING

This dressing is great with any greens—I especially like it drizzled over steamed asparagus or on a spinach salad. You can also use it as a sauce or dip for raw veggies or toasted pita.

1 cup raw, unsalted cashews
1 cup stemmed and quartered strawberries
2 tablespoons rice vinegar
Water (about ¼ cup)

Add first three ingredients to a blender or food processor (if using a food processor, you may want to soak the cashews for 15 to 45 minutes).
Add water, as needed, and blend to desired consistency.
Serve over a salad or over lightly steamed vegetables.

YIELD: 2 TO 4 SERVINGS

SESAME TAHINI DRESSING

This dressing is fantastic on salads but also serves as a great sauce on cooked vegetables and vegan burgers.

½ cup sesame tahini
Juice of 1 lemon
2 teaspoons vegan mayonnaise
1½ tablespoons sesame oil
¼ teaspoon garlic powder
¼ teaspoon onion salt
⅛ cup water

Simply mix all the ingredients in a bowl or in a blender. You can increase or decrease the amount of water for a thinner dressing or a thicker sauce. Cook's choice!

YIELD: 1 CUP

CASHEW-ALMOND-ORANGE DRESSING

This nut-based dressing gets a citrus kick from fresh orange juice. Not just for salads, this dressing makes a great chip or vegetable dip.

¼ cup raw, unsalted cashews
¼ cup raw, unsalted almonds
2–3 tablespoons sesame seeds
1 small clove garlic, quartered
¼ cup fresh orange juice
½ teaspoon agave syrup (optional)
⅛–¼ cup water
Iodized sea salt (optional)

Soak cashews and almonds in room-temperature water for 20 minutes.

Begin blending the cashews, almonds, sesame seeds, garlic, orange juice, and optional agave syrup in a blender or food processor.

Add water as needed to achieve a creamy salad dressing consistency.

Taste before adding salt.

YIELD: 1 CUP

TANGY TOMATO DRESSING

Tomatoes plus jalapeño peppers provide lots of vitamin C to enhance absorption of iron from iron-rich greens like spinach. For a vegan slaw toss with shredded cabbage and carrots.

½ cup cashews
1 medium tomato, diced
½ jalapeño, diced
¼ cup diced red onion
1 clove garlic, finely diced
1 lemon, peeled and quartered
1 teaspoon coconut aminos (raw) or Bragg Liquid Aminos (or soy sauce)
¼ cup water (for desired consistency)
Salt

Place all ingredients in a blender or food processor and blend to a desired consistency.

YIELD: 2 CUPS

CHEESY DRESSING
WITH CASHEWS AND CAPERS

While I call this recipe a dressing, it's quite thick and I like to use it as a vegetable dip. If you prefer a thinner dressing simply use more lemon juice or water.

1 cup raw, unsalted cashews
½ cup fresh lemon juice
½ cup chopped onion

¼ cup capers
1½ cups coarsely chopped red tomato
2 tablespoons nutritional yeast (I prefer the powder form of
  nutritional yeast, versus flakes, in this recipe)
1 cup coarsely chopped yellow pepper
½ teaspoon iodized sea salt (optional)

Blend all ingredients in a blender or food processor to a
desired consistency.

YIELD: 2½ CUPS

BRAZIL NUT AND ALMOND PÂTÉ

This is a great spread for vegetables, crackers, or sandwiches, and
Brazil nuts are a good source of the mineral selenium for vegans.
Try spreading this flavorful pâté on a large collard green, roll it up,
and eat as a sandwich wrap.

½ cup Brazil nuts
¼ cup chopped raw, unsalted almonds
¼ cup chopped red onion
1 clove garlic
Juice of half a lemon
1 teaspoon coconut aminos (raw) or Bragg Liquid Aminos

Soak Brazil nuts in room-temperature water for 20 minutes;
rinse and drain.
Add the Brazil nuts along with all the other ingredients to a
food processor and pulse to a spreadable consistency.

YIELD: 1 CUP

RED HUMMUS

This bean dip is a twist on a traditional chickpea hummus. Serve on crackers and as a dip for raw vegetables, or spread it on a whole wheat wrap and add your favorite toppings to enjoy as a sandwich.

2 cups red kidney beans (home-cooked or canned)
½ cup sundried tomatoes, soaked for 1 hour and drained
  (or oil-packed sundried tomatoes, no soaking required)
1 jalapeño, seeded and diced
1–2 cloves garlic, finely diced (garlic fans, use 3 cloves)
Juice of half a lime
½ teaspoon taco seasoning
¼ cup extra-virgin olive oil (or soak water from the sundried
  tomatoes)
½ teaspoon iodized sea salt

Place all the ingredients, except the olive oil and sea salt, in the food processor, (use the S blade).

Begin pulsing the ingredients; add olive oil or soak water from the top until you reach desired consistency. You may find you need a bit more oil or water, especially if you like it to be a thinner consistency.

Salt to taste.

YIELD: 2 CUPS

CURRY CASHEW BUTTER

Nut butters are all the rage—and they are so simple to make from scratch: put nuts in a food processor and blend for 12 minutes—scraping down the sides at 6 minutes. That's it. The surprise ingredient curry offers an extra kick. This is great on celery but consider making a nontraditional peanut butter and jelly sandwich by using this nut butter with chutney.

1½ cups raw, unsalted cashews
¼ teaspoon pink Himalayan salt
½ teaspoon curry powder
½ teaspoon coconut oil
½ teaspoon extra-virgin olive oil

Soak cashews in water for at least 20 minutes. Rinse and drain.

Place cashews in a food processor, using the S blade, and process for 6 minutes.

At 6 minutes, scrape down the sides, add the remaining ingredients, and process for another 6 minutes.

Add additional coconut oil if the nut butter appears too dry.

YIELD: 1½ CUPS

 # GARLIC ALMOND COLLARDS

Collard greens plus almonds make this dish an easy and delicious way to boost your calcium intake.

1 large bunch collard greens, washed and dried (use a salad
   spinner or pat with a paper towel)
1 teaspoon extra-virgin olive oil
3 (or 4!) cloves of garlic, minced
1 teaspoon Bragg Liquid Aminos (or a couple pinches of
   sea salt)
Slivered almonds (about ¼ cup)

To prepare the collard greens, remove the center stem by slicing along either side of the stem with your knife, cutting the leaf in half while removing the stem. Then cut the leaves into ¼-inch strips.

Heat the olive oil on medium-high heat in a large skillet. Add the garlic and quickly sauté for a few minutes.

Add the collard greens and a bit of Bragg Liquid Aminos to taste. Stir and cover.

Reduce the heat to low, keeping the skillet covered. Keep an eye on the collard greens—they will wilt down perfectly in just a few minutes.

Remove the cover and stir in the almond slivers.

YIELD: 6 SERVINGS

VARIATION: Substitute kale, Swiss chard, or cabbage for the collard greens.

KALE-CABBAGE-LEEK GRILL MIX

I never really considered grilling vegetables, other than kabobs, until I went vegan. I haven't met a vegetable I'm not willing to put onto the grill now! This is one vegetable mix that I happen to love—have fun with it and grill your favorite greens!

3 kale leaves, removed from stems and chopped
1 cup chopped cabbage
1 leek, sliced (soak the leek before slicing to remove all dirt and sand, and remove the dark green parts before slicing the tender, white part of the leek)
1 teaspoon sesame oil
Pinch of sea salt
1 teaspoon Sriracha or other hot sauce (optional)

Rinse and drain the first three ingredients and place them in a large bowl.

Drizzle with oil and add sea salt.

Massage the oil and salt into the vegetables with your hands.

Add the Sriracha and toss.

Grill for 8 minutes on an indoor/outdoor grill (such as a George Foreman) or a grill skillet on the stove. You can also make this on a gas or charcoal grill by simply wrapping the vegetables in foil and placing on the grill for 12 to 15 minutes.

YIELD: 2 SERVINGS

MEDITERRANEAN BEANS
WITH GREENS

Beans, tomatoes, greens, and a dash of extra-virgin olive oil make this the perfect healthy Mediterranean meal. I think you will enjoy the simplicity of the preparation and the intensity of flavor in this recipe, which has become a dinner staple in my house.

1 (14.5-ounce) can diced tomatoes, seasoned with basil,
  garlic, and oregano
1 (15-ounce) can cannellini beans, rinsed and drained
⅛ cup diced green olives
¼–½ cup vegetable broth
1 teaspoon extra-virgin olive oil
2 cloves garlic, finely diced
4 cups loosely packed arugula (5 ounces)
¼ cup fresh lemon juice
1–2 olives, sliced (for garnish)

In a saucepan bring the tomatoes, beans, olives, and broth to a boil.

Reduce the heat and simmer for about 5 minutes.

In a skillet, heat the extra-virgin olive oil on medium-high heat. Add the garlic and sauté until the garlic begins to brown.

Add the arugula and lemon juice. Stir, cover, and reduce the heat to low. Simmer for 3 to 5 minutes.

Serve beans over the greens and garnish with olive slices.

YIELD: 2 SERVINGS

SOUPS AND CHILI

CHIK'N LENTIL NOODLE SOUP

This soup is a reader favorite on my blog. I suspect because it is reminiscent of a childhood favorite for many of us—and because it's incredibly easy to prepare and delicious! The "chicken" flavoring is simply seasoning. I use Butler Chik-Style seasoning, though your favorite brand should do just fine. This is rich in protein and packed with healthy vegetables.

1 teaspoon extra-virgin olive oil
3 cloves garlic, finely diced
1 large onion, diced
2 cups bite-size pieces green beans (fresh or frozen)
1 cup chopped carrots
1 cup chopped celery
2 teaspoons vegan chicken-style seasoning
1 bay leaf
½ teaspoon dried sage
1 cup brown lentils, rinsed and drained
4 ounces soba noodles
4 cups vegetable broth (I used a vegan chicken-style broth)

PRESSURE COOKER INSTRUCTIONS:

Heat the olive oil on medium-high heat in an uncovered pressure cooker.

Sauté the garlic, onion, green beans, carrots, and celery for about 3 minutes.

Add the vegan chicken-style seasoning, bay leaf, and sage.

Add the lentils, noodles, and vegetable broth to the pressure cooker.

Cover the pressure cooker, locking the lid in place.

Bring to pressure, then reduce the heat low enough to maintain pressure (a gentle rocking motion of the jiggly top) for 8 minutes.

After 8 minutes, remove the pressure cooker from the heat and release the pressure with the quick-release method (still covered, hold the pressure cooker under cold running water).

Once the pressure is released, remove the lid, away from you.

Sample both the lentils and the noodles. If not quite done enough, simmer, on low, in the uncovered pressure cooker.

SOUP POT INSTRUCTIONS:

Heat the olive oil on medium-high heat in a soup pot.

Sauté the garlic, onion, green beans, carrots, and celery for about 3 minutes.

Add the vegan chicken-style seasoning, bay leaf, and sage.

Add the lentils and broth to the pot and bring to a boil.

Reduce the heat to medium-low and cook for 15 minutes.

Increase the heat to medium-high, to a light boil, and add the soba noodles.

Cook for 3 to 4 minutes, then taste noodles for doneness.

Reduce heat to medium-low and cook for 10 to 12 minutes.

YIELD: 4 SERVINGS

CREAMY KALE MISO SOUP

With just six ingredients, a saucepan, and a blender you will be enjoying a delicious, super-healthy soup in 20 minutes! Be sure to use a low-sodium vegetable broth, since the miso has a very salty flavor.

32-ounces (4 cups) low-sodium vegetable broth (low-sodium is
  very important!)
1 cup coarsely diced yellow onion
1 tablespoon coarsely chopped fresh garlic
1 (14-ounce) package soft (not silken) tofu, pressed and drained
4 cups loosely packed kale (curly and red Russian kale are
  great in this soup)
¼ cup yellow miso
Pieces of raw kale, chopped, for garnish

Bring the vegetable stock, onions, and garlic to a boil in a
large saucepan.
    Cube the pressed tofu, add it to the saucepan, and bring the
mixture back to a boil.
    Add the kale (torn into large pieces), stir, cover, and simmer
on low for 5 minutes.
    Remove the saucepan from the heat and stir in the miso—it's
okay if it doesn't all dissolve because you will soon be blending it.
    Transfer the soup from the saucepan to a blender, cover tightly,
and blend for 30 seconds to a minute, 3 cups at a time (or to the
half-full point of your particular blender). If you have an immersion blender, blend in the pot (cover with a dishtowel to prevent
hot splatters).
    Spoon into a bowl and garnish with a few pieces of raw kale.

YIELD: 6 SERVINGS

**NOTE: *Never fill a blender more than half full with hot li-
quid, as the liquid expands. As an added precaution, place a
towel over the top of the blender when using hot liquids.***

 ## CREAMY SQUASH AND APPLE SOUP

Great any time of year, this soup is particularly pleasing during the
fall—or whenever butternut squash is in season where you live.
Granny Smith or Honey Crisp apples are a terrific pairing with the
squash. Use fortified almond milk for a calcium-rich soup.

1 cup water

½ teaspoon sea salt

1 (2-pound) butternut squash, peeled and diced (about 20 ounces)

2 apples, cored, quartered, and diced

½ teaspoon ground cinnamon

½ teaspoon nutmeg

2 cups almond milk

PRESSURE COOKER INSTRUCTIONS:

Add water and salt to the pressure cooker and place a vegetable tray in the bottom.

Bring the water to a boil (uncovered).

Add squash, apples, and spices.

Cover and bring to pressure.

Cook at pressure for 3 minutes.

Use the quick-release method (still covered, hold the pressure cooker under cold running water). Once pressure is released, remove the lid, away from you.

STOVE TOP INSTRUCTIONS:

Add the water and salt to a large saucepan or soup pot.

Bring the water to a boil.

Add the squash, apples, and spices. If not covered, add more water.

Bring to a boil.

Cover, turn the heat down to a simmer, and cook for 30 minutes or until squash and apples soften.

TO PUREE (STOVE TOP AND PRESSURE COOKER):

Transfer cooked squash and apple to a blender or food processor (or use an immersion blender in the pot).

Add almond milk.

Blend to a puree (see note).

Serve with a dash of cinnamon.

YIELD: 2 TO 4 SERVINGS

> NOTE: *Never fill a blender more than half full with hot liquid as it expands. As an added precaution, place a towel over the top of the blender when using hot liquids. Similarly, if you are using an immersion blender, be sure to cover the pot with a dishtowel.*

EASY TOFU PUMPKIN SOUP

I make this in a measuring cup. Seriously. If you have a microwave, this single-serving soup is super-easy and delicious. Making it on the stove top requires slightly more time—with all of the flavor intact.

2 cups firmly packed chopped kale
¼ cup canned pumpkin
3 ounces extra-firm tofu, pressed, drained, and diced
¼ red pepper, diced
½ teaspoon Bragg Liquid Aminos
Pinch of hot curry powder
2 tablespoons cooked quinoa
1 cup vegetable broth

Steam the kale in a covered, microwave-safe dish, with a splash of water, for 1 minute in the microwave.
Place all the ingredients in a 2-cup measuring cup.
Cover with a piece of wax paper and microwave for 3 minutes. Stir and serve.

YIELD: 1 SERVING

VARIATION: If you would prefer to make this soup on the stove, simply steam the kale in a covered saucepan for one minute, add the remaining ingredients, bring to a boil and serve immediately.

PORTOBELLO MUSHROOM AND BARLEY SOUP

Soups are one of my very favorite hearty vegan meals. Adding a grain makes all the difference. Here, I've used barley, a great source of "slow carbs." You can make this soup using a pressure cooker or a soup pot.

1 teaspoon avocado or extra-virgin olive oil (you can
  substitute water or vegetable broth for the oil)
2 cloves garlic, minced
½ cup yellow diced onion
3 celery stalks, diced
2 carrots, diced
2 large portobello mushrooms (6 ounces), julienned and then
  chopped
1 tomato, diced
¾ cup pearled barley (dry), rinsed and drained
3 cups vegetable stock
4 cups water
2 thyme sprigs
Iodized sea salt and ground black pepper, to taste

PRESSURE COOKER INSTRUCTIONS:
  Heat the oil (or water/vegetable broth) in an uncovered pressure cooker.
  Add the garlic and onions and sauté for a few minutes.
  Add the celery and carrots and sauté for 3 to 5 minutes.
  Stir in the mushrooms, tomato, barley, stock, water, and thyme.
  Cover and bring to pressure.
  Cook at pressure for 20 minutes.
  Remove from the heat and allow the pressure to release naturally.
  Salt and pepper to taste.

STOVE TOP INSTRUCTIONS:
  Heat oil in a large pot.
  Add the garlic and onions and sauté for a few minutes.
  Add the celery and carrots and sauté for 3 to 5 minutes.
  Add the water and stock and bring to a boil.
  Add the mushrooms, tomato, barley, and thyme to the boiling water/stock and stir together.
  Cover the pot with a lid and reduce the heat to low for 35 to 40 minutes.
  Sea salt and pepper to taste.

YIELD: 6 TO 8 SERVINGS

ASIAN CROCKPOT CHILI

The Japanese adzuki bean (also known as aduki or azuki) cooks up quickly, without presoaking, in the crockpot, but you can also create this quickly on the stove if you prepare the beans ahead of time (see directions). These little red beans are especially rich in potassium, a mineral that can fall short in all kinds of diets.

2 tablespoons extra-virgin olive oil
1 cup vegetable broth (optional)
4 cups water (or 5 cups if you do not use the vegetable broth)
1 (15-ounce) can fire roasted diced tomatoes
2 tablespoons tomato paste
2 cloves garlic, finely chopped
2 carrots, diced
1 small onion, diced
1½ cups dried adzuki beans (rinsed and drained, no need
  to soak)
½ teaspoon Herbamere (or sea salt)
2 teaspoons Sriracha (or other red hot sauce)
1 tablespoon Bragg Liquid Aminos (or low-sodium soy sauce)
½ teaspoon dulse flakes (optional, but recommended!)
2 cups chopped cabbage (green or red)

CROCKPOT INSTRUCTIONS:
   Add all ingredients except the cabbage to the crockpot.
   Cook on high for 5 hours, adding the cabbage three hours into cooking.

SOUP POT INSTRUCTIONS:
   Soak the beans overnight.
   Place the beans, broth (if using), and water in a pot and bring to a boil.
   Reduce the heat and simmer on medium-low heat for 30 minutes.
   Add the remaining ingredients and simmer for an additional 30 to 40 minutes (or until the beans are tender).

YIELD: 4 TO 6 SERVINGS

LENTIL AND MILLET CHILI

This chili pulls together the three vegan meal essentials: beans, greens, and grains. Summer vegetables fresh from the garden and light lentils with quick-to-cook millet make this chili perfect year round.

2 tablespoons extra-virgin olive oil
1 cup chopped yellow onion
2 cloves garlic, finely diced
1 jalapeño, finely diced
½ teaspoon cinnamon
1 teaspoon chili powder
1 teaspoon ground cumin
½ cup diced, lightly peeled summer squash
2 cups tightly packed kale, torn into pieces
4 cups diced tomatoes
1 cup brown lentils, rinsed and drained
1 cup millet, rinsed and drained
1 bay leaf
2 cups low-sodium vegetable stock or broth
4 cups water
Juice of 1 lemon
1 tablespoon chopped fresh sweet basil (optional)
½ teaspoon iodized sea salt
Fresh basil for garnish

PRESSURE COOKER INSTRUCTIONS:
Heat the olive oil in a 6-quart (or larger) pressure cooker. Add the onions, stirring for a few minutes, add the garlic, stir, then add the jalapeño, cinnamon, chili powder, and cumin and cook, for a total of 5 minutes of sautéing.

Add the squash, kale, tomatoes, lentils, millet, bay leaf, vegetable stock, and water.

Close the pressure cooker lid tightly. Bring the chili to high pressure (this will take a while because the pressure cooker is loaded with veggies, lentils, grains, and liquid).

Once high pressure is achieved, lower the heat so that the pressure regulator continues to rock heartily. Cook at pressure for 8 minutes.

Remove from the burner and let the pressure release naturally.

Once the pressure is released, carefully remove the pressure cooker lid, away from you.

Place the pressure cooker back on the burner on simmer and add the lemon juice, basil (if using), and salt. Stir and let simmer for a few minutes.

Garnish with fresh basil and enjoy!

STOVE TOP INSTRUCTIONS:

Heat the olive oil in a large pot.

Add the onions, stirring for a few minutes, add the garlic, stir, add the jalapeño and cinnamon, chili powder, and cumin and cook, for a total of 5 minutes of sautéing.

Add the squash, kale, tomatoes, lentils, millet, bay leaf, vegetable stock, and water and bring to a boil.

Cover, reduce to a simmer, and cook for 20 to 25 minutes.

Stir in the lemon juice, basil (if using), and salt and simmer for a few more minutes.

Garnish with fresh basil and enjoy!

YIELD: 6 TO 8 SERVINGS

SANDWICHES AND BURGERS

 ## SWEET TEMPEH BACON SANDWICH

Tempeh, made from fermented soybeans, is an important source of protein in Indonesian diets. Some people don't take to it right away. In this recipe I use a steaming method, which isn't necessary, but does make the "bacon" particularly succulent.

4-ounce package tempeh
2–3 tablespoons maple syrup
¼ teaspoon liquid smoke
½ teaspoon cayenne pepper
1 tablespoon extra-virgin olive oil (or use water or
  vegetable broth)
4 pieces bread, toasted
Vegan mayonnaise

Lettuce
1 small tomato, sliced

Slice the tempeh lengthwise into ten strips.

Steam the tempeh for 5 to 10 minutes (I steam mine for 6 minutes in an electric steamer; you can also steam it in a covered skillet or saucepan with a bit of water for up to 10 minutes).

While the tempeh is steaming, mix the maple syrup, liquid smoke, and cayenne pepper.

Heat the oil in a skillet on high.

Add the steamed tempeh to the skillet, reduce the heat to medium-high, and drizzle half of the syrup mixture over the tempeh.

Cook for 5 minutes, flip the tempeh strips, drizzle the remaining syrup over the tempeh, and cook for an additional 3 to 5 minutes.

Assemble your sandwich with toasted bread, vegan mayonnaise, lettuce, tomato, and tempeh.

YIELD: 2 SANDWICHES

SLOPPY JOE SANDWICH WITH PORTOBELLO MUSHROOMS AND QUINOA

I grew up with tomato-based Sloppy Joe sandwiches—some people called them "loose meat" sandwiches. Our local mall in the Midwest had a Maid-Rite Sandwich shop, serving up loose meat sandwiches with a cream of mushroom base. This recipe merges both concepts. Is it a Sloppy Joe? A Maid-Rite? I say it's a sloppy sandwich made just right!

2 large portobello mushroom caps, coarsely chopped
¼ cup coarsely chopped green pepper
¼ cup coarsely chopped red onion
1 teaspoon avocado oil
2 cloves garlic, minced

½ cup cooked quinoa
¾ cup marinara sauce
¼ teaspoon iodized sea salt
½ teaspoon chipotle powder
½ teaspoon taco seasoning
Whole wheat bun
Sliced red onion
Yellow mustard
Dill pickles

Pulse mushrooms, green pepper, and onions in a food processor—do this one ingredient at a time—you want each to be finely diced but not so processed that it becomes water—set each ingredient aside. The mushrooms should look finely crumbled.

Heat the oil in the skillet on medium-high heat and quickly sauté the garlic.

Add the mushrooms, pepper, and onions and sauté on high heat for a few minutes.

Add the quinoa and sauté, still on high heat, for a few more minutes.

Add the marinara sauce, salt, and spices and bring the mixture to a boil. Stir frequently for 5 minutes.

Reduce the heat and simmer for 10 minutes.

Serve on a toasted whole wheat bun with sliced red onion, yellow mustard, and dill pickles.

YIELD: 6 TO 8 SANDWICHES

NOTE: Make the quinoa in homemade or store-bought low-sodium vegetable broth for an extra bit of flavor.

CHICKPEA SALAD SANDWICH

This sandwich is a nod to the tuna salad sandwich. While the dulse flakes are optional, this seaweed provides a fishlike aroma and taste that is familiar and flavorful. This is also delicious over a chopped lettuce, meal-size salad.

1 can chickpeas, rinsed and drained
¼ cup diced tomato
2 tablespoons finely diced Vidalia onion
⅛ teaspoon black salt (or salt of your choice; black salt—which
   is actually pink—provides an egglike aroma and taste)
⅛ teaspoon dulse flakes (optional)
1 tablespoon vegan mayonnaise
1 tablespoon sweet relish
½ cup finely diced celery
Bread, toasted
Lettuce leaves (for the sandwich)

Place the chickpeas in a food processor and pulse to small chunks (which will be somewhat flaky).

Transfer the chickpeas to a mixing bowl.

Mix in the tomato, onions, salt, dulse flakes, vegan mayonnaise, relish, and celery.

Serve on toast with vegan mayonnaise and lettuce leaves.

YIELD: 3 TO 4 SERVINGS

SOY CURL PAPRIKASH SANDWICH

Soy curls are a new soyfood made from the whole bean—so they have lots of isoflavones and protein. I had my first soy curls at Homegrown Smokers in Portland, Oregon. Their Macnocheeto—a burrito stuffed with soy curls, beans, grains, and barbeque sauce—is vegan junk food at its finest. A healthier take, this "meaty" recipe will make two loaded sandwiches, so grab a fork and knife!

½ bag Butler Soy Curls
½ teaspoon vegan butter
1 tablespoon chicken-style seasoning (try Butler Chik-Style)

1 teaspoon paprika
¼ cup sauerkraut
¼ cup vegan sour cream
Ground black pepper
Sourdough bread

Soak the soy curls in warm water for 5 minutes and drain.
Heat the vegan butter in a skillet on medium heat.
Add the soy curls, sautéing for 3 to 5 minutes.
Add the chicken-style seasoning and paprika.
Mix in the sauerkraut and simmer on low for 5 minutes.
Stir in the vegan sour cream (to taste, enough to cover the curls and sauerkraut and make a nice, creamy consistency).
Cover, simmer on low for a few more minutes.
Add pepper, to taste.
Toast the sourdough bread and spread vegan butter on each slice.
Spoon the paprikash onto the toasted slices and serve.

YIELD: 2 SANDWICHES

QUINOA DAIYA BURGER

Vegan burgers can be fun to make—there are so many great things you can include—but can be challenging to grill. I always opt for grilling on foil on a charcoal or gas grill, to avoid losing any of the burger, or frying on a grill skillet. The surprise in this vegan burger is the Daiya vegan cheese—one of the latest on the market that melts—in the middle; if you can't find Daiya, use your favorite vegan cheese.

½ cup TVP (texturized vegetable protein)
½ cup vegetable broth
1 teaspoon hot sauce
2½ tablespoons ground flaxseeds

3 tablespoons water
¾ cup red kidney beans (home-cooked or canned)
½ cup cooked quinoa
1 clove of garlic, quartered
½ teaspoon Herbamere (or salt)
¾ cup Daiya shredded vegan cheese (I like a mix of
    mozzarella and cheddar)

Mix the TVP, vegetable broth, and hot sauce in a large bowl and let it sit for 20 minutes.

Whisk the flaxseeds and water together in a small bowl and set aside (this is an egg replacer).

In the food processor, pulse the TVP, flaxseed, beans, quinoa, garlic, and Herbamere for 20 seconds; scrape the sides and pulse for another 20 seconds.

Form the TVP into eight thin patties. Layer a thin pattie with ¼ of the shredded cheese and place another thin pattie on top of the cheese. Press and pinch the sides closed. Repeat to make four cheese-filled patties.

On the grill, heat a piece of foil. When heated, spread olive oil over the foil. Grill the burgers for 20 minutes (10 minutes on each side); if you're not using a grill, pan fry, using spray oil to avoid sticking, for 8 to 10 minutes each side.

YIELD: 4 BURGERS

CHICKPEA-TVP BURGERS

TVP—textured vegetable protein—is super-rich in protein and also provides isoflavones, calcium, and fiber. It is also a great binder when making vegan burgers. I particularly love how it absorbs the flavor of the spices.

1½ cups chickpeas (home-cooked or canned)
½ cup TVP
½ cup low-sodium vegetable broth

¼ cup bread crumbs
¼ cup ground flaxseeds
¼ teaspoon liquid smoke
½ teaspoon chili powder
½ teaspoon cayenne pepper
Iodized sea salt and ground black pepper

If using cooked chickpeas, bring to room temperature (or, if cooked in advance and refrigerated, set out for 30 to 60 minutes to come to room temperature before using),

Combine the TVP and vegetable broth in a bowl and let it sit for 20 minutes.

In a food processor, using the S blade, quickly pulse the chickpeas (leave some chunk). Add the TVP and all the remaining ingredients and pulse until well combined.

Form into patties and refrigerate for a few hours (or overnight) or place in the freezer for 20 minutes. Set out at room temperature for about 30 minutes before grilling.

Grill on a George Foreman–type grill for 7 to 8 minutes on each side. You can also use a grill skillet on the stove.

YIELD: 6 BURGERS

TEMPEH PATTIES

If you're on the fence about the texture of tempeh you simply must try this! Serve the patties on whole grain buns or over steamed greens.

8 ounces tempeh
1 tablespoon water (more if needed, for consistency)
2 tablespoons nutritional yeast (I use powder; fortified with B vitamins)
¼ teaspoon black salt
1 tablespoon avocado oil (or other vegetable oil)

Soak the tempeh in water for 15 minutes.

Remove the tempeh from the bowl of water and place it in a food processor.

Using the "S" blade, pulse for a few seconds to break up the tempeh.

Add the nutritional yeast and salt and pulse, checking for consistency. Add 2 teaspoons of water (if needed).

Heat the avocado oil in the skillet.

Roll the tempeh mixture into a ball and flatten into two patties.

Fry the patties for 5 minutes on medium-high heat, flip, reduce the heat to medium, and fry for 3 to 4 minutes.

YIELD: 2 PATTIES

VARIATION: Consider adding 1 teaspoon of any of the following: chili powder, paprika, or taco seasoning.

TEMPEH TOSTADAS

A healthy twist on a traditional Mexican tostada, this is a fast and delicious way to boost protein intake (from the tempeh) and calcium (from the kale).

8 ounces tempeh
About ¼ cup vegetable broth (just enough to cover the bottom of the skillet)
½ teaspoon chili powder
¼ teaspoon garlic salt
¼ cup diced red onion
1 stalk celery, chopped
½ cup fresh salsa
Vegetable oil spray
6 to 8 small corn tortillas
1 tablespoon avocado oil (or other vegetable oil)
4 cups chopped kale

Sea salt
Vegan sour cream (optional)
Hot sauce (optional)

Preheat the oven to 400°F degrees (for the tortillas).

Cut the tempeh into four equal pieces and boil for 10 minutes. Drain and set aside.

In a skillet, cover the bottom of the skillet with vegetable broth and heat on medium-high.

When the broth begins to boil add the chili powder and garlic salt, to taste. Add the onions and celery and sauté for a few minutes.

Add the tempeh to the skillet and crumble into small bits.

Stir in the fresh salsa, cover, and lower the heat to simmer for 8 to 10 minutes.

Spray the vegetable oil on each side of the corn tortillas, place on a baking sheet, and bake for approximately 8 minutes.

While the tempeh is simmering and the tortillas are baking, pour a small amount of avocado oil over the kale, lightly salt, and massage the salt and oil into the kale with your hands.

To assemble, place a bed of massaged kale over a crispy corn tortilla, spoon tempeh over the kale and, if desired, top off with vegan sour cream and hot sauce.

YIELD: 6 TO 8 TOSTADAS

VARIATION: For an alternative to baking the tortilla, try frying them. Heat vegetable oil in a skillet and place the tortillas in the hot oil. Fry for just 2 to 3 minutes, flip and fry for another 3 minutes.

TOFU TACOS

Another spin on a traditional food, tofu, red wine, and shallots make this unlike any taco I have ever eaten. If you're looking to increase your intake of isoflavones—to counter hot flashes or smooth your skin—this is a fun way to do it.

6 ounces extra-firm tofu, pressed and drained
1 teaspoon avocado or extra-virgin olive oil (optional)
¼ cup red wine
⅛ cup diced shallots
1 clove garlic, finely diced
1 teaspoon Sriracha (or other hot sauce)
Iodized sea salt and ground black pepper
Avocado or extra-virgin olive oil spray (optional)
2 white corn tortillas
3 handfuls baby spinach
Vegan sour cream

Preheat the oven to 400°F degrees.

Slice half a block of tofu into four pieces and place in a shallow dish.

In a small bowl whisk the marinade: avocado oil (if using), red wine, shallots, garlic, Sriracha, salt, and pepper.

Pour the marinade over the tofu and let sit for 30 minutes.

Bake the tofu for 30 minutes on a baking sheet (at 15 minutes, flip the tofu).

During the final 15 minutes of baking the tofu, heat a skillet on medium-high and spray with oil (if using) and place the white corn tortillas in the hot skillet. Let the tortilla heat for 2 to 3 minutes before flipping. After another 2 to 3 minutes, fold the tortillas to a taco shape.

Let the tortillas cool and toss 3 handfuls of baby spinach in the hot skillet. Reduce heat to low and cover for just a few minutes.

Remove the tofu from the oven and slice into strips. Assemble the taco: spinach, tofu, and a dollop of vegan sour cream.

YIELD: 2 TACOS

SPICY WHITE BEAN–TVP MEATBALLS

Athletes and women over fifty who are looking for ways to pack in the protein will love this dish, which uses beans plus textured vegetable protein. The flaxseeds add omega-3. Serve these meatballs over buckwheat pasta with a simple marinara sauce and a dash of oregano.

½ cup TVP
½ cup vegetable stock
1½ cups white beans (home-cooked or canned)
¼ cup ground flaxseeds
2 tablespoons sesame seeds
2 tablespoons stone-ground wheat flour
1 teaspoon iodized sea salt
2 tablespoons nutritional yeast flakes
1 teaspoon sweet basil
½ teaspoon ground thyme
1 teaspoon Sriracha, or other hot sauce (if you like spicy, add more!)

Preheat the oven to 375°F.

Rehydrate the TVP in the vegetable stock for about 10 minutes.

Place all the ingredients in a food processor and pulse to the desired consistency.

Spoon about 1.5 tablespoons of mixture per meatball, rolling in the palm of your hands (you may want to wet your hands to keep the mixture from sticking).

Place the meatballs on a cookie sheet lined with parchment paper.

Bake for 15 minutes, turn, and bake for an additional 15 minutes.

Let meatballs sit for at least 15 minutes before serving.

YIELD: 12 TO 14 MEATBALLS

PIZZA AND PASTA

 ## PEPPERONI SAUSAGE

This vegan, seitan (also known as "wheat meat"), alternative to a favorite pizza topping can be made quickly and easily in the pressure cooker, but, if I haven't yet convinced you to use one, I offer stove top instructions, too. You can cut thicker slices and serve as a sausage patty with breakfast, dice up and serve in cooked beans, or even serve on crackers for an appetizer. In this recipe I suggest that you make four smaller sausages and one larger one so that you have some alternatives. You can slice the larger seitan cutlet into breakfast patties and you can slice the smaller sausages to make pepperoni slices for pizza.

Cooking broth: 3 cups water, 3 cups vegetable broth, and ¼
    cup low-sodium soy sauce
1½ cups vital wheat gluten
¼ cup garbanzo bean flour

2 tablespoons nutritional yeast

½ teaspoon allspice (or a mix of nutmeg, cinnamon, and clove
to equal ½ teaspoon)

½ teaspoon paprika

½ teaspoon anise seed, crumbled between your fingers or
rubbed in the palms of your hands

½ teaspoon crumbled fennel seed

½ teaspoon red pepper flakes

½ teaspoon garlic powder

½ teaspoon ground black pepper

1 cup vegetable broth (add more if too dry)

1 teaspoon extra-virgin olive oil

½ teaspoon liquid smoke

½ teaspoon vegan Worcestershire sauce

2 tablespoons Bragg Liquid Aminos (or soy sauce)

PRESSURE COOKER INSTRUCTIONS:

Bring the cooking broth ingredients to a boil in an uncovered pressure cooker.

Mix the dry ingredients together in a stand mixer bowl.

Mix the wet ingredients in a small bowl.

Add the wet ingredients to the dry, mix well, then knead with the dough hook of the mixer for 5 minutes.

Break the dough into half. From half of the dough, roll four small sausages and wrap individually in cheesecloth, tying the ends with string. Take the remaining half and roll into a larger sausage and wrap in cheesecloth, tying the ends with string.

Place in the boiling cooking broth, cover the pressure cooker, and bring to pressure.

Cook at pressure for 30 minutes.

Allow for a natural release.

Remove the sausages from the broth to cool before handling or serving.

STOVE TOP INSTRUCTIONS:

Bring the cooking broth ingredients to a boil in a large pot.

Mix the dry ingredients together in a stand mixer bowl

Mix the wet ingredients in a small bowl.

Add the wet ingredients to the dry, mix well, then knead with the dough hook of the mixer for 5 minutes.

Break the dough into half. From half of the dough, roll four small sausages and wrap individually in cheesecloth, tying the ends with string. Take the remaining half and roll into a larger sausage and wrap in cheesecloth, tying the ends with string.

Place in a large pot with cooking broth.

Bring almost to a boil, then reduce the heat to a simmer and cook for 1 hour.

Let the seitan cool to room temperature in the broth.

FOR PEPPERONI SLICES:

Freeze the sausage overnight and then use a food processor (use the slicing disc) for nice, thin spicy pieces of sausage. (Note: One tester indicated trouble doing this with her food processor, if you're concerned about slicing a frozen food in your food processor let the sausage thaw for awhile before slicing. I should note that I sliced the sausage straight out of the freezer with no problems—but being cautious is always a good thing!)

Store the whole sausage, in the cooking broth, in an airtight container in the refrigerator or in a sturdy bag in the freezer.

YIELD 8 TO 10 SERVINGS

VEGAN PEPPERONI PIZZA

Yes, even vegans want pepperoni pizza! Start with a store-bought whole wheat or whole-grain pizza dough and you'll be enjoying this pizza in no time.

1 teaspoon extra-virgin olive oil
2 cloves garlic, finely diced
1 package or roll of whole wheat pizza dough
½ cup tomato sauce
½ cup diced onion
1 cup shredded vegan mozzarella cheese
1 cup Pepperoni Sausage (page 287) or store bought
Red pepper flakes
2 tablespoons finely chopped fresh oregano

Preheat the oven to 500°F degrees.

Heat the olive oil and garlic in a cast-iron skillet, on medium-low heat, on the stove.

Remove the skillet from the heat.

Press the pizza dough into the skillet, and flip so that both sides are rubbed into the oil and garlic (the garlic will end up pressed into the dough).

Spread the sauce over the dough, add the onions, and sprinkle ½ to ¾ cup of the vegan mozzarella over the top.

Bake in the skillet for 15 minutes on the lowest rack in the oven.

Reduce the oven heat to 400°F, then remove the skillet from the oven to add the pepperoni, red pepper flakes to taste, oregano, and a bit more mozzarella.

Return the skillet to the oven and bake for an additional 15 to 18 minutes.

YIELD: 2 TO 4 SERVINGS

Note: Baking times may vary—following the baking instructions on the pizza dough package.

BLACK-EYED PEA AND COLLARD GREEN PIZZA

Pizza is always fun, and this one—with the addition of some rather unusual toppings—is loaded with good southern-style nutrition. Black-eyed peas add protein and collard greens provide calcium.

1 teaspoon extra-virgin olive oil
2 large whole wheat tortillas or wraps (standard or large size)
6 collard greens
¼ cup vegetable broth
1 clove garlic, finely diced
1 teaspoon taco seasoning
½ teaspoon ground cumin

1 cup black-eyed peas (home-cooked or canned)
½ cup tomato sauce
Vegan Parmesan cheese
½ cup sliced (half-moons) onion

Preheat the oven to 400°F.

Spread the oil over the tortillas and bake for about 5 minutes (I placed the tortillas directly on the oven rack). Remove from the oven.

Halve each collard leaf lengthwise with kitchen shears or a sharp knife, cutting out and discarding the center ribs. Stack the leaves and cut crosswise into ¼-inch-wide strips.

Heat the vegetable broth in a skillet over medium-high heat. Add the garlic, taco seasoning, and cumin.

Stir in the collard green strips, cover, reduce to simmer, and steam for 3 minutes.

Add the black-eyed peas and simmer for another few minutes.

Spread half the tomato sauce over each baked wrap.

Add half the cooked collard greens and black-eyed peas to each.

Sprinkle vegan Parmesan over each pizza.

Top off each pizza with a sprinkling of onions.

Bake for 10 minutes.

YIELD: 2 PIZZAS

VARIATION: Substitute a blend of oregano and basil for the taco seasoning or use chili powder for a little kick.

SOCCA PIZZA

Socca, a thin pancake, is made with garbanzo bean flour and produces a nutrient-rich crust with more protein, iron, and zinc than other pizzas. It's a great alternative to a heavier pizza crust.

1¼ cups water
1 cup chickpea (garbanzo bean) flour

1 tablespoon avocado oil (or extra-virgin olive oil)

1 clove garlic, diced

½ teaspoon iodized sea salt

Vegetable oil spray

½ cup diced onion

1 tablespoon chopped fresh chives

2 tablespoons tomato sauce

½ cup sliced baby bella mushrooms

Shredded vegan cheese

1 teaspoon dried oregano

Iodized sea salt and ground black pepper, to taste

Add water, flour, oil, garlic, and salt to a high-speed blender and blend for less than 30 seconds. Leave the batter in the blender for 30 minutes.

Place a 9-inch cast-iron skillet in the oven and preheat the skillet and oven to 450°F.

After at least 30 minutes, blend the batter again for 5 seconds (just flip the blender on and off to mix it a bit).

Remove the skillet from the oven and spray with a vegetable oil spray.

Add ¼ cup of the onions and the chives to the batter and pour into the skillet. Place the skillet back in the oven and bake for 15 minutes.

Remove the skillet from the oven. Layer the tomato sauce, mushrooms, the remaining onions, vegan cheese, oregano, salt, and pepper on the socca.

Return the skillet to the oven, reduce the heat to 425°F and bake for 7 to 9 minutes.

Remove the skillet from the oven and let the pizza sit for at least 10 minutes before slicing.

YIELD: 2 SERVINGS

VARIATION: Add your favorite vegan pizza toppings! Consider crumbled seitan, spinach, black olives, vegan pepperoni, and so on.

"Meaty" Lentil and Veggie Mac

Just like ground beef, Tofurky's veggie "beef" is packed with protein. What's missing is all the saturated fat, making this a deliciously healthy version of old-time comfort food. Serve with a side salad and you have a balanced and fun meal!

4 ounces elbow macaroni
1 teaspoon extra-virgin olive oil
1 cup diced mixed red and green pepper
¼ cup diced onion
Red pepper flakes and dried rosemary and oregano, to taste
²/₃ cup Tofurky "Ground Beef Style"
2 cups lentils (home-cooked or canned)
Vegan Parmesan cheese, to garnish

Cook the pasta according to the box directions.

In a skillet, heat the olive oil on medium-high heat. Sauté the peppers and onions for a few minutes.

Add the red pepper flakes, oregano, and rosemary to taste.

Crumble the Tofurky ground "beef" into the skillet and sauté for a minute or so.

Add the lentils, stir, cover, and simmer on low for 3 to 5 minutes.

Spoon over pasta in a bowl, top with Parma (or your favorite vegan Parmesan cheese), and stir.

YIELD: 2 SERVINGS

Spinach Bow Tie Pasta Salad

The creamy "green" sauce—featuring spinach and tofu—makes this vegan pasta salad a nutritional powerhouse! Be sure to chill for the recommended time to ensure a flavorful experience.

4 ounces Hodgson Mill Whole Wheat Whole-Grain Bow
  Tie Pasta
2 cups vegetable broth
Onion, diced in big chunks (I use half a small red onion)
2 cloves of garlic, diced in big chunks
6 ounces extra-firm tofu, pressed, drained, and cubed
2 handfuls baby spinach
½ teaspoon salt
½ teaspoon dill weed, plus a pinch for garnish
⅛ cup diced red onion
4 ounces finely diced haricots verts
Dash of dill weed
Ground black pepper
Chopped baby spinach leaves, for garnish

Cook the pasta according to the directions on the package. When finished, drain, rinse in cold water, drain again, and set aside.

Begin making the "cream" sauce by bringing the vegetable broth, onions, and garlic to a boil in a medium saucepan.

Add the tofu and bring back to a boil.

Add the spinach, cover, and simmer for 5 minutes.

Transfer the cooked tofu and spinach mixture from the saucepan to a blender (I use a Vitamix) or food processor, cover tightly, and blend for 30 seconds to a minute. (If you double and/or increase this recipe, be sure to blend in small batches, 2 to 3 cups at a time.) Store the leftover sauce in an airtight container in the refrigerator for 3 to 5 days.

This will make about 3 cups of sauce. Pour 2 cups of sauce over the cooked, rinsed, and drained pasta. Stir in the salt, dill, onions, and haricots vert.

Add a pinch of dill weed, pour into a bowl with an airtight lid, and refrigerator for at least two hours.

Once chilled, serve with fresh ground black pepper and garnish with a few chopped baby spinach leaves.

YIELD: 2 ENTREE SERVINGS OR 4 SIDE SERVINGS

QUINOA-MILLET VEGGIE BOWL

You can make this grain and vegetable dish easily in your rice cooker (set it up to start cooking before you get home from work!) or in minutes on the stove.

1 teaspoon vegetable oil (optional)
½ teaspoon whole, dried rosemary crumbled with fingers
½ cup diced zucchini
1 stalk diced celery
¼ cup diced onion
½ cup millet, rinsed and drained
2¼ cups water
1 cup quinoa, rinsed and drained
Iodized sea salt and ground black pepper

Rice cooker instructions:

Add all the ingredients to a rice cooker, stir, and cook on brown rice setting.

Stove top instructions:

Sauté the oil, rosemary, zucchini, celery, and onions in a large saucepan. (If you are not using oil, simply dry-sauté the ingredients.)

Add the millet and water to the saucepan and bring to a boil. Cover, reduce to simmer, and cook for 10 minutes.

Add the quinoa and bring back to a boil. Cover, reduce to simmer, and cook for 10 to 15 more minutes. (Begin checking on it at 10 minutes; it is done when all the liquid is absorbed.)

Remove the saucepan from the heat and let stand, covered, for 5 minutes.

Fluff, salt and pepper to taste, and serve.

YIELD: 2 ENTREE SERVINGS; 4 SIDE SERVINGS

VARIATION: Serve this in a squash for an even heartier meal—perfect in the fall and winter. Slice an acorn squash in half, remove the seeds, and place face down on a baking sheet lined with parchment paper. Bake for 30 minutes at 350°F. Serve the Quinoa-Millet in the acorn squash "bowl."

Turmeric, Cumin, and Ginger Tofu

Marinating tofu is pretty easy. I typically use a fat (olive or sesame oil), an acid (vinegar or citrus juice), and spices to start. Ume plum vinegar gives this a nice burst of umami. Tofu provides isoflavones, calcium, and lots of protein. I serve this with steamed vegetables and cinnamon mashed sweet potatoes.

1 (14-ounce) package extra-firm tofu, pressed, drained, and cubed
1 teaspoon toasted sesame oil

2 tablespoons ume plum vinegar

1 tablespoon low-sodium soy sauce

½ teaspoon ground ginger

1 teaspoon turmeric

½ teaspoon cumin

3 cloves garlic, minced

1 teaspoon maple syrup

Place the cubed tofu in a shallow baking pan suitable for marinating.

In a small bowl, whisk together the oil, vinegar, and soy sauce.

Add the ginger, turmeric, and cumin and whisk again.

Stir in the garlic and then pour the mixture over the cubed tofu.

Toss the tofu in the marinade, coating each piece well.

Drizzle maple syrup over the tofu, cover, and refrigerate for several hours (or overnight).

To cook, heat a nonstick pan (sprayed lightly with oil) on medium-high. Add the tofu and fry for 5 minutes. Turn the tofu pieces and cook for another 3 to 5 minutes.

YIELD: 4 SERVINGS

CINNAMON TOFU

While the star here is cinnamon—a spice with healing powers, especially for people with diabetes—Herbamere—a blend of sea salt and herbs and spices and a great alternative to table salt—adds additional flavor to this dish. If you do not have Herbamere, simply use half a teaspoon of salt and a blend of your favorite herbs. Serve with your favorite sautéed leafy greens and brown rice or serve cold over a salad.

6 ounces extra-firm tofu (half a typical package of tofu), pressed and drained

1 tablespoon sesame oil

2 tablespoons rice vinegar

2 cloves garlic, finely diced

1 teaspoon Herbamere

½ teaspoon ground cinnamon

Slice the tofu into five pieces and place in a shallow dish.

Whisk the remaining ingredients in a small bowl and pour over the tofu. Marinade for 2 hours (but for as long as 24 hours, if you like).

Grill on an indoor/outdoor grill—or a grill skillet—for 8 minutes (turn at 4 minutes).

YIELD: 2 TO 3 SERVINGS

 ## CASHEW CREAM TOFU

I like to think of this as an "alfredo" tofu; the cashews provide a plant-based creaminess that is thick with a nutty flavor. I serve it over toast (reminiscent of a creamed chipped beef toast meal I grew up with) or with steamed asparagus.

½ cup raw, unsalted cashews

¾ cup water

2 cloves garlic

2 tablespoons red wine vinegar

1 (14-ounce) package extra firm tofu, pressed and drained

⅛–¼ cup chopped cashews

Iodized sea salt and ground black pepper, to taste

Place the first four ingredients in a blender or food processor and blend to a creamy consistency.

Slice the tofu into six cutlets and arrange them in a shallow baking dish.

Preheat the oven to 400°F.

Pour the cashew cream over the tofu, cover, and let sit while preparing a side dish and allowing the oven to preheat.

Place the tofu cutlets on a baking sheet (lined with parchment paper) and press half of the chopped cashew pieces on top.

Bake for 10 minutes.

Flip the tofu, pour the remaining cashew cream over it, and press the remaining cashew pieces on top.

Return the cutlets to the oven and bake for another 10 minutes.

Salt and pepper to taste and serve.

YIELD: 4 SERVINGS

CINNAMON-GINGER SEITAN

Seitan, also known as "wheat meat," can take on a variety of flavors simply by changing up the spices and seasoning. Follow this recipe, but swap out the ginger, cinnamon, and cumin for three spices of your choice and you change the flavor but not the texture!

1½ cups vital wheat gluten
¼ cup garbanzo bean flour
2 tablespoons nutritional yeast
½ teaspoon garlic powder
½ teaspoon ground black pepper
½ teaspoon each ground ginger, cinnamon, and cumin
1 cup vegetable broth
1 teaspoon avocado oil
1 teaspoon blackstrap molasses
2 tablespoons Bragg Liquid Aminos (or soy sauce)
Cooking broth: 3 cups water, 3 cups vegetable broth, and
  ¼ cup low-sodium soy sauce

PRESSURE COOKER INSTRUCTIONS:

Combine the first six ingredients (dry) in a medium bowl (or a Kitchen Aid bowl).

Whisk together the wet ingredients (not the cooking broth) in a small bowl.

Add the wet ingredients to the dry ingredients and stir until well combined.

Knead for 5 minutes (I highly recommend using the dough hook of a Kitchen Aid, or similar appliance).

Pull the dough apart to form six cutlets. Set aside.

Bring the broth ingredients to a boil in the uncovered pressure cooker.

Add the cutlets to the boiling water and lock the pressure cooker cover in place.

Bring to pressure, cook at low pressure for 30 minutes.

Remove from the heat and allow for a natural release.

Remove the cutlets from the broth to cool before handling or serving.

Store the cutlets, in the cooking broth, in an airtight container in the refrigerator or in a sturdy bag in the freezer.

STOVE TOP INSTRUCTIONS:

Follow the first five instructions above.

Bring the cooking broth ingredients to a boil in a large pot.

Place the cutlets in the boiling broth.

Bring almost to a boil, then reduce the heat to a simmer and cook for 1 hour.

Let the seitan cool to room temperature in the broth.

YIELD: 8 TO 10 SERVINGS

Soy Curl Cacciatore

One of the challenges when beginning to cook or eat vegan is replacing meat. I find soy curls to be an excellent substitute. Here soy curls replace the typical chicken in a modified cacciatore recipe.

1 teaspoon extra-virgin olive oil (or vegetable broth or water)
1 clove garlic, finely diced
½ cup diced onion
½ cup chopped red pepper
Half bag Butler Soy Curls, rehydrated
1 tablespoon "chicken-style" seasoning
½ teaspoon dried oregano
1 cup sliced baby bella mushrooms
¼ cup marinara sauce
2 cups loosely packed baby spinach
Vegan Parmesan cheese
Sea salt, to taste
Ground black pepper, to taste

Heat the olive oil in a skillet.

On medium-high heat sauté the garlic, onions, and red pepper for about 3 minutes.

Add the soy curls, "chicken-style" seasoning, and oregano and sauté for about 5 minutes.

Add the mushrooms and continue sautéing for a few more minutes.

Add the marinara sauce and spinach, stir and cover.

Reduce the heat and simmer for 5 minutes.

Serve with vegan Parmesan cheese, salt, and pepper.

Yield: 2 servings

DESSERTS

Banana Butter, page 302
Cinnamon and Walnut Banana Bread, page 303
Coconut-Gingered Black Bean Brownies, page 304

BANANA BUTTER

This Banana Butter is a kid-friendly recipe that your children will love to cook . . . and eat! Serve it over toast for an extra-special breakfast or as a sauce over a warm piece of cake or banana bread.

2 tablespoons vegan butter
1 tablespoon unsweetened coconut milk
1 ripe banana
2 tablespoons jumbo raisins
Dash of ground cinnamon

Heat the butter and coconut milk in a small saucepan.
Mash the banana and add the raisins, mashing together.
Add the banana mixture to the saucepan and simmer for a few minutes.
Stir in the cinnamon.
Serve over warm slices of bread or toast.

YIELD: 2 SERVINGS

CINNAMON AND
WALNUT BANANA BREAD

With the healing power of cinnamon and plant-based omega-3 essential fatty acids from walnuts, this flavorful loaf of bread is a terrific dessert (serve it warm with the Banana Butter recipe!) and is great toasted for breakfast.

Extra-virgin olive oil or avocado oil spray
⅓ cup almond milk, plus 1 tablespoon
1 tablespoon apple cider vinegar
2 Ener-G Egg Replacer "eggs"
½ cup melted vegan margarine
1 teaspoon vanilla extract
1½ cups mashed banana (about 3 bananas)
½ teaspoon iodized sea salt
1 cup Sucanat
1 teaspoon ground cinnamon
¾ teaspoon baking powder
1 teaspoon baking soda
1 cup unbleached all-purpose bread flour
1 cup buckwheat flour
⅔ cup chopped walnuts (optional)

Preheat the oven to 350°F.

Lightly grease (I use avocado oil spray) a 9 x 5-inch loaf pan.

In a small bowl, whisk the almond milk and vinegar and allow to settle (curdle) for about 5 minutes.

Prepare the Energ-G Egg replacers according to the package instructions (I use a blender).

Pour the almond milk mixture and the "eggs" into a large mixing bowl.

Add the vegan margarine, vanilla extract, and bananas. Mix well.

Add the salt, Sucanat, and cinnamon. Mix well.

Sprinkle the baking powder and baking soda into the bowl. Mix well.

Fold in the all-purpose flour and buckwheat flour and mix well.
Add walnuts (if using).

Pour the batter into the greased loaf pan.

Bake for 50 minutes.

Cool on a rack.

Remove the bread from the pan and slice to serve.

YIELD: 1 LOAF

COCONUT-GINGERED
BLACK BEAN BROWNIES

Black bean brownies are not a new concept, but it took a while for
me to fall in love with them. I decided to experiment with subtle,
less "sweet" flavors—and bring my love of using my pressure
cooker for homemade beans into play. These brownies are not
sweet, so consider serving them with your favorite vegan ice
cream or Banana Butter (page 302). Athletes enjoy them as a post-
workout recovery snack.

For the beans:

1½–2 cups dried black beans, soaked overnight (rinse and
   drain; weigh the beans after the overnight soak—use 15
   ounces)

2 tablespoons date syrup (or brown rice or maple syrup)

1 (13.5 ounce) can organic light coconut milk

Additional ingredients for the brownies:

¾ cup no-sugar added applesauce

2 teaspoons vanilla extract

1 tablespoon grated fresh ginger (or 1 teaspoon powdered
   ginger)

¼ cup date syrup (if you prefer a sweeter dessert, you may
   want to increase this a bit)

½ cup cacao powder (I used 100 percent organic and raw)
½ cup millet flour
⅛ cup chopped into chunky pieces, dark chocolate
¼ cup chopped walnuts

PRESSURE COOKER BEANS:
Place the black beans (rinsed and drained), date syrup, and coconut milk in a pressure cooker (see below for cooking beans on the stove top).

Lock the lid into place and bring to pressure.

Cook at pressure for 12 minutes.

Allow for a natural release.

Once pressure is released, remove the lid, away from you, and taste the beans for doneness.

If necessary, simmer, lightly covered (do not lock lid in place) for 5 to 10 minutes.

STOVE TOP BEANS:
Place the black beans (rinsed and drained), date syrup, and coconut milk in a pot.

Bring the pot of beans to a gentle boil and let them cook until they're tender. Keep testing the beans for doneness.

After the beans have finished cooking, remove them from the heat and drain them.

FOR THE BROWNIES:
Preheat the oven to 350°F

Pour the cooked beans into a food processor fitted with an S blade and pulse to chop up the beans.

Add the applesauce, vanilla extract, ginger, and date syrup and blend until smooth.

Add the dry ingredients, cacao powder and millet flour, and blend until smooth, resembling a cake batter.

Add half the dark chocolate and half the chopped walnuts to the food processor and quickly pulse (don't blend) so the pieces are mixed in but still chunky.

Pour the batter into 9 x 9-inch baking dish, lined with parchment paper. Sprinkle the remaining chocolate and walnut pieces on top.

Bake for 40 to 50 minutes.

Remove the brownies and the parchment paper from the baking dish and let them cool on a rack for 20 minutes.

YIELD: 12 BROWNIES

METRIC CONVERSION CHART

- The recipes in this book have not been tested with metric measurements, so some variations might occur.
- Remember that the weight of dry ingredients varies according to the volume or density factor: 1 cup of flour weighs far less than 1 cup of sugar, and 1 tablespoon doesn't necessarily hold 3 teaspoons.

General Formulas for Metric Conversion

Ounces to grams	➡ ounces × 28.35 = grams
Grams to ounces	➡ grams × 0.035 = ounces
Pounds to grams	➡ pounds × 453.5 = grams
Pounds to kilograms	➡ pounds × 0.45 = kilograms
Cups to liters	➡ cups × 0.24 = liters
Fahrenheit to Celsius	➡ (°F − 32) × 5 ÷ 9 = °C
Celsius to Fahrenheit	➡ (°C × 9) ÷ 5 + 32 = °F

Linear Measurements

½ inch	=	1½ cm
1 inch	=	2½ cm
6 inches	=	15 cm
8 inches	=	20 cm
10 inches	=	25 cm
12 inches	=	30 cm
20 inches	=	50 cm

Volume (Dry) Measurements

¼ teaspoon = 1 milliliter
½ teaspoon = 2 milliliters
¾ teaspoon = 4 milliliters
1 teaspoon = 5 milliliters
1 tablespoon = 15 milliliters
¼ cup = 59 milliliters
⅓ cup = 79 milliliters
½ cup = 118 milliliters
⅔ cup = 158 milliliters
¾ cup = 177 milliliters
1 cup = 225 milliliters
4 cups or 1 quart = 1 liter
½ gallon = 2 liters
1 gallon = 4 liters

Volume (Liquid) Measurements

1 teaspoon = ⅙ fluid ounce = 5 milliliters
1 tablespoon = ½ fluid ounce = 15 milliliters
2 tablespoons = 1 fluid ounce = 30 milliliters
¼ cup = 2 fluid ounces = 60 milliliters
⅓ cup = 2⅔ fluid ounces = 79 milliliters
½ cup = 4 fluid ounces = 118 milliliters
1 cup or ½ pint = 8 fluid ounces = 250 milliliters
2 cups or 1 pint = 16 fluid ounces = 500 milliliters
4 cups or 1 quart = 32 fluid ounces = 1,000 milliliters
1 gallon = 4 liters

Oven Temperature Equivalents, Fahrenheit (F) and Celsius (C)

100°F = 38°C
200°F = 95°C
250°F = 120°C
300°F = 150°C
350°F = 180°C
400°F = 205°C
450°F = 230°C

Weight (Mass) Measurements

1 ounce = 30 grams
2 ounces = 55 grams
3 ounces = 85 grams
4 ounces = ¼ pound = 125 grams
8 ounces = ½ pound = 240 grams
12 ounces = ¾ pound = 375 grams
16 ounces = 1 pound = 454 grams

Acknowledgments

From Ginny and JL

We could not have asked for a more supportive, insightful, and encouraging team of experts than the ones we found at Da Capo. Thank you especially to Renée Sedliar for her skillful editing and patient guidance. And to senior project editor Cisca Schreefel, copyeditor Martha Whitt, and designer Linda Mark. And a special thank you to our agent Angela Miller for her enthusiastic and expert support and guidance through development and submission of our proposal, and her continued support through every step of the writing and publishing process.

From Ginny

Asking JL Fields to write this book with me is one of the smartest things I've ever done. I expected her contributions to be brilliant, but she has brought joy and energy to this project beyond what I ever imagined and has also given me a new best friend for life. Thank you, JL, for joining me on this adventure!

What a gift it was to find Ari Evergreen of Shirari Industries to design the food guide for this book. Not only is she a talented artist but she is also a vegan and a rescuer of feral cats.

I feel a debt of gratitude to so many people who have supported, mentored, and guided me through the years, both in the field of nutrition and also through our shared work on behalf of farmed and companion animals. Jack Norris, RD, and Reed Mangels, PhD, RD, are my go-to vegan nutrition experts. I'm grateful for their unfailing generosity in sharing their knowledge, as well as their friendship, wisdom, humor, and their commitment to scientific integrity and to advocacy for animals.

My long-time colleague Dr. Enette Larson-Meyer, RD, gave me many helpful suggestions regarding vegan diets for female athletes. Over two decades in this field, I've worked with and been inspired by many other professionals in the field of vegan dietetics—experts who promote dietary practices that underscore not just health but also compassion. Thank you to my long time friends Brenda Davis, RD; Vesanto Melina, MS, RD; and Dr. Suzanne Havala-Hobbs, MS, RD; and to Matt Ruscigno, MPH, RD; Mark Rifkin, MS, RD; and Dina Aronson, MS, RD. I continue to be inspired as well by a wonderful new generation of dietitians like Ed Coffin, RD, and Carolyn Tampe, MS, RD, who are changing the world for people and animals.

Erik Marcus is among my oldest and dearest friends in the vegan community, long a source of encouragement and inspiration and always a source of moral support.

Charles Stahler and Debra Wasserman of the Vegetarian Resource Group and Dr. Neal Barnard of PCRM gave me opportunities to develop my skills and knowledge in the field of vegan nutrition. They were all instrumental in pointing me toward a career that I might not otherwise have envisioned.

I am inspired every day by activists who advocate for animals from a position of compassion, wisdom, and integrity and whose support for my own work and efforts means more to me than they could possibly know. Thank you to David Sutherland and Debra Stephens of Vegan Chicago; Unny Nambudiripad and Dave Rolsky of Compassionate Action for Animals; Jon Camp of Vegan Outreach, Jasmin Singer and Mariann Sullivan of Our Hen House, and Dustin Rhodes and Lee Hall of Friends of Animals.

Matt Ball and Anne Green of Vegan Outreach remain among my personal heroes for the wisdom, compassion, and insight they bring to animal activism.

Writer Hillary Rettig brings vast knowledge and kindness to her work in helping activists stay focused and productive. She has generously coached me through career- and activism-related bumps and challenges.

Dr. Michael Greger is a fount of nutrition information with a gift for making it fun. He's also a much-appreciated friend and the only person to ever send me a package of purple sweet potatoes in the mail.

Lisa Herzstein, who shares my passions for books, veganism, and animals, is proof positive that social networking can provide meaningful and affirming friendships.

Phyllis Becker and Paul Becker are two of my local heroes. They traded in a well-deserved retirement for full-time animal rescue. Phyllis is the best friend a feral cat could ever have, and she is also an inspired vegan cook.

My friend Kate Schumann has collaborated with me on projects over the years related to vegan nutrition and companion animals. She never runs out of ideas for ways to help animals and, after twenty-five years, each collaboration feels as fresh and fun as the first.

My cats' veterinarian, Dr. Ginny Johnson of Hadlock Veterinary Clinic, is tireless in her efforts to help rescued animals and the people and organizations who advocate for them. She is one of the most generous people I know.

Louise Holton, founder of Alley Cat Rescue, remains my model for compassion and selflessness in her advocacy for homeless cats and all animals.

Landing in a great family is a matter of pure luck, and I am very, very lucky. I have the two best brothers, Bill Kisch and Steve Kisch, and am also blessed by my wonderful sisters-in-law Irma Kisch and Agnes Kisch, nieces Sarah Gorden, Christen Kisch and Heather Kisch; nephews Noah Gordon, BJ Kisch, and Chris Kisch, plus adorable little Reid Ellie Kisch and brand-new Bradley Gavin Kisch.

Willie Schrenk Kisch and Bill Kisch are forever in my heart.

My friends are among my most treasured sources of happiness and comfort. Thank you for always being by my side to Joan Petrokofsky, Lynn Myhal Zornetzer, Diana Longo, Paige Pettit, and Debbi Zabel.

I could get twice as much work done in half as much time if I weren't always maneuvering around a pile of cats, but I wouldn't have it any other way. Thank you Blackberry, Bamboo, Nicholas, Phoebe, and Juniper for being good company, for reminding me when it's time to take a break, and for the comfort and humor you bring into my life.

Finally, I am the luckiest and most blessed person in the world to be married to Mark Messina. He still holds me accountable for every single thing I say about nutrition, makes me laugh, and continues to (almost) never complain when I bring home stray cats.

FROM JL

Ginny Messina made a lifelong dream come true when she wrote an e-mail asking "Write a book with me?" My mentor from afar became my mentor in real life, my dearest friend, my coauthor, and my sister in the quest to encourage women to be compassionate to themselves and to others.

I am forever indebted to the nameless goat I met in Africa. His loss of life was the beginning of my compassionate journey.

To vegan bloggers, far too many to name, who dared to think people were actually interested in pictures of their vegan food, I was, and you helped me learn to eat and cook vegan.

Christina Pirello and the instructors at Organic Avenue and the Natural Gourmet Institute educated me on the basics of vegan cooking, taught me to think intuitively in the kitchen, and gave me enough skills to keep this home cook from burning down her house.

Jasmin Singer and Mariann Sullivan of Our Hen House and the volunteers and animals (special shout-out to Clover the goat) at the Woodstock Farm Animal Sanctuary have taught me that veganism extends beyond the plate.

Victoria Moran, who is creating a peaceful army of vegan lifestyle coaches through the Main Street Vegan Academy, taught me that you can be fiercely ethical and incredibly gentle while working to change the hearts of humans and save animals' lives.

To women over forty who know that every decade is a new opportunity, not a lost chapter, I thank you.

My recipe testers Amanda, Ashley, Aviv, Cassandra, Erica, Gayle, Jamie, Jared, Jennifer, Megan, Sabrina, Terri, and Regina supported me, a fellow home cook, from day one. A special thanks to Melissa who tested every single recipe!

My husband and I opted for a furry family. Our hearts still ache for our dog Abby and cat Matisse. Our hearts overflow with love for our current feline companions CK and Ernie.

Aunt Candy—what can I say? She still thinks I could be president of the United States.

Janice and Larry Fields, my parents, have always been so incredibly proud and supportive of their somewhat odd and loud daughter. Their support is why I'm still odd and still loud. Who could ask for more from parents?

My husband, Dave Burgess, is my biggest fan. And I am his. How lucky that we have become two entirely different people from when we first met and laugh louder and love harder than ever.

Resources for Vegan Women

Our Blogs

Ginny: www.TheVeganRD.com
JL: www.JLGoesVegan.com

Online Vegan Communities and Discussion Boards

http://forum.theppk.com/
www.veggieboards.com/f/

Vegan Nutrition

Websites

www.jacknorrisrd.com
http://nutritionfacts.org/
www.TheVeganRD.com
www.veganhealth.org
www.vegetariannutrition.net
www.vrg.org

Books

Becoming Vegan, by Brenda Davis and Vesanto Melina (Summertown, TN: Book Publishing, 2013)

Defeating Diabetes, by Brenda Davis and Tom Barnard (Summertown, TN: Healthy Living Publications, 2003)

Plant Powered Diet, by Sharon Palmer (New York: The Experiment, 2012)

Simply Vegan, 5th edition, by Debra Wasserman and Reed Mangels (Baltimore, MD: The Vegetarian Resource Group, 2012)

Vegan for Life, by Jack Norris and Virginia Messina (Cambridge, MA: Da Capo Press, 2011)

Women's Health (Not Vegan)

Change Your Menopause, by Dr. Wulf Utian (Beachwood, OH: Utian Press, 2011)

The Fertility Diet, by Jorge E Chavarro, Walter Willet, and Patrick J Skerrett (New York: McGraw Hill, 2008)

Dr. Susan Love's Breast Book, by Susan Love (Cambridge, MA: Da Capo Press, 2000)

Nutrition for Pregnancy and Breastfeeding

The Everything Vegan Pregnancy Book, by Reed Mangels (Avon, MA: Adams Media, 2011)

Vegan Pregnancy Survival Guide, by Sayward Rebhal (Portland, OR: Herbivore Books, 2011)

Sports Nutrition

Vegan Bodybuilding and Fitness, by Robert Cheeke (Summertown, TN: Book Publishing, 2010)

Vegetarian Sports Nutrition, by D. Enette Larson-Meyer (Champaign, IL: Human Kinetics, 2007)

Health and Happiness Beyond the Scale

Websites

www.bodypositive.com/
www.choosingraw.com (for vegans recovering from eating disorders)
www.haescommunity.org/
www.sizediversityandhealth.org
www.StopChasingSkinny.com

Books

Health at Every Size, by Linda Bacon (Dallas, TX: BenBella, 2008)

Intuitive Eating, by Evelyn Tribole and Elyse Resch (New York: St. Martin's Press, 2012)

A Few of Our Favorite Vegan Cookbooks

Big Vegan, by Robin Asbell (San Francisco: Chronicle Books, 2011)

Blissful Bites, by Christy Morgan (Dallas, TX: BenBella Books, 2011)

The Blooming Platter, by Betsy DiJulio (Woodstock, VA: Vegan Heritage Press, 2011)

Great Vegetarian Cooking Under Pressure, by Lorna Sass (New York: William Morrow Cookbooks, 1994)

Let Them Eat Vegan, by Dreena Burton (Cambridge, MA: Da Capo Press, 2012)

The New Fast Food: The Veggie Queen Pressure Cooks Whole Food Meals in Less Than 30 Minutes, by Jill Nussinow (Santa Rosa, CA: Vegetarian Connection Press, 2012)

Tofu Cookery, 25th Anniversary Edition, by Louise Hagler (Summertown, TN: Book Publishing, 2008)

The Urban Vegan, by Dynise Balcavage (Guilford, CT: Globe Pequot Press, 2010)

Vegan Comfort Food, by Alicia Simpson (New York: The Experiment, 2009)

Vegan Diner, by Julie Hasson (Philadelphia: Running Press, 2011)

Vegan Eats World, by Terry Hope Romero (Cambridge, MA: Da Capo Press, 2012)

Vegan on the Cheap, by Robin Robertson (Hoboken, NJ: John Wiley & Sons, 2010)

Veganomicon, by Isa Chandra Moskowitz and Terry Hope Romero (Cambridge, MA: Da Capo Press, 2007)

World Vegan Feast, by Bryanna Clark Grogan (Woodstock, VA: Vegan Heritage Press, 2011)

LIVING THE VEGAN LIFE

Books

Living Among Meateaters: The Vegetarian's Survival Handbook, by Carol J. Adams (New York: Continuum, 2003)

Main Street Vegan, by Victoria Moran (New York: Penguin, 2012)

Sistah Vegan: Black Female Vegans Speak out on Food, Identity, Health and Society, by Breeze Harper (Brooklyn, NY: Lantern Books, 2010)

30-Day Vegan Challenge, by Colleen Patrick-Goudreau (New York: Ballantine Books, 2011)

The Ultimate Vegan Guide, by Erik Marcus (Santa Cruz, CA: Vegan.com, 2009) Also online for free, download at www.www.vegan.com/ultimate-vegan -guide/

Website

www.vegnews.com

ONLINE SHOPPING

http://vegancuts.com/
www.alternativeoutfitters.com/herbivore
www.compassioncoutureshop.com/vegan cuts
www.cosmosveganshoppe.com/
www.healthy-eating.com
www.herbivoreclothing.com/
www.veganessentials.com
www.veganstore.com
www.thevegetariansite.com

Vegan Fashion and Style Consulting

http://totalimageconsultants.com/

LGBT Vegans

http://queerveganfood.com/
https://www.facebook.com/groups/90514461349/ (Gay Vegan Network on Facebook)
www.lgbtcompassion.org/

Vegetarian Feminist Theory

Books

Defiant Daughters: 21 Women on Art, Activism, Animals, and the Sexual Politics of Meat, edited by Kara Davis and Wendy Lee (New York: Lantern Books, 2013)

The Feminist Care Tradition in Animal Ethics, edited by Josephine Donovan and Carol Adams (New York: Columbia University Press, 2007)

Sexual Politics of Meat, by Carol J Adams (New York: Continuum Publishing, 1992)

Website

http://veganfeministagitator.blogspot.com/

Vegan Activism

Books

The Animal Activist's Handbook, by Matt Ball and Bruce Friedrich (New York: Lantern Books, 2009)

Animal Impact: Secrets Proven to Achieve Results and Move the World, by Caryn Ginsberg (Arlington, VA: Priority Ventures Group, LLC, 2011)

Change of Heart, by Nick Cooney (New York: Lantern Books, 2011)

The Lifelong Activist, by Hillary Rettig (Brooklyn, NY: Lantern Books, 2006)

Strategic Action for Animals, by Melanie Joy (New York: Lantern Books, 2008)

Striking at the Roots, by Mark Hawthorne (Winchester, UK: O Books, 2008)

Websites

www.OurHenHouse.org
www.veganoutreach.org

Appendix A:
Be a Healthy
Vegan Woman for Life

- Get regular exercise—both aerobic and strengthening exercise.
- Manage stress and depression.
- Stay socially and mentally active.
- If you smoke, take steps to quit.
- Use a sunscreen that protects against UVA and UVB rays.
- Take supplements of vitamin B_{12}, vitamin D, and the omega-3 fats DHA and EPA.
- Eat plenty of calcium-rich foods: calcium-set tofu, fortified plant milks and juices, leafy greens like kale, collard greens, and turnip greens.
- Eat several servings of legumes every day.
- Eat traditional soyfoods like tofu, soymilk, tempeh, and miso.
- Eat generous amounts of fruits and vegetables. Choose a variety, including leafy greens and good sources of vitamin C. Choose both cooked and raw vegetables.
- Include a serving or two of nuts or seeds in your daily menu.
- Choose a daily source of essential omega-3 fats—walnuts, flaxseeds, chia seeds, or canola oil.
- Use vegetable oils with a light hand and choose extra-virgin olive oil most of the time.
- Choose slow carbs most often—sweet potatoes, oats, pasta, and barley.

- Use moist cooking methods like braising, simmering, and—best of all—steaming. When you bake, roast, or grill, marinate the food in acidic sauces first, like those made from lemon juice, tomatoes, or vinegar.
- If you drink, choose red wine most of the time and keep intake moderate.
- Minimize processed foods to keep your sodium intake in check. When you add salt to foods, choose iodized salt.
- Eat healthy whole plant foods most of the time, but enjoy some treats, too.
- Eat mindfully, paying attention to hunger signals.
- Choose foods for pleasure and health rather than weight reduction.
- Celebrate your vegan lifestyle—one that brings benefits well beyond health.

APPENDIX B: FOOD SOURCES OF NUTRIENTS THAT ARE IMPORTANT IN WOMEN'S HEALTH

	Protein	Iron	Vitamin C	Zinc	Folate	Calcium	Potassium	Vitamin K	Magnesium
How It Affects Women's Health	For strong muscles and bones	For healthy blood, immunity, and hair	Important for iron absorption, healthy skin and bones, and chronic disease prevention	Supports healthy hair and skin	Crucial in early pregnancy and may play a role in fertility	Supports bone health	Supports heart and bone health	Supports bone health	May reduce symptoms of PMS, important in diabetes
RDA for Women	46 grams	8–18 grams	75 milligrams	8–12 milligrams	400 micrograms	1000–1200 milligrams	4700 milligrams	90 micrograms	310–320 milligrams
LEGUMES (½ cup)									
Adzuki beans	8.6	2.3		2.0	140	32	611		60
Black beans	7.6	2.6		0.7	80	51	400		45
Chickpeas	7.5	2.4		1.2		40	239		39
Great northern beans	7.4	1.9		0.78	90	60	346		44
Kidney beans	8.1	2.0		0.9	115	25	358		37
Lentils	8.9	3.3		1.3	179		365		
Lima beans	7.3	2		0.9	136		365		48
Navy beans	7.5	2.3		0.9		63	354		48
Peanuts, ¼ cup	9.4	1.7		1.2	88		257		62
Peanut butter, 2 tbsp	8	0.6		0.9	24		238		51
Pinto beans	7.7	2.2		0.8	147	40	373		43
Vegetarian baked beans	6	1.7		2.9		43	284		34

— continues —

APPENDIX B *continued*

	Protein	Iron	Vitamin C	Zinc	Folate	Calcium	Potassium	Vitamin K	Magnesium
SOYFOODS AND SEITAN									
Soybeans	14.3	4.4		1.0	46	87	443		74
Soybeans, immature (edamame)	11	2.2	15	0.8	100	130	485		54
Soy curls	6.6	1.8					340		56
Soymilk, fortified	5–10	1.1–1.8		0.6		250–300	299		39
Soynuts, ¼ cup	17	1.7		2.0	88	60	586		98
Tempeh	15.5	1.3		1.0	20	55			67
Textured Vegetable Protein	11	1.4				85			
Tofu, firm	10–20	2.0		1.1		150–300	186		47
Tofu, soft	8–10			0.8	54	100–150*	149		33
Veggie meats, 1 ounce	6–18	0.8–2.1		1.4–1.8					
Seitan, 3 ounces	22	1.7							
NUTS AND SEEDS									
Almonds, ¼ cup	7.3	1.3		1.1		24	252		98
Almond butter, 2 tbsp	7.0	1.1		1.0		86	243		97
Brazil nuts, 4 pieces	2.8	0.5	0.8	0.7		15	130		74
Cashews, ¼ cup	5.2	2.0		0.9			187		83
Pecans, ¼ cup	2.5	0.7		1.1			101		30
Pistachios, ¼ cup	6.4	1.1		0.6			285		31
Pumpkin seeds, 2 tbsp	4.4	0.25		1.1			250		74

— *continues* —

APPENDIX B *continued*

	Protein	Iron	Vitamin C	Zinc	Folate	Calcium	Potassium	Vitamin K	Magnesium
Sunflower seeds, 2 tbsp	3.1	1.1		0.9	40		139		21
Tahini, 2 tbsp	5.0	0.75		1.4	29	128	124		29
Walnuts, ¼ cup	4.4	0.8		0.9	28		125		45
VEGETABLES (½ cup cooked)									
Avocado, ¼ cup					30		182		11
Beet greens	1.8	1.4	18				654		49
Bok choy	1.3	0.9	22		35	79	315		
Broccoli	1.8		51		84	31	229	110	
Brussels sprouts	2.0	0.9	48		47		247	109	
Butternut squash	0.9		15			46	291		30
Collards	2.0	1.1	17		88	133	110	418	
Kale	1.3		26			47		531	
Peas	3.4	1.2	12		35		102		18
Pepper	0.6		60				130		
Potato	1.8	0.8	6				378		20
Spinach	2.6	3.2	9		131		419	444	78
Sweet potato	2.2	1.2	21		10	45	377		29
Swiss chard	1.6	2.0	16				480	286	75
Tomato juice, 1 cup			44		51		556		
Turnip greens	0.8	0.6	20		85	98	146	265	16
FRUITS									
Dried figs		1.5				120	506		51
Banana			10		24		422		32
Blueberries									
Cantaloupe			59		34		213		

— continues —

APPENDIX B *continued*

	Protein	Iron	Vitamin C	Zinc	Folate	Calcium	Potassium	Vitamin K	Magnesium
Grapefruit			39				180		
Grapefruit juice, 6 ounces			67				300		22
Guava, ½ cup			188		40		344		18
Kiwi			64				215		12
Orange, 1 medium			83		48	60	232		15
Orange juice, fortified			84		47	300	443		27
Papaya, 1 medium			188				131		15
Pineapple			39						
Prunes, ¼ cup		1.2							
Strawberries			49						
GRAINS (½ cup cooked)									
Barley	1.7	1.0							32
Oatmeal	3.0	1.0		1.2					21
Pasta, whole wheat	4.0	0.7			137				
Pasta, white enriched	4.0	0.8							12
Quinoa	4.0	1.4		1.0	39		159		59
Brown rice	2.5	0.5		0.6					43
Whole wheat bread	2–6	0.9							23
FATS (1 teaspoon)									

REFERENCES

CHAPTER 1: GOING VEGAN: AN EASY TRANSITION

1. Haverstock K, Forgays DK. To eat or not to eat. A comparison of current and former animal product limiters. *Appetite* 2012;58:1030.

CHAPTER 2: VEGAN NUTRITION: A PRIMER

1. Hu FB, Stampfer MJ, Manson JE, et al. Frequent nut consumption and risk of coronary heart disease in women: prospective cohort study. *BMJ* 1998;317:1341–5.

2. Ellsworth JL, Kushi LH, Folsom AR. Frequent nut intake and risk of death from coronary heart disease and all causes in postmenopausal women: the Iowa Women's Health Study. *Nutr Metab Cardiovasc Dis* 2001;11:372–7.

3. McManus K, Antinoro L, Sacks F. A randomized controlled trial of a moderate-fat, low-energy diet compared with a low fat, low-energy diet for weight loss in overweight adults. *Int J Obes Relat Metab Disord* 2001;25:1503–11.

4. Alper CM, Mattes RD. Effects of chronic peanut consumption on energy balance and hedonics. *Int J Obes Relat Metab Disord* 2002;26:1129–37.

5. Sanders TA. DHA status of vegetarians. *Prostaglandins Leukot Essent Fatty Acids* 2009;81:137–41.

6. Savage DG, Lindenbaum J. Neurological complications of acquired cobalamin deficiency: clinical aspects. *Baillieres Clin Haematol* 1995;8:657–78.

7. Skarupski KA, Tangney C, Li H, Ouyang B, Evans DA, Morris MC. Longitudinal association of vitamin B-6, folate, and vitamin B-12 with depressive symptoms among older adults over time. *Am J Clin Nutr* 2010;92:330–5.

8. Antoniades C, Antonopoulos AS, Tousoulis D, Marinou K, Stefanadis C. Homocysteine and coronary atherosclerosis: from folate fortification to the recent clinical trials. *Eur Heart J* 2009;30:6–15.

9. Janssen I, Shepard DS, Katzmarzyk PT, Roubenoff R. The healthcare costs of sarcopenia in the United States. *J Am Geriatr Soc* 2004;52:80–5.

10. Campbell WW. Synergistic use of higher-protein diets or nutritional supplements with resistance training to counter sarcopenia. *Nutr Rev* 2007;65:416–22.

11. Mithal A, Bonjour JP, Boonen S, et al. Impact of nutrition on muscle mass, strength, and performance in older adults. *Osteoporos Int* 2012.

12. Millward DJ. Sufficient protein for our elders? *Am J Clin Nutr* 2008;88:1187–8.

13. Gaffney-Stomberg E, Insogna KL, Rodriguez NR, Kerstetter JE. Increasing dietary protein requirements in elderly people for optimal muscle and bone health. *J Am Geriatr Soc* 2009;57:1073–9.

14. Campbell WW, Trappe TA, Wolfe RR, Evans WJ. The recommended dietary allowance for protein may not be adequate for older people to maintain skeletal muscle. *J Gerontol A Biol Sci Med Sci* 2001;56:M373–80.

15. Houston DK, Nicklas BJ, Ding J, et al. Dietary protein intake is associated with lean mass change in older, community-dwelling adults: the Health, Aging, and Body Composition (Health ABC) Study. *Am J Clin Nutr* 2008;87:150–5.

16. Scott D, Blizzard L, Fell J, Giles G, Jones G. Associations between dietary nutrient intake and muscle mass and strength in community-dwelling older adults: the Tasmanian Older Adult Cohort Study. *J Am Geriatr Soc* 2010;58:2129–34.

17. Knight EL, Stampfer MJ, Hankinson SE, Spiegelman D, Curhan GC. The impact of protein intake on renal function decline in women with normal renal function or mild renal insufficiency. *Ann Intern Med* 2003;138:460–7.

18. Kim MH, Bae YJ. Postmenopausal vegetarians' low serum ferritin level may reduce the risk for metabolic syndrome. *Biol Trace Elem Res* 2012;149:34–41.

CHAPTER 3: BEYOND NUTRIENTS: ONE HEALTHY DIET

1. Bacon L, Aphramor L. Weight science: evaluating the evidence for a paradigm shift. *Nutr J* 2011;10:9.

2. Valachovicova M, Krajcovicova-Kudlackova M, Blazicek P, Babinska K. No evidence of insulin resistance in normal weight vegetarians. A case control study. *Eur J Nutr* 2006;45:52–4.

3. Hung CJ, Huang PC, Li YH, Lu SC, Ho LT, Chou HF. Taiwanese vegetarians have higher insulin sensitivity than omnivores. *Br J Nutr* 2006;95:129–35.

4. Kuo CS, Lai NS, Ho LT, Lin CL. Insulin sensitivity in Chinese ovo-lactovegetarians compared with omnivores. *Eur J Clin Nutr* 2004;58:312–6.

5. Goff LM, Bell JD, So PW, Dornhorst A, Frost GS. Veganism and its relationship with insulin resistance and intramyocellular lipid. *Eur J Clin Nutr* 2005;59:291–8.

6. Waldmann A, Strohle A, Koschizke JW, Leitzmann C, Hahn A. Overall glycemic index and glycemic load of vegan diets in relation to plasma lipoproteins and triacylglycerols. *Ann Nutr Metab* 2007;51:335–44.

7. Yudkin JS, Stehouwer CD, Emeis JJ, Coppack SW. C-reactive protein in healthy subjects: associations with obesity, insulin resistance, and endothelial dysfunction: a potential role for cytokines originating from adipose tissue? *Arterioscler Thromb Vasc Biol* 1999;19:972–8.

8. Calder PC, Ahluwalia N, Brouns F, et al. Dietary factors and low-grade inflammation in relation to overweight and obesity. *Br J Nutr* 2011;106 Suppl 3:S5–78.

9. Krajcovicova-Kudlackova M, Blazicek P. C-reactive protein and nutrition. *Bratisl Lek Listy* 2005;106:345–7.

10. Szeto YT, Kwok TC, Benzie IF. Effects of a long-term vegetarian diet on biomarkers of antioxidant status and cardiovascular disease risk. *Nutrition* 2004;20:863–6.

11. Paalani M, Lee JW, Haddad E, Tonstad S. Determinants of inflammatory markers in a bi-ethnic population. *Ethn Dis* 2011;21:142–9.

12. Esposito K, Ciotola M, Giugliano D. Mediterranean diet, endothelial function and vascular inflammatory markers. *Public Health Nutr* 2006;9:1073–6.

13. Kelly KR, Haus JM, Solomon TP, et al. A low-glycemic index diet and exercise intervention reduces TNF (alpha) in isolated mononuclear cells of older, obese adults. *J Nutr* 2011;141:1089–94.

14. Pitsavos C, Panagiotakos DB, Tzima N, et al. Diet, exercise, and C-reactive protein levels in people with abdominal obesity: the ATTICA epidemiological study. *Angiology* 2007;58:225–33.

15. Pischon T, Hankinson SE, Hotamisligil GS, Rifai N, Willett WC, Rimm EB. Habitual dietary intake of n-3 and n-6 fatty acids in relation to inflammatory markers among US men and women. *Circulation* 2003;108:155–60.

16. Johnson GH, Fritsche K. Effect of dietary linoleic acid on markers of inflammation in healthy persons: a systematic review of randomized controlled trials. *J Acad Nutr Diet* 2012;112:1029–41 e15.

17. Levitan EB, Cook NR, Stampfer MJ, et al. Dietary glycemic index, dietary glycemic load, blood lipids, and C-reactive protein. *Metabolism* 2008;57:437–43.

18. Lopez-Garcia E, Schulze MB, Meigs JB, et al. Consumption of trans fatty acids is related to plasma biomarkers of inflammation and endothelial dysfunction. *J Nutr* 2005;135:562–6.

19. Blokhina O, Virolainen E, Fagerstedt KV. Antioxidants, oxidative damage and oxygen deprivation stress: a review. *Ann Bot* 2003;91 Spec No:179–94.

20. Ames BN, Gold LS, Willett WC. The causes and prevention of cancer. *Proc Natl Acad Sci U S A* 1995;92:5258–65.

21. Diaz MN, Frei B, Vita JA, Keaney JF, Jr. Antioxidants and atherosclerotic heart disease. *N Engl J Med* 1997;337:408–16.

22. Ceriello A, Bortolotti N, Motz E, et al. Meal-induced oxidative stress and low-density lipoprotein oxidation in diabetes: the possible role of hyperglycemia. *Metabolism* 1999;48:1503–8.

23. Carlsen MH, Halvorsen BL, Holte K, et al. The total antioxidant content of more than 3100 foods, beverages, spices, herbs and supplements used worldwide. *Nutr J* 2010;9:3.

24. Uribarri J, Tuttle KR. Advanced glycation end products and nephrotoxicity of high-protein diets. *Clin J Am Soc Nephrol* 2006;1:1293–9.

25. Ahmed N. Advanced glycation endproducts—role in pathology of diabetic complications. *Diabetes Res Clin Pract* 2005;67:3–21.

26. Uribarri J, Cai W, Peppa M, et al. Circulating glycotoxins and dietary advanced glycation endproducts: two links to inflammatory response, oxidative stress, and aging. *J Gerontol A Biol Sci Med Sci* 2007;62:427–33.

27. Vlassara H, Cai W, Crandall J, et al. Inflammatory mediators are induced by dietary glycotoxins, a major risk factor for diabetic angiopathy. *Proc Natl Acad Sci U S A* 2002;99:15596–601.

28. Sims TJ, Rasmussen LM, Oxlund H, Bailey AJ. The role of glycation cross-links in diabetic vascular stiffening. *Diabetologia* 1996;39:946–51.

29. Cruz-Sanchez FF, Girones X, Ortega A, Alameda F, Lafuente JV. Oxidative stress in Alzheimer's disease hippocampus: a topographical study. *J Neurol Sci* 2010;299:163–7.

30. Haus JM, Carrithers JA, Trappe SW, Trappe TA. Collagen, crosslinking, and advanced glycation end products in aging human skeletal muscle. *J Appl Physiol* 2007;103:2068–76.

31. Koschinsky T, He CJ, Mitsuhashi T, et al. Orally absorbed reactive

glycation products (glycotoxins): an environmental risk factor in diabetic nephropathy. *Proc Natl Acad Sci U S A* 1997;94:6474–9.

32. Wu CH, Yen GC. Inhibitory effect of naturally occurring flavonoids on the formation of advanced glycation endproducts. *J Agric Food Chem* 2005;53:3167–73.

33. Dearlove RP, Greenspan P, Hartle DK, Swanson RB, Hargrove JL. Inhibition of protein glycation by extracts of culinary herbs and spices. *J Med Food* 2008;11:275–81.

34. Uribarri J, Woodruff S, Goodman S, et al. Advanced glycation end products in foods and a practical guide to their reduction in the diet. *J Am Diet Assoc* 2010;110:911–16 e12.

35. Yoshikawa T, Miyazaki A, Fujimoto S. Decrease in serum levels of advanced glycation end-products by short-term lifestyle modification in non-diabetic middle-aged females. *Med Sci Monit* 2009;15:PH65–73.

CHAPTER 5: DIET AND HORMONES THROUGHOUT A WOMAN'S LIFE

1. Messina M, Nagata C, Wu AH. Estimated Asian adult soy protein and isoflavone intakes. *Nutr Cancer* 2006;55:1–12.

2. Messina M. Investigating the optimal soy protein and isoflavone intakes for women: a perspective. *Womens Health (Lond Engl)* 2008;4:337–56.

3. Barnard ND, Scialli AR, Hurlock D, Bertron P. Diet and sex-hormone binding globulin, dysmenorrhea, and premenstrual symptoms. *Obstet Gynecol* 2000;95:245–50.

4. Bennett FC, Ingram DM. Diet and female sex hormone concentrations: an intervention study for the type of fat consumed. *Am J Clin Nutr* 1990;52:808–12.

5. Aubertin-Leheudre M, Hamalainen E, Adlercreutz H. Diets and hormonal levels in postmenopausal women with or without breast cancer. *Nutr Cancer* 2011;63:514–24.

6. Quaranta S, Buscaglia MA, Meroni MG, Colombo E, Cella S. Pilot study of the efficacy and safety of a modified-release magnesium 250 mg tablet (Sincromag) for the treatment of premenstrual syndrome. *Clin Drug Investig* 2007;27:51–8.

7. Wyatt KM, Dimmock PW, Jones PW, Shaughn O'Brien PM. Efficacy of vitamin B-6 in the treatment of premenstrual syndrome: systematic review. *BMJ* 1999;318:1375–81.

8. Kim HW, Kwon MK, Kim NS, Reame NE. Intake of dietary soy isoflavones in relation to perimenstrual symptoms of Korean women living in the USA. *Nurs Health Sci* 2006;8:108–13.

9. Deutch B. Menstrual pain in Danish women correlated with low n-3 polyunsaturated fatty acid intake. *Eur J Clin Nutr* 1995;49:508–16.

10. Thys-Jacobs S, Starkey P, Bernstein D, Tian J. Calcium carbonate and the premenstrual syndrome: effects on premenstrual and menstrual symptoms. Premenstrual Syndrome Study Group. *Am J Obstet Gynecol* 1998;179:444–52.

11. Whelan AM, Jurgens TM, Naylor H. Herbs, vitamins and minerals in the treatment of premenstrual syndrome: a systematic review. *Can J Clin Pharmacol* 2009;16:e407–29.

12. Murakami K, Sasaki S, Takahashi Y, et al. Dietary glycemic index is associated with decreased premenstrual symptoms in young Japanese women. *Nutrition* 2008;24:554–61.

13. Gonzalez F. Inflammation in Polycystic Ovary Syndrome: underpinning of insulin resistance and ovarian dysfunction. *Steroids* 2012;77:300–5.

14. Moran LJ, Noakes M, Clifton PM, Wittert GA, Williams G, Norman RJ. Short-term meal replacements followed by dietary macronutrient restriction enhance weight loss in polycystic ovary syndrome. *Am J Clin Nutr* 2006;84:77–87.

15. Ehrmann DA. Polycystic ovary syndrome. *N Engl J Med* 2005;352:1223–36.

16. Khani B, Mehrabian F, Khalesi E, Eshraghi A. Effect of soy phytoestrogen on metabolic and hormonal disturbance of women with polycystic ovary syndrome. *J Res Med Sci* 2011;16:297–302.

17. Romualdi D, Costantini B, Campagna G, Lanzone A, Guido M. Is there a role for soy isoflavones in the therapeutic approach to polycystic ovary syndrome? Results from a pilot study. *Fertil Steril* 2008;90:1826–33.

18. Tremellen K, Pearce K. Dysbiosis of Gut Microbiota (DOGMA)—a novel theory for the development of Polycystic Ovarian Syndrome. *Med Hypotheses* 2012;79:104–12.

19. Rushton DH. Nutritional factors and hair loss. *Clin Exp Dermatol* 2002;27:396–404.

20. Goldberg LJ, Lenzy Y. Nutrition and hair. *Clin Dermatol* 2010;28:412–9.

21. Jacquet A, Coolen V, Vandermander J. Effect of dietary supplementation with INVERSION Femme on slimming, hair loss, and skin and nail parameters in women. *Adv Ther* 2007;24:1154–71.

22. Shojania AM, Wylie B. The effect of oral contraceptives on vitamin B12 metabolism. *Am J Obstet Gynecol* 1979;135:129–34.

23. Gardyn J, Mittelman M, Zlotnik J, Sela BA, Cohen AM. Oral contraceptives can cause falsely low vitamin B(12) levels. *Acta Haematol* 2000;104:22–4.

24. Smith RN, Mann NJ, Braue A, Makelainen H, Varigos GA. A low-glycemic-load diet improves symptoms in acne vulgaris patients: a randomized controlled trial. *Am J Clin Nutr* 2007;86:107–15.

25. Kwon HH, Yoon JY, Hong JS, Jung JY, Park MS, Suh DH. Clinical and histological effect of a low glycaemic load diet in treatment of acne vulgaris in Korean patients: a randomized, controlled trial. *Acta Derm Venereol* 2012;92:241–6.

26. Ciotta L, Calogero AE, Farina M, De Leo V, La Marca A, Cianci A. Clinical, endocrine and metabolic effects of acarbose, an alpha-glucosidase inhibitor, in PCOS patients with increased insulin response and normal glucose tolerance. *Hum Reprod* 2001;16:2066–72.

27. Armstrong BK, Brown JB, Clarke HT, et al. Diet and reproductive hormones: a study of vegetarian and nonvegetarian postmenopausal women. *J Natl Cancer Inst* 1981;67:761–7.

28. Hartmann S, Steinhart H. Natural occurrence of steroid hormones in food. *Food Chem* 1998;62:7–20.

29. Darling JA, Laing AH, Harkness RA. A survey of the steroids in cows' milk. *J Endocrinol* 1974;62:291–7.

30. Adebamowo CA, Spiegelman D, Danby FW, Frazier AL, Willett WC, Holmes MD. High school dietary dairy intake and teenage acne. *J Am Acad Dermatol* 2005;52:207–14.

31. Arbesman H. Dairy and acne—the iodine connection. *J Am Acad Dermatol* 2005;53:1102.

32. El-Akawi Z, Abdel-Latif N, Abdul-Razzak K. Does the plasma level of vitamins A and E affect acne condition? *Clin Exp Dermatol* 2006;31:430–4.

33. Amer M, Bahgat MR, Tosson Z, Abdel Mowla MY, Amer K. Serum zinc in acne vulgaris. *Int J Dermatol* 1982;21:481–4.

34. Fraser GE, Shavlik DJ. Ten years of life: is it a matter of choice? *Arch Intern Med* 2001;161:1645–52.

35. Avis NE, Brockwell S, Colvin A. A universal menopausal syndrome? *Am J Med* 2005;118 Suppl 12B:37–46.

36. Martin MC, Block JE, Sanchez SD, Arnaud CD, Beyene Y. Menopause without symptoms: the endocrinology of menopause among

rural Mayan Indians. *Am J Obstet Gynecol* 1993;168:1839–43; discussion 1843–5.

37. Shultz TD, Leklem JE. Nutrient intake and hormonal status of premenopausal vegetarian Seventh-Day Adventists and premenopausal nonvegetarians. *Nutr Cancer* 1983;4:247–59.

38. Gold EB, Sternfeld B, Kelsey JL, et al. Relation of demographic and lifestyle factors to symptoms in a multi-racial/ethnic population of women 40–55 years of age. *Am J Epidemiol* 2000;152:463–73.

39. Taku K, Melby MK, Kronenberg F, Kurzer MS, Messina M. Extracted or synthesized soybean isoflavones reduce menopausal hot flash frequency and severity: systematic review and meta-analysis of randomized controlled trials. *Menopause* 2012;19:776–90.

CHAPTER 6: A PLANT-BASED PLAN TO ENHANCE FERTILITY

1. Chavarro JE, Rich-Edwards JW, Rosner BA, Willett WC. Diet and lifestyle in the prevention of ovulatory disorder infertility. *Obstet Gynecol* 2007;110:1050–8.

2. Chavarro JE, Rich-Edwards JW, Rosner BA, Willett WC. A prospective study of dietary carbohydrate quantity and quality in relation to risk of ovulatory infertility. *Eur J Clin Nutr* 2009;63:78–86.

3. Hjollund NH, Jensen TK, Bonde JP, Henriksen TB, Andersson AM, Skakkebaek NE. Is glycosylated haemoglobin a marker of fertility? A follow-up study of first-pregnancy planners. *Hum Reprod* 1999;14:1478–82.

4. Chavarro JE, Rich-Edwards JW, Rosner BA, Willett WC. Dietary fatty acid intakes and the risk of ovulatory infertility. *Am J Clin Nutr* 2007;85:231–7.

5. Missmer SA, Chavarro JE, Malspeis S, et al. A prospective study of dietary fat consumption and endometriosis risk. *Hum Reprod* 2010;25:1528–35.

6. Morrison JA, Glueck CJ, Wang P. Dietary trans fatty acid intake is associated with increased fetal loss. *Fertil Steril* 2008;90:385–90.

7. Gillingham LG, Harris-Janz S, Jones PJ. Dietary monounsaturated fatty acids are protective against metabolic syndrome and cardiovascular disease risk factors. *Lipids* 2011;46:209–28.

8. Chavarro JE, Rich-Edwards JW, Rosner BA, Willett WC. Protein intake and ovulatory infertility. *Am J Obstet Gynecol* 2008;198:210 e1–7.

9. Anderson K, Nisenblat V, Norman R. Lifestyle factors in people seeking infertility treatment—a review. *Aust N Z J Obstet Gynaecol* 2010;50:8–20.

10. Parazzini F, Chiaffarino F, Surace M, et al. Selected food intake and risk of endometriosis. *Hum Reprod* 2004;19:1755–9.

11. Visioli F, Hagen TM. Antioxidants to enhance fertility: role of eNOS and potential benefits. *Pharmacol Res* 2011;64:431–7.

12. Chavarro JE, Rich-Edwards JW, Rosner BA, Willett WC. Caffeinated and alcoholic beverage intake in relation to ovulatory disorder infertility. *Epidemiology* 2009;20:374–81.

13. Rich-Edwards JW, Spiegelman D, Garland M, et al. Physical activity, body mass index, and ovulatory disorder infertility. *Epidemiology* 2002;13:184–90.

14. Kiddy DS, Hamilton-Fairley D, Bush A, et al. Improvement in endocrine and ovarian function during dietary treatment of obese women with polycystic ovary syndrome. *Clin Endocrinol (Oxf)* 1992;36:105–11.

15. Wong WY, Merkus HM, Thomas CM, Menkveld R, Zielhuis GA, Steegers-Theunissen RP. Effects of folic acid and zinc sulfate on male factor subfertility: a double-blind, randomized, placebo-controlled trial. *Fertil Steril* 2002;77:491–8.

16. Olsen J, Bolumar F, Boldsen J, Bisanti L. Does moderate alcohol intake reduce fecundability? A European multicenter study on infertility and subfecundity. European Study Group on Infertility and Subfecundity. *Alcohol Clin Exp Res* 1997;21:206–12.

17. Frey KA, Navarro SM, Kotelchuck M, Lu MC. The clinical content of preconception care: preconception care for men. *Am J Obstet Gynecol* 2008;199:S389–95.

18. Tremellen K. Oxidative stress and male infertility—a clinical perspective. *Hum Reprod Update* 2008;14:243–58.

19. Barr SI, Janelle KC, Prior JC. Vegetarian vs nonvegetarian diets, dietary restraint, and subclinical ovulatory disturbances: prospective 6-mo study. *Am J Clin Nutr* 1994;60:887–94.

20. Karelis AD, Fex A, Filion ME, Adlercreutz H, Aubertin-Leheudre M. Comparison of sex hormonal and metabolic profiles between omnivores and vegetarians in pre- and post-menopausal women. *Br J Nutr* 2010;104:222–6.

21. Barnard ND, Scialli AR, Hurlock D, Bertron P. Diet and sex-hormone binding globulin, dysmenorrhea, and premenstrual symptoms. *Obstet Gynecol* 2000;95:245–50.

22. Toledo E, Lopez-del Burgo C, Ruiz-Zambrana A, et al. Dietary patterns and difficulty conceiving: a nested case-control study. *Fertil Steril* 2011;96:1149–53.

23. Verkasalo PK, Appleby PN, Davey GK, Key TJ. Soy milk intake and plasma sex hormones: a cross-sectional study in pre- and postmenopausal women (EPIC-Oxford). *Nutr Cancer* 2001;40:79–86.

24. Hooper L, Ryder JJ, Kurzer MS, et al. Effects of soy protein and isoflavones on circulating hormone concentrations in pre- and post-menopausal women: a systematic review and meta-analysis. *Hum Reprod Update* 2009;15:423–40.

25. Kurzer MS. Hormonal effects of soy in premenopausal women and men. *J Nutr* 2002;132:570S-3S.

26. Tsuchiya M, Miura T, Hanaoka T, et al. Effect of soy isoflavones on endometriosis: interaction with estrogen receptor 2 gene polymorphism. *Epidemiology* 2007;18:402–8.

27. Chu M, Seltzer TF. Myxedema coma induced by ingestion of raw bok choy. *N Engl J Med* 2010;362:1945–6.

28. Hamilton-Reeves JM, Vazquez G, Duval SJ, Phipps WR, Kurzer MS, Messina MJ. Clinical studies show no effects of soy protein or isoflavones on reproductive hormones in men: results of a meta-analysis. *Fertil Steril* 2009;94:997–1007.

29. Messina M. Soybean isoflavone exposure does not have feminizing effects on men: a critical examination of the clinical evidence. *Fertil Steril* 2010;93:2095–104.

30. Mitchell JH, Cawood E, Kinniburgh D, Provan A, Collins AR, Irvine DS. Effect of a phytoestrogen food supplement on reproductive health in normal males. *Clin Sci (Lond)* 2001;100:613–8.

31. Beaton LK, McVeigh BL, Dillingham BL, Lampe JW, Duncan AM. Soy protein isolates of varying isoflavone content do not adversely affect semen quality in healthy young men. *Fertil Steril* 2009.

32. Messina M, Watanabe S, Setchell KD. Report on the 8th International Symposium on the Role of Soy in Health Promotion and Chronic Disease Prevention and Treatment. *J Nutr* 2009;139:796S–802S.

33. Casini ML, Gerli S, Unfer V. An infertile couple suffering from oligospermia by partial sperm maturation arrest: can phytoestrogens play a therapeutic role? A case report study. *Gynecol Endocrinol* 2006;22:399–401.

CHAPTER 7: GROWING NEW VEGANS:
NUTRITION FOR PREGNANCY AND BREASTFEEDING

1. Carter JP, Furman T, Hutcheson HR. Preeclampsia and reproductive performance in a community of vegans. *South Med J* 1987;80:692–7.

2. Thomas J, Ellis FR. The health of vegans during pregnancy. *Proc Nutr Soc* 1977;36:46A.

3. Dagnelie PC, van Staveren WA, Vergote FJ, et al. Nutritional status of infants aged 4 to 18 months on macrobiotic diets and matched omnivorous

control infants: a population-based mixed-longitudinal study. II. Growth and psychomotor development. *Eur J Clin Nutr* 1989;43:325–38.

4. Shull MW, Reed RB, Valadian I, Palombo R, Thorne H, Dwyer JT. Velocities of growth in vegetarian preschool children. *Pediatrics* 1977;60:410–7.

5. Caudill MA. Folate bioavailability: implications for establishing dietary recommendations and optimizing status. *Am J Clin Nutr* 2010;91:1455S–1460S.

6. Carlson SE. Docosahexaenoic acid supplementation in pregnancy and lactation. *Am J Clin Nutr* 2009;89:678S–84S.

7. Simopoulos AP, Leaf A, Salem N, Jr. Workshop on the Essentiality of and Recommended Dietary Intakes for Omega-6 and Omega-3 Fatty Acids. *J Am Coll Nutr* 1999;18:487–9.

8. Nishiyama S, Mikeda T, Okada T, Nakamura K, Kotani T, Hishinuma A. Transient hypothyroidism or persistent hyperthyrotropinemia in neonates born to mothers with excessive iodine intake. *Thyroid* 2004;14:1077–83.

9. Tan PC, Omar SZ. Contemporary approaches to hyperemesis during pregnancy. *Curr Opin Obstet Gynecol* 2011;23:87–93.

10. Steele NM, French J, Gatherer-Boyles J, Newman S, Leclaire S. Effect of acupressure by Sea-Bands on nausea and vomiting of pregnancy. *J Obstet Gynecol Neonatal Nurs* 2001;30:61–70.

11. Matthews A, Dowswell T, Haas DM, Doyle M, O'Mathuna DP. Interventions for nausea and vomiting in early pregnancy. *Cochrane Database Syst Rev* 2010:CD007575.

12. Sanders TA, Reddy S. The influence of a vegetarian diet on the fatty acid composition of human milk and the essential fatty acid status of the infant. *J Pediatr* 1992;120:S71–7.

13. Cunnane SC, Francescutti V, Brenna JT, Crawford MA. Breast-fed infants achieve a higher rate of brain and whole body docosahexaenoate accumulation than formula-fed infants not consuming dietary docosahexaenoate. *Lipids* 2000;35:105–11.

14. Jensen CL, Voigt RG, Prager TC, et al. Effects of maternal docosahexaenoic acid intake on visual function and neurodevelopment in breastfed term infants. *Am J Clin Nutr* 2005;82:125–32.

15. Hergenrather J, Hlady G, Wallace B, Savage E. Pollutants in breast milk of vegetarians. *N Engl J Med* 1981;304:792.

16. North K, Golding J. A maternal vegetarian diet in pregnancy is associated with hypospadias. The ALSPAC Study Team. Avon Longitudinal Study of Pregnancy and Childhood. *BJU Int* 2000;85:107–13.

17. Carmichael SL, Ma C, Feldkamp ML, et al. Nutritional factors and hypospadias risks. *Paediatr Perinat Epidemiol* 2012;26:353–60.

18. Pierik FH, Burdorf A, Deddens JA, Juttmann RE, Weber RF. Maternal and paternal risk factors for cryptorchidism and hypospadias: a case-control study in newborn boys. *Environ Health Perspect* 2004;112:1570–6.

Chapter 8: Powered by Plants:
The Vegan Female Athlete

1. Powers SK, DeRuisseau KC, Quindry J, Hamilton KL. Dietary antioxidants and exercise. *J Sports Sci* 2004;22:81–94.

2. Atalay M, Lappalainen J, Sen CK. Dietary antioxidants for the athlete. *Curr Sports Med Rep* 2006;5:182–6.

3. Dusek T. Influence of high intensity training on menstrual cycle disorders in athletes. *Croat Med J* 2001;42:79–82.

4. Hubert P, King NA, Blundell JE. Uncoupling the effects of energy expenditure and energy intake: appetite response to short-term energy deficit induced by meal omission and physical activity. *Appetite* 1998;31:9–19.

5. Warren MP, Chua AT. Exercise-induced amenorrhea and bone health in the adolescent athlete. *Ann N Y Acad Sci* 2008;1135:244–52.

6. Zanker CL, Cooke CB. Energy balance, bone turnover, and skeletal health in physically active individuals. *Med Sci Sports Exerc* 2004;36:1372–81.

7. Manore MM. Dietary recommendations and athletic menstrual dysfunction. *Sports Med* 2002;32:887–901.

8. Barnard ND, Scialli AR, Turner-McGrievy G, Lanou AJ, Glass J. The effects of a low-fat, plant-based dietary intervention on body weight, metabolism, and insulin sensitivity. *Am J Med* 2005;118:991–7.

9. Toth MJ, Poehlman ET. Sympathetic nervous system activity and resting metabolic rate in vegetarians. *Metabolism* 1994;43:621–5.

10. Phillips SM, Atkinson SA, Tarnopolsky MA, MacDougall JD. Gender differences in leucine kinetics and nitrogen balance in endurance athletes. *J Appl Physiol* 1993;75:2134–41.

11. Phillips SM, Moore DR, Tang JE. A critical examination of dietary protein requirements, benefits, and excesses in athletes. *Int J Sport Nutr Exerc Metab* 2007;17 Suppl:S58–76.

12. Rodriguez NR, DiMarco NM, Langley S. Position of the American Dietetic Association, Dietitians of Canada, and the American College of Sports Medicine: Nutrition and athletic performance. *J Am Diet Assoc* 2009;109:509–27.

13. Romijn JA, Coyle EF, Sidossis LS, Rosenblatt J, Wolfe RR. Substrate metabolism during different exercise intensities in endurance-trained women. *J Appl Physiol* 2000;88:1707–14.

14. Larson-Meyer DE, Newcomer BR, Hunter GR. Influence of endurance running and recovery diet on intramyocellular lipid content in women: a 1H NMR study. *Am J Physiol Endocrinol Metab* 2002;282:E95–E106.

15. Laughlin GA, Yen SS. Nutritional and endocrine-metabolic aberrations in amenorrheic athletes. *J Clin Endocrinol Metab* 1996;81:4301–9.

16. Balsom PD, Soderlund K, Ekblom B. Creatine in humans with special reference to creatine supplementation. *Sports Med* 1994;18:268–80.

17. Burke DG, Chilibeck PD, Parise G, Candow DG, Mahoney D, Tarnopolsky M. Effect of creatine and weight training on muscle creatine and performance in vegetarians. *Med Sci Sports Exerc* 2003;35:1946–55.

18. Delanghe J, De Slypere JP, De Buyzere M, Robbrecht J, Wieme R, Vermeulen A. Normal reference values for creatine, creatinine, and carnitine are lower in vegetarians. *Clin Chem* 1989;35:1802–3.

19. Shomrat A, Weinstein Y, Katz A. Effect of creatine feeding on maximal exercise performance in vegetarians. *Eur J Appl Physiol* 2000;82:321–5.

20. Krajcovicova-Kudlackova M, Simoncic R, Bederova A, Babinska K, Beder I. Correlation of carnitine levels to methionine and lysine intake. *Physiol Res* 2000;49:399–402.

21. Lombard KA, Olson AL, Nelson SE, Rebouche CJ. Carnitine status of lactoovovegetarians and strict vegetarian adults and children. *Am J Clin Nutr* 1989;50:301–6.

22. Rebouche CJ, Bosch EP, Chenard CA, Schabold KJ, Nelson SE. Utilization of dietary precursors for carnitine synthesis in human adults. *J Nutr* 1989;119:1907–13.

CHAPTER 9: HEALTH AND HAPPINESS BEYOND THE SCALE

1. Hill JO, Wyatt HR, Peters JC. Energy balance and obesity. *Circulation* 2012;126:126–32.

2. Elobeid MA, Padilla MA, Brock DW, Ruden DM, Allison DB. Endocrine disruptors and obesity: an examination of selected persistent organic pollutants in the NHANES 1999–2002 data. *Int J Environ Res Public Health* 2010;7:2988–3005.

3. Power ML, Schulkin J. Sex differences in fat storage, fat metabolism, and the health risks from obesity: possible evolutionary origins. *Br J Nutr* 2008;99:931–40.

4. Carnell S, Wardle J. Appetitive traits in children. New evidence for associations with weight and a common, obesity-associated genetic variant. *Appetite* 2009;53:260–3.

5. Cecil JE, Tavendale R, Watt P, Hetherington MM, Palmer CN. An obesity-associated FTO gene variant and increased energy intake in children. *N Engl J Med* 2008;359:2558–66.

6. Taheri S, Lin L, Austin D, Young T, Mignot E. Short sleep duration is associated with reduced leptin, elevated ghrelin, and increased body mass index. *PLoS Med* 2004;1:e62.

7. Spencer EA, Appleby PN, Davey GK, Key TJ. Diet and body mass index in 38000 EPIC-Oxford meat-eaters, fish-eaters, vegetarians and vegans. *Int J Obes Relat Metab Disord* 2003;27:728–34.

8. Tonstad S, Butler T, Yan R, Fraser GE. Type of vegetarian diet, body weight, and prevalence of type 2 diabetes. *Diabetes Care* 2009;32:791–6.

9. Janelle KC, Barr SI. Nutrient intakes and eating behavior scores of vegetarian and nonvegetarian women. *J Am Diet Assoc* 1995;95:180–6, 189, quiz 187–8.

10. Thomas EL, Frost G, Barnard ML, et al. An in vivo 13C magnetic resonance spectroscopic study of the relationship between diet and adipose tissue composition. *Lipids* 1996;31:145–51.

11. Anderson JW, Baird P, Davis RH, Jr, et al. Health benefits of dietary fiber. *Nutr Rev* 2009;67:188–205.

12. Willett WC. Is dietary fat a major determinant of body fat? [see comments] [published erratum appears in *Am J Clin Nutr* 1999 Aug;70(2):304]. *Am J Clin Nutr* 1998;67:556S–562S.

13. Ludwig DS. Dietary glycemic index and obesity. *J Nutr* 2000;130:280S–283S.

14. Roberts SB. High-glycemic index foods, hunger, and obesity: is there a connection? *Nutr Rev* 2000;58:163–9.

15. Santacruz A, Marcos A, Warnberg J, et al. Interplay between weight loss and gut microbiota composition in overweight adolescents. *Obesity (Silver Spring)* 2009;17:1906–15.

16. Fischer-Posovszky P, Kukulus V, Tews D, et al. Resveratrol regulates human adipocyte number and function in a Sirt1-dependent manner. *Am J Clin Nutr* 2010;92:5–15.

17. Chantre P, Lairon D. Recent findings of green tea extract AR25 (Exolise) and its activity for the treatment of obesity. *Phytomedicine* 2002;9:3–8.

18. Yoshioka M, Lim K, Kikuzato S, et al. Effects of red-pepper diet on the energy metabolism in men. *J Nutr Sci Vitaminol (Tokyo)* 1995;41:647–56.

19. Bes-Rastrollo M, Wedick NM, Martinez-Gonzalez MA, Li TY, Sampson L, Hu FB. Prospective study of nut consumption, long-term weight change, and obesity risk in women. *Am J Clin Nutr* 2009;89:1913–9.

20. McManus K, Antinoro L, Sacks F. A randomized controlled trial of a moderate-fat, low-energy diet compared with a low-fat, low-energy diet for weight loss in overweight adults. *Int J Obes Relat Metab Disord* 2001;25:1503–11.

21. Alper CM, Mattes RD. Effects of chronic peanut consumption on energy balance and hedonics. *Int J Obes Relat Metab Disord* 2002;26:1129–37.

22. O'Neil CE, Keast DR, Nicklas TA, Fulgoni VL, 3rd. Nut consumption is associated with decreased health risk factors for cardiovascular disease and metabolic syndrome in U.S. adults: NHANES 1999–2004. *J Am Coll Nutr* 2011;30:502–10.

23. Flynn MM, Reinert SE. Comparing an olive oil–enriched diet to a standard lower-fat diet for weight loss in breast cancer survivors: a pilot study. *J Womens Health (Larchmt)* 2010;19:1155–61.

24. Weigle DS, Cummings DE, Newby PD, et al. Roles of leptin and ghrelin in the loss of body weight caused by a low fat, high carbohydrate diet. *J Clin Endocrinol Metab* 2003;88:1577–86.

25. Beasley JM, Ange BA, Anderson CA, et al. Associations between macronutrient intake and self-reported appetite and fasting levels of appetite hormones: results from the Optimal Macronutrient Intake Trial to Prevent Heart Disease. *Am J Epidemiol* 2009;169:893–900.

26. Beavers KM, Lyles MF, Davis CC, Wang X, Beavers DP, Nicklas BJ. Is lost lean mass from intentional weight loss recovered during weight regain in postmenopausal women? *Am J Clin Nutr* 2011;94:767–74.

27. Rosenbaum M, Leibel RL. Adaptive thermogenesis in humans. *Int J Obes (Lond)* 2010;34 Suppl 1:S47–55.

28. Maclean PS, Bergouignan A, Cornier MA, Jackman MR. Biology's response to dieting: the impetus for weight regain. *Am J Physiol Regul Integr Comp Physiol* 2011;301:R581–600.

29. Korner J, Aronne LJ. Pharmacological approaches to weight reduction: therapeutic targets. *J Clin Endocrinol Metab* 2004;89:2616–21.

30. Wing RR, Hill JO. Successful weight loss maintenance. *Annu Rev Nutr* 2001;21:323–41.

31. Ogden LG, Stroebele N, Wyatt HR, et al. Cluster analysis of the national weight control registry to identify distinct subgroups maintaining successful weight loss. *Obesity (Silver Spring)* 2012;20:2039–47.

32. Hamer M, Stamatakis E. Metabolically healthy obesity and risk of all-cause and cardiovascular disease mortality. *J Clin Endocrinol Metab* 2012.

33. Brochu M, Tchernof A, Dionne IJ, et al. What are the physical characteristics associated with a normal metabolic profile despite a high level of obesity in postmenopausal women? *J Clin Endocrinol Metab* 2001;86:1020–5.

34. Messier V, Karelis AD, Prud'homme D, Primeau V, Brochu M, Rabasa-Lhoret R. Identifying metabolically healthy but obese individuals in sedentary postmenopausal women. *Obesity (Silver Spring)* 2010;18:911–7.

35. Bacon L, Stern JS, Keim NL, Van Loan MD. Low bone mass in premenopausal chronic dieting obese women. *Eur J Clin Nutr* 2004;58:966–71.

36. Strohacker K, McFarlin BK. Influence of obesity, physical inactivity, and weight cycling on chronic inflammation. *Front Biosci (Elite Ed)* 2010;2:98–104.

37. Schulz M, Liese AD, Boeing H, Cunningham JE, Moore CG, Kroke A. Associations of short-term weight changes and weight cycling with incidence of essential hypertension in the EPIC-Potsdam Study. *J Hum Hypertens* 2005;19:61–7.

38. Diaz VA, Mainous AG, 3rd, Everett CJ. The association between weight fluctuation and mortality: results from a population-based cohort study. *J Community Health* 2005;30:153–65.

39. Lissner L, Odell PM, D'Agostino RB, et al. Variability of body weight and health outcomes in the Framingham population. *N Engl J Med* 1991;324:1839–44.

40. Puhl RM, Andreyeva T, Brownell KD. Perceptions of weight discrimination: prevalence and comparison to race and gender discrimination in America. *Int J Obes (Lond)* 2008;32:992–1000.

41. Klein S, Burke LE, Bray GA, et al. Clinical implications of obesity with specific focus on cardiovascular disease: a statement for professionals from the American Heart Association Council on Nutrition, Physical Activity, and Metabolism: endorsed by the American College of Cardiology Foundation. *Circulation* 2004;110:2952–67.

42. Bacon L, Stern JS, Van Loan MD, Keim NL. Size acceptance and intuitive eating improve health for obese, female chronic dieters. *J Am Diet Assoc* 2005;105:929–36.

43. Appel LJ, Moore TJ, Obarzanek E, et al. A clinical trial of the effects of dietary patterns on blood pressure. DASH Collaborative Research Group. *N Engl J Med* 1997;336:1117–24.

44. Mathieu J. What should you know about mindful and intuitive eating? *J Am Diet Assoc* 2009;109:1982–7.

45. Kristeller JL, Hallett CB. An exploratory study of a meditation-based intervention for binge eating disorder. *J Health Psychol* 1999;4:357–63.

46. Abete I, Goyenechea E, Zulet MA, Martinez JA. Obesity and metabolic syndrome: Potential benefit from specific nutritional components. *Nutr Metab Cardiovasc Dis* 2011.

47. Tappy L. Thermic effect of food and sympathetic nervous system activity in humans. *Reprod Nutr Dev* 1996;36:391–7.

48. Mojtahedi MC, Thorpe MP, Karampinos DC, et al. The effects of a higher protein intake during energy restriction on changes in body composition and physical function in older women. *J Gerontol A Biol Sci Med Sci* 2011;66:1218–25.

49. Morenga LT, Williams S, Brown R, Mann J. Effect of a relatively high-protein, high-fiber diet on body composition and metabolic risk factors in overweight women. *Eur J Clin Nutr* 2010;64:1323–31.

50. Abete I, Parra D, Martinez JA. Legume-, fish-, or high-protein-based hypocaloric diets: effects on weight loss and mitochondrial oxidation in obese men. *J Med Food* 2009;12:100–8.

51. Hermsdorff HH, Zulet MA, Abete I, Martinez JA. A legume-based hypocaloric diet reduces proinflammatory status and improves metabolic features in overweight/obese subjects. *Eur J Nutr* 2010.

52. Spiegel K, Leproult R, L'Hermite-Baleriaux M, Copinschi G, Penev PD, Van Cauter E. Leptin levels are dependent on sleep duration: relationships with sympathovagal balance, carbohydrate regulation, cortisol, and thyrotropin. *J Clin Endocrinol Metab* 2004;89:5762–71.

53. Chaput JP, Despres JP, Bouchard C, Tremblay A. Short sleep duration is associated with reduced leptin levels and increased adiposity: Results from the Quebec family study. *Obesity (Silver Spring)* 2007;15:253–61.

54. Kilpelainen TO, Qi L, Brage S, et al. Physical activity attenuates the influence of FTO variants on obesity risk: a meta-analysis of 218,166 adults and 19,268 children. *PLoS Med* 2011;8:e1001116.

55. Mangweth-Matzek B, Rupp CI, Hausmann A, et al. Never too old for eating disorders or body dissatisfaction: a community study of elderly women. *Int J Eat Disord* 2006;39:583–6.

56. Bacon L, Aphramor L. Weight science: evaluating the evidence for a paradigm shift. *Nutr J* 2011;10:9.

57. Martins Y, Pliner P, O'Connor R. Restrained eating among vegetarians: does a vegetarian eating style mask concerns about weight? *Appetite* 1999;32:145–54.

58. O'Connor MA, Touyz SW, Dunn SM, Beumont PJ. Vegetarianism in anorexia nervosa? A review of 116 consecutive cases. *Med J Aust* 1987;147:540–2.

59. Robinson-O'Brien R, Perry CL, Wall MM, Story M, Neumark-Sztainer D. Adolescent and young adult vegetarianism: better dietary intake and weight outcomes but increased risk of disordered eating behaviors. *J Am Diet Assoc* 2009;109:648–55.

60. Fisak B, Jr, Peterson RD, Tantleff-Dunn S, Molnar JM. Challenging previous conceptions of vegetarianism and eating disorders. *Eat Weight Disord* 2006;11:195–200.

61. Forestell CA, Spaeth AM, Kane SA. To eat or not to eat red meat. A closer look at the relationship between restrained eating and vegetarianism in college females. *Appetite* 2012;58:319–25.

62. Perry CL, McGuire MT, Neumark-Sztainer D, Story M. Characteristics of vegetarian adolescents in a multiethnic urban population. *J Adolesc Health* 2001;29:406–16.

CHAPTER 10: HEALTHY AGING

1. Krajcovicova-Kudlackova M, Valachovicova M, Paukova V, Dusinska M. Effects of diet and age on oxidative damage products in healthy subjects. *Physiol Res* 2008;57:647–51.

2. Glem P, Beeson WL, Fraser GE. The incidence of dementia and intake of animal products: preliminary findings from the Adventist Health Study. *Neuroepidemiology* 1993;12:28–36.

3. Sofi F, Cesari F, Abbate R, Gensini GF, Casini A. Adherence to Mediterranean diet and health status: meta-analysis. *BMJ* 2008;337:a1344.

4. Sartori AC, Vance DE, Slater LZ, Crowe M. The impact of inflammation on cognitive function in older adults: implications for healthcare practice and research. *J Neurosci Nurs* 2012;44:206–217.

5. Candela P, Gosselet F, Saint-Pol J, et al. Apical-to-basolateral transport of amyloid-beta peptides through blood-brain barrier cells is mediated by the receptor for advanced glycation end-products and is restricted by P-glycoprotein. *J Alzheimers Dis* 2010;22:849–59.

6. Cruz-Sanchez FF, Girones X, Ortega A, Alameda F, Lafuente JV. Oxidative stress in Alzheimer's disease hippocampus: a topographical study. *J Neurol Sci* 2010;299:163–7.

7. Luchsinger JA, Tang MX, Shea S, Mayeux R. Hyperinsulinemia and risk of Alzheimer disease. *Neurology* 2004;63:1187–92.

8. Stampfer MJ. Cardiovascular disease and Alzheimer's disease: common links. *J Intern Med* 2006;260:211–23.

9. Farkas E, De Vos RA, Jansen Steur EN, Luiten PG. Are Alzheimer's disease, hypertension, and cerebrocapillary damage related? *Neurobiol Aging* 2000;21:235–43.

10. Rigaud AS, Seux ML, Staessen JA, Birkenhager WH, Forette F. Cerebral complications of hypertension. *J Hum Hypertens* 2000;14:605–616.

11. Pohjasvaara T, Mantyla R, Salonen O, et al. MRI correlates of dementia after first clinical ischemic stroke. *J Neurol Sci* 2000;181:111–7.

12. Wolozin B, Kellman W, Ruosseau P, Celesia GG, Siegel G. Decreased prevalence of Alzheimer disease associated with 3-hydroxy-3-methyglutaryl coenzyme A reductase inhibitors. *Arch Neurol* 2000;57:1439–43.

13. Fonseca AC, Resende R, Oliveira CR, Pereira CM. Cholesterol and statins in Alzheimer's disease: current controversies. *Exp Neurol* 2009:223:282–93.

14. Naqvi AZ, Harty B, Mukamal KJ, Stoddard AM, Vitolins M, Dunn JE. Monounsaturated, trans, and saturated fatty acids and cognitive decline in women. *J Am Geriatr Soc* 2011;59:837–43.

15. Devore EE, Stampfer MJ, Breteler MM, et al. Dietary fat intake and cognitive decline in women with type 2 diabetes. *Diabetes Care* 2009;32:635–40.

16. Morris MC, Evans DA, Bienias JL, et al. Dietary fats and the risk of incident Alzheimer disease. *Arch Neurol* 2003;60:194–200.

17. Morris MC, Evans DA, Bienias JL, et al. Consumption of fish and n-3 fatty acids and risk of incident Alzheimer disease. *Arch Neurol* 2003;60:940–6.

18. Schaefer EJ, Bongard V, Beiser AS, et al. Plasma phosphatidylcholine docosahexaenoic acid content and risk of dementia and Alzheimer disease: the Framingham heart study. *Arch Neurol* 2006;63:1545–50.

19. Beydoun MA, Kaufman JS, Satia JA, Rosamond W, Folsom AR. Plasma n-3 fatty acids and the risk of cognitive decline in older adults: the Atherosclerosis Risk in Communities Study. *Am J Clin Nutr* 2007;85:1103–11.

20. Duron E, Hanon O. Vascular risk factors, cognitive decline, and dementia. *Vasc Health Risk Manag* 2008;4:363–81.

21. Middleton LE, Yaffe K. Promising strategies for the prevention of dementia. *Arch Neurol* 2009;66:1210–5.

22. Haan MN, Miller JW, Aiello AE, et al. Homocysteine, B vitamins, and the incidence of dementia and cognitive impairment: results from the Sacramento Area Latino Study on Aging. *Am J Clin Nutr* 2007;85:511–7.

23. Morris MC, Evans DA, Bienias JL, et al. Dietary folate and vitamin B12 intake and cognitive decline among community-dwelling older persons. *Arch Neurol* 2005;62:641–5.

24. Shah RC, Wilson RS, Tang Y, Dong X, Murray A, Bennett DA. Relation of hemoglobin to level of cognitive function in older persons. *Neuroepidemiology* 2009;32:40–6.

25. Lovell MA, Robertson JD, Teesdale WJ, Campbell JL, Markesbery WR. Copper, iron and zinc in Alzheimer's disease senile plaques. *J Neurol Sci* 1998;158:47–52.

26. Dishman RK, Berthoud HR, Booth FW, et al. Neurobiology of exercise. *Obesity (Silver Spring)* 2006;14:345–56.

27. Yoshikawa T, Miyazaki A, Fujimoto S. Decrease in serum levels of advanced glycation end-products by short-term lifestyle modification in non-diabetic middle-aged females. *Med Sci Monit* 2009;15:PH65–73.

28. Wilson RS, Hoganson GM, Rajan KB, Barnes LL, Mendes de Leon CF, Evans DA. Temporal course of depressive symptoms during the development of Alzheimer disease. *Neurology* 2010;75:21–6.

29. Saczynski JS, Beiser A, Seshadri S, Auerbach S, Wolf PA, Au R. Depressive symptoms and risk of dementia: the Framingham Heart Study. *Neurology* 2010;75:35–41.

30. Dotson VM, Beydoun MA, Zonderman AB. Recurrent depressive symptoms and the incidence of dementia and mild cognitive impairment. *Neurology* 2010;75:27–34.

31. White LR, Petrovitch H, Ross GW, et al. Brain aging and midlife tofu consumption. *J Am Coll Nutr* 2000;19:242–55.

32. Woo J, Lynn H, Lau WY, et al. Nutrient intake and psychological health in an elderly Chinese population. *Int J Geriatr Psychiatry* 2006;21:1036–43.

33. Henderson VW, St John JA, Hodis HN, et al. Long-term soy isoflavone supplementation and cognition in women: a randomized, controlled trial. *Neurology* 2012;78:1841–8.

34. Rae C, Digney AL, McEwan SR, Bates TC. Oral creatine monohydrate supplementation improves brain performance: a double-blind, placebo-controlled, cross-over trial. *Proc Biol Sci* 2003;270:2147–50.

35. Benton D, Donohoe R. The influence of creatine supplementation on the cognitive functioning of vegetarians and omnivores. *Br J Nutr* 2011;105:1100–5.

36. Sies H, Stahl W. Nutritional protection against skin damage from sunlight. *Annu Rev Nutr* 2004;24:173–200.

37. Grove GL, Kligman AM. Age-associated changes in human epidermal cell renewal. *J Gerontol* 1983;38:137–42.

38. Nowson CA, Margerison C. Vitamin D intake and vitamin D status of Australians. *Med J Aust* 2002;177:149–52.

39. Binkley N, Novotny R, Krueger D, et al. Low vitamin D status despite abundant sun exposure. *J Clin Endocrinol Metab* 2007;92:2130–5.

40. Jacobs ET, Alberts DS, Foote JA, et al. Vitamin D insufficiency in southern Arizona. *Am J Clin Nutr* 2008;87:608–13.

41. Shapira N. Nutritional approach to sun protection: a suggested complement to external strategies. *Nutr Rev* 2010;68:75–86.

42. Rhie G, Shin MH, Seo JY, et al. Aging- and photoaging-dependent changes of enzymic and nonenzymic antioxidants in the epidermis and dermis of human skin in vivo. *J Invest Dermatol* 2001;117:1212–7.

43. Purba MB, Kouris-Blazos A, Wattanapenpaiboon N, et al. Skin wrinkling: can food make a difference? *J Am Coll Nutr* 2001;20:71–80.

44. Perugini P, Vettor M, Rona C, et al. Efficacy of oleuropein against UVB irradiation: preliminary evaluation. *Int J Cosmet Sci* 2008;30:113–20.

45. Owen RW, Giacosa A, Hull WE, et al. Olive-oil consumption and health: the possible role of antioxidants. *Lancet Oncol* 2000;1:107–12.

46. D'Angelo S, Ingrosso D, Migliardi V, et al. Hydroxytyrosol, a natural antioxidant from olive oil, prevents protein damage induced by long-wave ultraviolet radiation in melanoma cells. *Free Radic Biol Med* 2005;38:908–19.

47. Stahl W, Heinrich U, Aust O, Tronnier H, Sies H. Lycopene-rich products and dietary photoprotection. *Photochem Photobiol Sci* 2006;5:238–42.

48. Stahl W, Heinrich U, Wiseman S, Eichler O, Sies H, Tronnier H. Dietary tomato paste protects against ultraviolet light-induced erythema in humans. *J Nutr* 2001;131:1449–51.

49. Lee J, Jiang S, Levine N, Watson RR. Carotenoid supplementation reduces erythema in human skin after simulated solar radiation exposure. *Proc Soc Exp Biol Med* 2000;223:170–4.

50. Stephen ID CV, Perrett DI. Carotenoid and melanin pigment coloration affect perceived human health. *Evolution and Human Behavior* 2011;32:216–227.

51. Verbeke P, Siboska GE, Clark BF, Rattan SI. Kinetin inhibits protein oxidation and glycoxidation in vitro. *Biochem Biophys Res Commun* 2000;276:1265–70.

52. Wu CH, Yen GC. Inhibitory effect of naturally occurring flavonoids on the formation of advanced glycation endproducts. *J Agric Food Chem* 2005;53:3167–73.

53. Dearlove RP, Greenspan P, Hartle DK, Swanson RB, Hargrove JL. Inhibition of protein glycation by extracts of culinary herbs and spices. *J Med Food* 2008;11:275–81.

54. Verzijl N, DeGroot J, Oldehinkel E, et al. Age-related accumulation of Maillard reaction products in human articular cartilage collagen. *Biochem J* 2000;350 Pt 2:381–7.

55. Appleby PN, Allen NE, Key TJ. Diet, vegetarianism, and cataract risk. *Am J Clin Nutr* 2011;93:1128–35.

56. Cho E, Hung S, Willett WC, et al. Prospective study of dietary fat and the risk of age-related macular degeneration. *Am J Clin Nutr* 2001;73:209–18.

57. Moraes AB, Haidar MA, Soares Junior JM, Simoes MJ, Baracat EC, Patriarca MT. The effects of topical isoflavones on postmenopausal skin: double-blind and randomized clinical trial of efficacy. *Eur J Obstet Gynecol Reprod Biol* 2009;146:188–92.

58. Patriarca MT, Barbosa de Moraes AR, Nader HB, et al. Hyaluronic acid concentration in postmenopausal facial skin after topical estradiol and genistein treatment: a double-blind, randomized clinical trial of efficacy. *Menopause* 2012.

59. Accorsi-Neto A, Haidar M, Simoes R, Simoes M, Soares-Jr J, Baracat E. Effects of isoflavones on the skin of postmenopausal women: a pilot study. *Clinics (São Paulo)* 2009;64:505–10.

60. Izumi T, Saito M, Obata A, Arii M, Yamaguchi H, Matsuyama A. Oral intake of soy isoflavone aglycone improves the aged skin of adult women. *J Nutr Sci Vitaminol (Tokyo)* 2007;53:57–62.

61. Berg Rvd. Effect of a supplemented soy drink on skin aging of postmenopausal women. 11th Asian Congress of Nutrition. Singapore, 2011.

62. Wang F, Garza LA, Kang S, et al. In vivo stimulation of de novo collagen production caused by cross-linked hyaluronic acid dermal filler injections in photodamaged human skin. *Arch Dermatol* 2007;143:155–63.

63. Rubino C, Farace F, Dessy LA, Sanna MP, Mazzarello V. A prospective study of anti-aging topical therapies using a quantitative method of assessment. *Plast Reconstr Surg* 2005;115:1156–62; discussion 1163–4.

64. Gamble R, Dunn J, Dawson A, et al. Topical antimicrobial treatment of acne vulgaris: an evidence-based review. *Am J Clin Dermatol* 2012;13:141–52.

65. Kishimoto Y, Saito N, Kurita K, Shimokado K, Maruyama N, Ishigami A. Ascorbic acid enhances the expression of type 1 and type 4 collagen and SVCT2 in cultured human skin fibroblasts. *Biochem Biophys Res Commun* 2012.

66. Nagle DG, Ferreira D, Zhou YD. Epigallocatechin-3-gallate (EGCG): chemical and biomedical perspectives. *Phytochemistry* 2006;67:1849–55.

CHAPTER 11: PREVENTING BREAST CANCER

1. Blackwood MA, Weber BL. BRCA1 and BRCA2: from molecular genetics to clinical medicine. *J Clin Oncol* 1998;16:1969–77.

2. Colditz GA, Frazier AL. Models of breast cancer show that risk is set

by events of early life: prevention efforts must shift focus. *Cancer Epidemiol Biomarkers Prev* 1995;4:567–71.

3. Turner LB. A meta-analysis of fat intake, reproduction, and breast cancer risk: an evolutionary perspective. *Am J Hum Biol* 2011;23:601–8.

4. Colomer R, Lupu R, Papadimitropoulou A, et al. Giacomo Castelvetro's salads. Anti-HER2 oncogene nutraceuticals since the 17th century? *Clin Transl Oncol* 2008;10:30–4.

5. Tantamango-Bartley Y, Jaceldo-Siegl K, Fan J, Fraser G. Vegetarian diets and the incidence of cancer in a low-risk population. *Cancer Epidemiol Biomarkers Prev* 2012.

6. Goldin BR, Adlercreutz H, Gorbach SL, et al. Estrogen excretion patterns and plasma levels in vegetarian and omnivorous women. *N Engl J Med* 1982;307:1542–7.

7. Adlercreutz H, Fotsis T, Bannwart C, Hamalainen E, Bloigu S, Ollus A. Urinary estrogen profile determination in young Finnish vegetarian and omnivorous women. *J Steroid Biochem* 1986;24:289–96.

8. Barbosa JC, Shultz TD, Filley SJ, Nieman DC. The relationship among adiposity, diet, and hormone concentrations in vegetarian and nonvegetarian postmenopausal women [see comments]. *Am J Clin Nutr* 1990;51:798–803.

9. Rose DP, Goldman M, Connolly JM, Strong LE. High-fiber diet reduces serum estrogen concentrations in premenopausal women. *Am J Clin Nutr* 1991;54:520–5.

10. Vinnari M, Montonen J, Harkanen T, Mannisto S. Identifying vegetarians and their food consumption according to self-identification and operationalized definition in Finland. *Public Health Nutr* 2009;12:481–8.

11. Murtaugh MA, Sweeney C, Giuliano AR, et al. Diet patterns and breast cancer risk in Hispanic and non-Hispanic white women: the Four-Corners Breast Cancer Study. *Am J Clin Nutr* 2008;87:978–84.

12. Wu AH, Yu MC, Tseng CC, Stanczyk FZ, Pike MC. Dietary patterns and breast cancer risk in Asian American women. *Am J Clin Nutr* 2009;89:1145–54.

13. Jo EH, Kim SH, Ahn NS, et al. Efficacy of sulforaphane is mediated by p38 MAP kinase and caspase-7 activations in ER-positive and COX-2-expressed human breast cancer cells. *Eur J Cancer Prev* 2007;16:505–10.

14. Meng Q, Goldberg ID, Rosen EM, Fan S. Inhibitory effects of Indole-3-carbinol on invasion and migration in human breast cancer cells. *Breast Cancer Res Treat* 2000;63:147–52.

15. Senthilkumar K, Arunkumar R, Elumalai P, et al. Quercetin inhibits invasion, migration and signalling molecules involved in cell survival and

proliferation of prostate cancer cell line (PC-3). *Cell Biochem Funct* 2011;29:87–95.

16. Dong JY, He K, Wang P, Qin LQ. Dietary fiber intake and risk of breast cancer: a meta-analysis of prospective cohort studies. *Am J Clin Nutr* 2011.

17. Cade JE, Burley VJ, Greenwood DC. Dietary fibre and risk of breast cancer in the UK Women's Cohort Study. *Int J Epidemiol* 2007;36:431–8.

18. Travis RC, Allen NE, Appleby PN, Spencer EA, Roddam AW, Key TJ. A prospective study of vegetarianism and isoflavone intake in relation to breast cancer risk in British women. *Int J Cancer* 2008;122:705–10.

19. Messina M, Hilakivi-Clarke L. Early intake appears to be the key to the proposed protective effects of soy intake against breast cancer. *Nutr Cancer* 2009;61:792–8.

20. Holmes MD, Spiegelman D, Willett WC, et al. Dietary fat intake and endogenous sex steroid hormone levels in postmenopausal women [In Process Citation]. *J Clin Oncol* 2000;18:3668–76.

21. Prentice RL, Caan B, Chlebowski RT, et al. Low-fat dietary pattern and risk of invasive breast cancer: the Women's Health Initiative Randomized Controlled Dietary Modification Trial. *JAMA* 2006;295:629–42.

22. Lof M, Sandin S, Lagiou P, et al. Dietary fat and breast cancer risk in the Swedish women's lifestyle and health cohort. *Br J Cancer* 2007;97:1570–6.

23. Smith-Warner SA, Spiegelman D, Adami HO, et al. Types of dietary fat and breast cancer: a pooled analysis of cohort studies. *Int J Cancer* 2001;92:767–74.

24. Wang J, John EM, Horn-Ross PL, Ingles SA. Dietary fat, cooking fat, and breast cancer risk in a multiethnic population. *Nutr Cancer* 2008;60:492–504.

25. Martin-Moreno JM, Willett WC, Gorgojo L, et al. Dietary fat, olive oil intake and breast cancer risk. *Int J Cancer* 1994;58:774–80.

26. La Vecchia C, Negri E, Franceschi S, Decarli A, Giacosa A, Lipworth L. Olive oil, other dietary fats, and the risk of breast cancer (Italy). *Cancer Causes Control* 1995;6:545–50.

27. Trichopoulou A, Katsouyanni K, Stuver S, et al. Consumption of olive oil and specific food groups in relation to breast cancer risk in Greece. *J Natl Cancer Inst* 1995;87:110–6.

28. Demetriou CA, Hadjisavvas A, Loizidou MA, et al. The Mediterranean dietary pattern and breast cancer risk in Greek-Cypriot women: a case-control study. *BMC Cancer* 2012;12:113.

29. Pelucchi C, Bosetti C, Negri E, Lipworth L, La Vecchia C. Olive oil

and cancer risk: an update of epidemiological findings through 2010. *Curr Pharm Des* 2011;17:805–12.

30. Menendez JA, Vazquez-Martin A, Colomer R, et al. Olive oil's bitter principle reverses acquired autoresistance to trastuzumab (Herceptin) in HER2-overexpressing breast cancer cells. *BMC Cancer* 2007;7:80.

31. Holmes MD, Colditz GA, Hunter DJ, et al. Meat, fish and egg intake and risk of breast cancer. *Int J Cancer* 2003;104:221–7.

32. Taylor VH, Misra M, Mukherjee SD. Is red meat intake a risk factor for breast cancer among premenopausal women? *Breast Cancer Res Treat* 2009;117:1–8.

33. Pala V, Krogh V, Berrino F, et al. Meat, eggs, dairy products, and risk of breast cancer in the European Prospective Investigation into Cancer and Nutrition (EPIC) cohort. *Am J Clin Nutr* 2009;90:602–12.

34. Ferrucci LM, Cross AJ, Graubard BI, et al. Intake of meat, meat mutagens, and iron and the risk of breast cancer in the Prostate, Lung, Colorectal, and Ovarian Cancer Screening Trial. *Br J Cancer* 2009;101:178–84.

35. Cho E, Spiegelman D, Hunter DJ, et al. Premenopausal fat intake and risk of breast cancer. *J Natl Cancer Inst* 2003;95:1079–85.

36. Bessaoud F, Daures JP, Gerber M. Dietary factors and breast cancer risk: a case control study among a population in Southern France. *Nutr Cancer* 2008;60:177–87.

37. Voorrips LE, Brants HA, Kardinaal AF, Hiddink GJ, van den Brandt PA, Goldbohm RA. Intake of conjugated linoleic acid, fat, and other fatty acids in relation to postmenopausal breast cancer: the Netherlands Cohort Study on Diet and Cancer. *Am J Clin Nutr* 2002;76:873–82.

38. Samani AA, Yakar S, LeRoith D, Brodt P. The role of the IGF system in cancer growth and metastasis: overview and recent insights. *Endocr Rev* 2007;28:20–47.

39. Allen NE, Appleby PN, Davey GK, Kaaks R, Rinaldi S, Key TJ. The associations of diet with serum insulin-like growth factor I and its main binding proteins in 292 women meat-eaters, vegetarians, and vegans. *Cancer Epidemiol Biomarkers Prev* 2002;11:1441–8.

40. Allen NE, Appleby PN, Davey GK, Key TJ. Hormones and diet: low insulin-like growth factor-I but normal bioavailable androgens in vegan men. *Br J Cancer* 2000;83:95–7.

41. Key TJ, Appleby PN, Reeves GK, Roddam AW. Insulin-like growth factor 1 (IGF1), IGF binding protein 3 (IGFBP3), and breast cancer risk: pooled individual data analysis of 17 prospective studies. *Lancet Oncol* 2010;11:530–42.

42. Levi F, Pasche C, Lucchini F, Ghidoni R, Ferraroni M, La Vecchia C. Resveratrol and breast cancer risk. *Eur J Cancer Prev* 2005;14:139–42.

43. Linos E, Holmes MD, Willett WC. Diet and breast cancer. *Curr Oncol Rep* 2007;9:31–41.

44. Shu XO, Zheng Y, Cai H, et al. Soy food intake and breast cancer survival. *JAMA* 2009;302:2437–43.

45. Kang X, Zhang Q, Wang S, Huang X, Jin S. Effect of soy isoflavones on breast cancer recurrence and death for patients receiving adjuvant endocrine therapy. *CMAJ* 2010;182:1857–62.

46. Caan BJ, Natarajan L, Parker B, et al. Soy food consumption and breast cancer prognosis. *Cancer Epidemiol Biomarkers Prev* 2011;20:854–8.

47. Guha N, Kwan ML, Quesenberry CP, Jr, Weltzien EK, Castillo AL, Caan BJ. Soy isoflavones and risk of cancer recurrence in a cohort of breast cancer survivors: the Life After Cancer Epidemiology study. *Breast Cancer Res Treat* 2009;118:395–405.

48. Nechuta SJ, Caan BJ, Chen WY, et al. Soy food intake after diagnosis of breast cancer and survival: an in-depth analysis of combined evidence from cohort studies of US and Chinese women. *Am J Clin Nutr* 2012;96:123–32.

49. Jain M, Miller AB, To T. Premorbid diet and the prognosis of women with breast cancer. *J Natl Cancer Inst* 1994;86:1390–7.

50. Holmes MD, Stampfer MJ, Colditz GA, Rosner B, Hunter DJ, Willett WC. Dietary factors and the survival of women with breast carcinoma. *Cancer* 1999;86:826–35.

51. Pierce JP, Stefanick ML, Flatt SW, et al. Greater survival after breast cancer in physically active women with high vegetable-fruit intake regardless of obesity. *J Clin Oncol* 2007;25:2345–51.

52. Bertram LA, Stefanick ML, Saquib N, et al. Physical activity, additional breast cancer events, and mortality among early-stage breast cancer survivors: findings from the WHEL Study. *Cancer Causes Control* 2011;22:427–35.

53. Davaasambuu G, Cui X, Feskanich D, Hankinson SE, Willett WC. Milk, dairy intake and risk of endometrial cancer: A twenty-six-year follow-up. *Int J Cancer* 2011.

54. Faber MT, Jensen A, Sogaard M, et al. Use of dairy products, lactose, and calcium and risk of ovarian cancer-results from a Danish case-control study. *Acta Oncol* 2012;51:454–64.

55. Genkinger JM, Hunter DJ, Spiegelman D, et al. Dairy products and ovarian cancer: a pooled analysis of 12 cohort studies. *Cancer Epidemiol Biomarkers Prev* 2006;15:364–72.

56. Piyathilake CJ, Henao OL, Macaluso M, et al. Folate is associated with the natural history of high-risk human papillomaviruses. *Cancer Res* 2004;64:8788–93.

57. Henderson HJ. Why lesbians should be encouraged to have regular cervical screening. *J Fam Plann Reprod Health Care* 2009;35:49–52.

58. Korpela JT, Adlercreutz H, Turunen MJ. Fecal free and conjugated bile acids and neutral sterols in vegetarians, omnivores, and patients with colorectal cancer. *Scand J Gastroenterol* 1988;23:277–83.

59. Van Faassen A, Hazen MJ, van den Brandt PA, van den Bogaard AE, Hermus RJ, Janknegt RA. Bile acids and pH values in total feces and in fecal water from habitually omnivorous and vegetarian subjects. *Am J Clin Nutr* 1993;58:917–22.

60. Aries VG, Crowther JS, Drasar BS, Hill MJ, Ellis FR. The effect of a strict vegetarian diet on the faecal flora and faecal steroid concentration. *J Pathol* 1972;103:54–56.

61. Davey GK, Spencer EA, Appleby PN, Allen NE, Knox KH, Key TJ. EPIC-Oxford: lifestyle characteristics and nutrient intakes in a cohort of 33 883 meat-eaters and 31 546 non meat-eaters in the UK. *Public Health Nutr* 2003;6:259–69.

62. Tonstad S, Butler T, Yan R, Fraser GE. Type of vegetarian diet, body weight, and prevalence of type 2 diabetes. *Diabetes Care* 2009;32:791–6.

CHAPTER 12: EATING FOR A HEALTHY HEART

1. Thomas EL, Frost G, Barnard ML, et al. An in vivo 13C magnetic resonance spectroscopic study of the relationship between diet and adipose tissue composition. *Lipids* 1996;31:145–51.

2. Toohey ML, Harris MA, DeWitt W, Foster G, Schmidt WD, Melby CL. Cardiovascular disease risk factors are lower in African-American vegans compared to lacto-ovo-vegetarians [see comments]. *J Am Coll Nutr* 1998;17:425–34.

3. Li D, Sinclair A, Mann N, et al. The association of diet and thrombotic risk factors in healthy male vegetarians and meat-eaters. *Eur J Clin Nutr* 1999;53:612–9.

4. Su TC, Jeng JS, Wang JD, et al. Homocysteine, circulating vascular cell adhesion molecule and carotid atherosclerosis in postmenopausal vegetarian women and omnivores. *Atherosclerosis* 2006;184:356–62.

5. Haddad EH, Berk LS, Kettering JD, Hubbard RW, Peters WR. Dietary intake and biochemical, hematologic, and immune status of vegans compared with nonvegetarians. *Am J Clin Nutr* 1999;70:586S-593S.

6. Donaldson AN. The relation of protein foods to hypertension. *Calif West Med* 1926;24:328–331.

7. Fraser GE. Vegetarian diets: what do we know of their effects on common chronic diseases? *Am J Clin Nutr* 2009;89:1607S-1612S.

8. Appleby PN, Davey GK, Key TJ. Hypertension and blood pressure among meat eaters, fish eaters, vegetarians and vegans in EPIC-Oxford. *Public Health Nutr* 2002;5:645–54.

9. Booth GL, Kapral MK, Fung K, Tu JV. Relation between age and cardiovascular disease in men and women with diabetes compared with non-diabetic people: a population-based retrospective cohort study. *Lancet* 2006;368:29–36.

10. Kawachi I, Colditz GA, Speizer FE, et al. A prospective study of passive smoking and coronary heart disease. *Circulation* 1997;95:2374–9.

11. Rosenkranz MA, Davidson RJ, Maccoon DG, Sheridan JF, Kalin NH, Lutz A. A comparison of mindfulness-based stress reduction and an active control in modulation of neurogenic inflammation. *Brain Behav Immun* 2012.

12. Schneider RH, Grim CE, Rainforth MV, et al. Stress reduction in the secondary prevention of cardiovascular disease: randomized controlled trial of transcendental meditation and health education in blacks. *Circ Cardiovasc Qual Outcomes* 2012.

13. Manson JE, Hu FB, Rich-Edwards JW, et al. A prospective study of walking as compared with vigorous exercise in the prevention of coronary heart disease in women. *N Engl J Med* 1999;341:650–8.

14. Pearson TA, Mensah GA, Alexander RW, et al. Markers of inflammation and cardiovascular disease: application to clinical and public health practice: A statement for healthcare professionals from the Centers for Disease Control and Prevention and the American Heart Association. *Circulation* 2003;107:499–511.

15. Yamamoto K, Kawano H, Gando Y, et al. Poor trunk flexibility is associated with arterial stiffening. *Am J Physiol Heart Circ Physiol* 2009;297:H1314–8.

16. Thom T, Haase N, Rosamond W, et al. Heart disease and stroke statistics—2006 update: a report from the American Heart Association Statistics Committee and Stroke Statistics Subcommittee. *Circulation* 2006;113:e85–151.

17. Knopp RH, Zhu X, Bonet B. Effects of estrogens on lipoprotein metabolism and cardiovascular disease in women. *Atherosclerosis* 1994;110 Suppl:S83–91.

18. Gordon DJ, Knoke J, Probstfield JL, Superko R, Tyroler HA. High-

density lipoprotein cholesterol and coronary heart disease in hypercholesterolemic men: the Lipid Research Clinics Coronary Primary Prevention Trial. *Circulation* 1986;74:1217–25.

19. Krejza J, Arkuszewski M, Kasner SE, et al. Carotid artery diameter in men and women and the relation to body and neck size. *Stroke* 2006;37:1103–5.

20. McCredie RJ, McCrohon JA, Turner L, Griffiths KA, Handelsman DJ, Celermajer DS. Vascular reactivity is impaired in genetic females taking high-dose androgens. *J Am Coll Cardiol* 1998;32:1331–5.

21. New G, Timmins KL, Duffy SJ, et al. Long-term estrogen therapy improves vascular function in male to female transsexuals. *J Am Coll Cardiol* 1997;29:1437–44.

22. De Biase SG, Fernandes SF, Gianini RJ, Duarte JL. Vegetarian diet and cholesterol and triglycerides levels. *Arq Bras Cardiol* 2007;88:35–9.

23. Goff LM, Bell JD, So PW, Dornhorst A, Frost GS. Veganism and its relationship with insulin resistance and intramyocellular lipid. *Eur J Clin Nutr* 2005;59:291–8.

24. Phillips RL, Lemon FR, Beeson WL, Kuzma JW. Coronary heart disease mortality among Seventh-Day Adventists with differing dietary habits: a preliminary report. *Am J Clin Nutr* 1978;31:S191-S198.

25. Key TJ, Fraser GE, Thorogood M, et al. Mortality in vegetarians and nonvegetarians: detailed findings from a collaborative analysis of 5 prospective studies. *Am J Clin Nutr* 1999;70:516S-524S.

26. Key TJ, Appleby PN, Spencer EA, Travis RC, Roddam AW, Allen NE. Mortality in British vegetarians: results from the European Prospective Investigation into Cancer and Nutrition (EPIC-Oxford). *Am J Clin Nutr* 2009;89:1613S-1619S.

27. Antoniades C, Antonopoulos AS, Tousoulis D, Marinou K, Stefanadis C. Homocysteine and coronary atherosclerosis: from folate fortification to the recent clinical trials. *Eur Heart J* 2009;30:6–15.

28. Mann NJ, Li D, Sinclair AJ, et al. The effect of diet on plasma homocysteine concentrations in healthy male subjects. *Eur J Clin Nutr* 1999;53:895–9.

29. Herrmann W, Schorr H, Obeid R, Geisel J. Vitamin B-12 status, particularly holotranscobalamin II and methylmalonic acid concentrations, and hyperhomocysteinemia in vegetarians. *Am J Clin Nutr* 2003;78:131–6.

30. Keys A, Menotti A, Karvonen MJ, et al. The diet and 15-year death rate in the seven countries study. *Am J Epidemiol* 1986;124:903–15.

31. Mente A, de Koning L, Shannon HS, Anand SS. A systematic review of the evidence supporting a causal link between dietary factors and coronary heart disease. *Arch Intern Med* 2009;169:659–69.

32. Fung TT, Rexrode KM, Mantzoros CS, Manson JE, Willett WC, Hu FB. Mediterranean diet and incidence of and mortality from coronary heart disease and stroke in women. *Circulation* 2009;119:1093–100.

33. Kastorini CM, Milionis HJ, Esposito K, Giugliano D, Goudevenos JA, Panagiotakos DB. The effect of Mediterranean diet on metabolic syndrome and its components: a meta-analysis of 50 studies and 534,906 individuals. *J Am Coll Cardiol* 2011;57:1299–313.

34. Marin C, Ramirez R, Delgado-Lista J, et al. Mediterranean diet reduces endothelial damage and improves the regenerative capacity of endothelium. *Am J Clin Nutr* 2011;93:267–74.

35. Jones JL, Comperatore M, Barona J, et al. A Mediterranean-style, low-glycemic-load diet decreases atherogenic lipoproteins and reduces lipoprotein (a) and oxidized low-density lipoprotein in women with metabolic syndrome. *Metabolism* 2012;61:366–72.

36. Ornish D, Brown SE, Scherwitz LW, et al. Can lifestyle changes reverse coronary heart disease? The Lifestyle Heart Trial. *Lancet* 1990;336:129–33.

37. Howard BV, Van Horn L, Hsia J, et al. Low-fat dietary pattern and risk of cardiovascular disease: the Women's Health Initiative Randomized Controlled Dietary Modification Trial. *JAMA* 2006;295:655–66.

38. Hu FB, Stampfer MJ, Manson JE, et al. Dietary fat intake and the risk of coronary heart disease in women. *N Engl J Med* 1997;337:1491–9.

39. Oh K, Hu FB, Manson JE, Stampfer MJ, Willett WC. Dietary fat intake and risk of coronary heart disease in women: 20 years of follow-up of the nurses' health study. *Am J Epidemiol* 2005;161:672–9.

40. Barnard ND, Scialli AR, Bertron P, Hurlock D, Edmonds K, Talev L. Effectiveness of a low-fat vegetarian diet in altering serum lipids in healthy premenopausal women. *Am J Cardiol* 2000;85:969–72.

41. Jenkins DJ, Chiavaroli L, Wong JM, et al. Adding monounsaturated fatty acids to a dietary portfolio of cholesterol-lowering foods in hypercholesterolemia. *CMAJ* 2010.

42. Koba S, Hirano T, Kondo T, et al. Significance of small dense low-density lipoproteins and other risk factors in patients with various types of coronary heart disease. *Am Heart J* 2002;144:1026–35.

43. Bendinelli B, Masala G, Saieva C, et al. Fruit, vegetables, and olive oil

and risk of coronary heart disease in Italian women: the EPICOR Study. *Am J Clin Nutr* 2011;93:275–83.

44. Razquin C, Martinez JA, Martinez-Gonzalez MA, Mitjavila MT, Estruch R, Marti A. A 3 years follow-up of a Mediterranean diet rich in virgin olive oil is associated with high plasma antioxidant capacity and reduced body weight gain. *Eur J Clin Nutr* 2009;63:1387–93.

45. Masella R, Giovannini C, Vari R, et al. Effects of dietary virgin olive oil phenols on low density lipoprotein oxidation in hyperlipidemic patients. *Lipids* 2001;36:1195–202.

46. Pischon T, Hankinson SE, Hotamisligil GS, Rifai N, Willett WC, Rimm EB. Habitual dietary intake of n-3 and n-6 fatty acids in relation to inflammatory markers among US men and women. *Circulation* 2003;108:155–60.

47. Baer DJ, Judd JT, Clevidence BA, Tracy RP. Dietary fatty acids affect plasma markers of inflammation in healthy men fed controlled diets: a randomized crossover study. *Am J Clin Nutr* 2004;79:969–73.

48. Mennen L, de Maat M, Meijer G, et al. Factor VIIa response to a fat-rich meal does not depend on fatty acid composition: a randomized controlled trial. *Arterioscler Thromb Vasc Biol* 1998;18:599–603.

49. Mozaffarian D, Pischon T, Hankinson SE, et al. Dietary intake of trans fatty acids and systemic inflammation in women. *Am J Clin Nutr* 2004;79:606–12.

50. Mozaffarian D, Katan MB, Ascherio A, Stampfer MJ, Willett WC. Trans fatty acids and cardiovascular disease. *N Engl J Med* 2006;354:1601–13.

51. Siri-Tarino PW, Sun Q, Hu FB, Krauss RM. Meta-analysis of prospective cohort studies evaluating the association of saturated fat with cardiovascular disease. *Am J Clin Nutr* 2010;91:535–46.

52. Howard BV, Curb JD, Eaton CB, et al. Low-fat dietary pattern and lipoprotein risk factors: the Women's Health Initiative Dietary Modification Trial. *Am J Clin Nutr* 2010;91:860–74.

53. Pereira MA, O'Reilly E, Augustsson K, et al. Dietary fiber and risk of coronary heart disease: a pooled analysis of cohort studies. *Arch Intern Med* 2004;164:370–6.

54. Liu S, Manson JE, Stampfer MJ, et al. Whole grain consumption and risk of ischemic stroke in women: a prospective study. *JAMA* 2000;284:1534–40.

55. Taylor RS, Ashton KE, Moxham T, Hooper L, Ebrahim S. Reduced dietary salt for the prevention of cardiovascular disease: a meta-analysis of randomized controlled trials (Cochrane review). *Am J Hypertens* 2011;24:843–53.

56. Esmaillzadeh A, Azadbakht L. Legume consumption is inversely associated with serum concentrations of adhesion molecules and inflammatory biomarkers among Iranian women. *J Nutr* 2012;142:334–9.

57. Villegas R, Gao YT, Yang G, et al. Legume and soy food intake and the incidence of type 2 diabetes in the Shanghai Women's Health Study. *Am J Clin Nutr* 2008;87:162–7.

58. Bazzano LA, He J, Ogden LG, et al. Legume consumption and risk of coronary heart disease in US men and women: NHANES I Epidemiologic Follow-Up Study. *Arch Intern Med* 2001;161:2573–8.

59. Davy BM, Davy KP, Ho RC, Beske SD, Davrath LR, Melby CL. High-fiber oat cereal compared with wheat cereal consumption favorably alters LDL-cholesterol subclass and particle numbers in middle-aged and older men. *Am J Clin Nutr* 2002;76:351–8.

60. Jenkins DJ, Mirrahimi A, Srichaikul K, et al. Soy protein reduces serum cholesterol by both intrinsic and food displacement mechanisms. *J Nutr* 2010;140:2302S-2311S.

61. Jenkins DJ, Kendall CW, Faulkner D, et al. A dietary portfolio approach to cholesterol reduction: combined effects of plant sterols, vegetable proteins, and viscous fibers in hypercholesterolemia. *Metabolism* 2002;51:1596–604.

62. Li SH, Liu XX, Bai YY, et al. Effect of oral isoflavone supplementation on vascular endothelial function in postmenopausal women: a meta-analysis of randomized placebo-controlled trials. *Am J Clin Nutr* 2010;91:480–6.

63. Desroches S, Mauger JF, Ausman LM, Lichtenstein AH, Lamarche B. Soy protein favorably affects LDL size independently of isoflavones in hypercholesterolemic men and women. *J Nutr* 2004;134:574–9.

64. Zhang X, Shu XO, Gao YT, et al. Soy food consumption is associated with lower risk of coronary heart disease in Chinese women. *J Nutr* 2003;133:2874–8.

65. Hodis HN, Mack WJ, Kono N, et al. Isoflavone soy protein supplementation and atherosclerosis progression in healthy postmenopausal women: a randomized controlled trial. *Stroke* 2011;42:3168–75.

66. Sabate J, Oda K, Ros E. Nut consumption and blood lipid levels: a pooled analysis of 25 intervention trials. *Arch Intern Med* 2010;170:821–7.

67. Ros E, Nunez I, Perez-Heras A, et al. A walnut diet improves endothelial function in hypercholesterolemic subjects: a randomized crossover trial. *Circulation* 2004;109:1609–14.

68. Salas-Salvado J, Casas-Agustench P, Murphy MM, Lopez-Uriarte P, Bullo M. The effect of nuts on inflammation. *Asia Pac J Clin Nutr* 2008;17 Suppl 1:333–6.

69. Hu FB, Stampfer MJ, Manson JE, et al. Frequent nut consumption and risk of coronary heart disease in women: prospective cohort study. *BMJ* 1998;317:1341–5.

70. Ellsworth JL, Kushi LH, Folsom AR. Frequent nut intake and risk of death from coronary heart disease and all causes in postmenopausal women: the Iowa Women's Health Study. *Nutr Metab Cardiovasc Dis* 2001;11:372–7.

71. Cook NR, Obarzanek E, Cutler JA, et al. Joint effects of sodium and potassium intake on subsequent cardiovascular disease: the Trials of Hypertension Prevention follow-up study. *Arch Intern Med* 2009;169:32–40.

72. Mozaffarian D, Appel LJ, Van Horn L. Components of a cardioprotective diet: new insights. *Circulation* 2011;123:2870–91.

73. Rimm EB, Klatsky A, Grobbee D, Stampfer MJ. Review of moderate alcohol consumption and reduced risk of coronary heart disease: is the effect due to beer, wine, or spirits? *BMJ* 1996;312:731–6.

74. Baer DJ, Judd JT, Clevidence BA, et al. Moderate alcohol consumption lowers risk factors for cardiovascular disease in postmenopausal women fed a controlled diet. *Am J Clin Nutr* 2002;75:593–9.

75. Hooper L, Kay C, Abdelhamid A, et al. Effects of chocolate, cocoa, and flavan-3-ols on cardiovascular health: a systematic review and meta-analysis of randomized trials. *Am J Clin Nutr* 2012.

CHAPTER 13: STRONG BONES FOR LIFE

1. Sahi T. Genetics and epidemiology of adult-type hypolactasia. *Scand J Gastroenterol Suppl* 1994;202:7–20.

2. Ausman LM, Oliver LM, Goldin BR, Woods MN, Gorbach SL, Dwyer JT. Estimated net acid excretion inversely correlates with urine pH in vegans, lacto-ovo vegetarians, and omnivores. *J Ren Nutr* 2008;18:456–65.

3. Bow CH, Cheung E, Cheung CL, et al. Ethnic difference of clinical vertebral fracture risk. *Osteoporos Int* 2012;23:879–85.

4. Faulkner KG, Cummings SR, Black D, Palermo L, Gluer CC, Genant HK. Simple measurement of femoral geometry predicts hip fracture: the study of osteoporotic fractures. *J Bone Miner Res* 1993;8:1211–7.

5. Fenton TR, Lyon AW, Eliasziw M, Tough SC, Hanley DA. Meta-analysis of the effect of the acid-ash hypothesis of osteoporosis on calcium balance. *J Bone Miner Res* 2009;24:1835–40.

6. Kerstetter JE, O'Brien KO, Caseria DM, Wall DE, Insogna KL. The impact of dietary protein on calcium absorption and kinetic measures of bone turnover in women. *J Clin Endocrinol Metab* 2005;90:26–31.

7. Darling AL, Millward DJ, Torgerson DJ, Hewitt CE, Lanham-New SA.

Dietary protein and bone health: a systematic review and meta-analysis. *Am J Clin Nutr* 2009.

8. Fenton TR, Tough SC, Lyon AW, Eliasziw M, Hanley DA. Causal assessment of dietary acid load and bone disease: a systematic review and meta-analysis applying Hill's epidemiologic criteria for causality. *Nutr J* 2011;10:41.

9. Munger RG, Cerhan JR, Chiu BC. Prospective study of dietary protein intake and risk of hip fracture in postmenopausal women. *Am J Clin Nutr* 1999;69:147–52.

10. Promislow JH, Goodman-Gruen D, Slymen DJ, Barrett-Connor E. Protein consumption and bone mineral density in the elderly: the Rancho Bernardo Study. *Am J Epidemiol* 2002;155:636–44.

11. Devine A, Dick IM, Islam AF, Dhaliwal SS, Prince RL. Protein consumption is an important predictor of lower limb bone mass in elderly women. *Am J Clin Nutr* 2005;81:1423–8.

12. Schurch MA, Rizzoli R, Slosman D, Vadas L, Vergnaud P, Bonjour JP. Protein supplements increase serum insulin-like growth factor-I levels and attenuate proximal femur bone loss in patients with recent hip fracture. A randomized, double-blind, placebo-controlled trial. *Ann Intern Med* 1998;128:801–9.

13. Appleby P, Roddam A, Allen N, Key T. Comparative fracture risk in vegetarians and nonvegetarians in EPIC-Oxford. *Eur J Clin Nutr* 2007;61:1400–6.

14. Feskanich D, Weber P, Willett WC, Rockett H, Booth SL, Colditz GA. Vitamin K intake and hip fractures in women: a prospective study. *Am J Clin Nutr* 1999;69:74–9.

15. Booth SL, Broe KE, Gagnon DR, et al. Vitamin K intake and bone mineral density in women and men. *Am J Clin Nutr* 2003;77:512–6.

16. Ruiz-Ramos M, Vargas LA, Fortoul Van der Goes TI, Cervantes-Sandoval A, Mendoza-Nunez VM. Supplementation of ascorbic acid and alpha-tocopherol is useful to preventing bone loss linked to oxidative stress in elderly. *J Nutr Health Aging* 2010;14:467–72.

17. Appel LJ, Moore TJ, Obarzanek E, et al. A clinical trial of the effects of dietary patterns on blood pressure. DASH Collaborative Research Group. *N Engl J Med* 1997;336:1117–24.

18. Reginster JY, Strause L, Deroisy R, Lecart MP, Saltman P, Franchimont P. Preliminary report of decreased serum magnesium in postmenopausal osteoporosis. *Magnesium* 1989;8:106–9.

19. Tucker KL, Hannan MT, Chen H, Cupples LA, Wilson PW, Kiel DP.

Potassium, magnesium, and fruit and vegetable intakes are associated with greater bone mineral density in elderly men and women. *Am J Clin Nutr* 1999;69:727–36.

20. Kramer LB, Osis D, Coffey J, Spencer H. Mineral and trace element content of vegetarian diets. *J Am Coll Nutr* 1984;3:3–11.

21. Zhang X, Shu XO, Li H, et al. Prospective cohort study of soy food consumption and risk of bone fracture among postmenopausal women. *Arch Intern Med* 2005;165:1890–5.

22. Koh WP, Wu AH, Wang R, et al. Gender-specific associations between soy and risk of hip fracture in the Singapore Chinese Health Study. *Am J Epidemiol* 2009;170:901–9.

23. Matthews VL, Knutsen SF, Beeson WL, Fraser GE. Soy milk and dairy consumption is independently associated with ultrasound attenuation of the heel bone among postmenopausal women: the Adventist Health Study-2. *Nutr Res* 2011;31:766–75.

24. Kanis JA, Johansson H, Johnell O, et al. Alcohol intake as a risk factor for fracture. *Osteoporos Int* 2005;16:737–42.

25. Kato I, Toniolo P, Akhmedkhanov A, Koenig KL, Shore R, Zeleniuch-Jacquotte A. Prospective study of factors influencing the onset of natural menopause. *J Clin Epidemiol* 1998;51:1271–6.

26. Li L, Wu J, Pu D, et al. Factors associated with the age of natural menopause and menopausal symptoms in Chinese women. *Maturitas* 2012.

27. Teucher B, Dainty JR, Spinks CA, et al. Sodium and bone health: impact of moderately high and low salt intakes on calcium metabolism in postmenopausal women. *J Bone Miner Res* 2008;23:1477–85.

28. van der Voort DJ, Geusens PP, Dinant GJ. Risk factors for osteoporosis related to their outcome: fractures. *Osteoporos Int* 2001;12:630–8.

29. Armamento-Villareal R, Sadler C, Napoli N, et al. Weight loss in obese older adults increases serum sclerostin and impairs hip geometry but both are prevented by exercise training. *J Bone Miner Res* 2012;27:1215–21.

CHAPTER 14: FIGHTING PAIN WITH PLANT FOODS

1. Skoldstam L, Hagfors L, Johansson G. An experimental study of a Mediterranean diet intervention for patients with rheumatoid arthritis. *Ann Rheum Dis* 2003;62:208–14.

2. McKellar G, Morrison E, McEntegart A, et al. A pilot study of a Mediterranean-type diet intervention in female patients with rheumatoid arthritis living in areas of social deprivation in Glasgow. *Ann Rheum Dis* 2007;66:1239–43.

3. Hanninen O, Kaartinen K, Rauma AL, et al. Antioxidants in vegan diet and rheumatic disorders. *Toxicology* 2000;155:45–53.

4. Hanninen O, Rauma AL, Kaartinen K, Nenonen M. Vegan diet in physiological health promotion. *Acta Physiol Hung* 1999;86:171–80.

5. Nenonen MT, Helve TA, Rauma AL, Hanninen OO. Uncooked, lactobacilli-rich, vegan food and rheumatoid arthritis. *Br J Rheumatol* 1998;37:274–81.

6. Peltonen R, Nenonen M, Helve T, Hanninen O, Toivanen P, Eerola E. Faecal microbial flora and disease activity in rheumatoid arthritis during a vegan diet. *Br J Rheumatol* 1997;36:64–8.

7. Ebringer A, Rashid T. Rheumatoid arthritis is an autoimmune disease triggered by Proteus urinary tract infection. *Clin Dev Immunol* 2006;13:41–8.

8. Darlington LG, Ramsey NW, Mansfield JR. Placebo-controlled, blind study of dietary manipulation therapy in rheumatoid arthritis. *Lancet* 1986;1:236–8.

9. Darlington LG, Ramsey NW. Review of dietary therapy for rheumatoid arthritis. *Br J Rheumatol* 1993;32:507–14.

10. Hafstrom I, Ringertz B, Spangberg A, et al. A vegan diet free of gluten improves the signs and symptoms of rheumatoid arthritis: the effects on arthritis correlate with a reduction in antibodies to food antigens. *Rheumatology (Oxford)* 2001;40:1175–9.

11. Leventhal LJ, Boyce EG, Zurier RB. Treatment of rheumatoid arthritis with gammalinolenic acid. *Ann Intern Med* 1993;119:867–73.

12. Brennan P, Bankhead C, Silman A, Symmons D. Oral contraceptives and rheumatoid arthritis: results from a primary care-based incident case-control study. *Semin Arthritis Rheum* 1997;26:817–23.

13. Lahiri M, Morgan C, Symmons DP, Bruce IN. Modifiable risk factors for RA: prevention, better than cure? *Rheumatology (Oxford)* 2012;51:499–512.

14. Lu H, Sun T, Yao L, Zhang Y. Role of protein tyrosine kinase in IL-1 beta induced activation of mitogen-activated protein kinase in fibroblast-like synoviocytes of rheumatoid arthritis. *Chin Med J (Engl)* 2000;113:872–6.

15. Dijsselbloem N, Vanden Berghe W, De Naeyer A, Haegeman G. Soy isoflavone phyto-pharmaceuticals in interleukin-6 affections. Multi-purpose nutraceuticals at the crossroad of hormone replacement, anti-cancer and anti-inflammatory therapy. *Biochem Pharmacol* 2004;68:1171–85.

16. Costenbader KH, Karlson EW. Cigarette smoking and autoimmune disease: what can we learn from epidemiology? *Lupus* 2006;15:737–45.

17. Criswell LA, Merlino LA, Cerhan JR, et al. Cigarette smoking and the

risk of rheumatoid arthritis among postmenopausal women: results from the Iowa Women's Health Study. *Am J Med* 2002;112:465–71.

18. Henrotin Y, Kurz B, Aigner T. Oxygen and reactive oxygen species in cartilage degradation: friends or foes? *Osteoarthritis Cartilage* 2005;13:643–54.

19. McAlindon TE, Jacques P, Zhang Y, et al. Do antioxidant micronutrients protect against the development and progression of knee osteoarthritis? *Arthritis Rheum* 1996;39:648–56.

20. Blotman F, Maheu E, Wulwik A, Caspard H, Lopez A. Efficacy and safety of avocado/soybean unsaponifiables in the treatment of symptomatic osteoarthritis of the knee and hip. A prospective, multicenter, three-month, randomized, double-blind, placebo-controlled trial. *Rev Rhum Engl Ed* 1997;64:825–34.

21. Appelboom T, Schuermans J, Verbruggen G, Henrotin Y, Reginster JY. Symptoms modifying effect of avocado/soybean unsaponifiables (ASU) in knee osteoarthritis. A double blind, prospective, placebo-controlled study. *Scand J Rheumatol* 2001;30:242–7.

22. Lequesne M, Maheu E, Cadet C, Dreiser RL. Structural effect of avocado/soybean unsaponifiables on joint space loss in osteoarthritis of the hip. *Arthritis Rheum* 2002;47:50–8.

23. Towheed TE, Maxwell L, Anastassiades TP, et al. Glucosamine therapy for treating osteoarthritis. *Cochrane Database Syst Rev* 2005:CD002946.

24. Reginster JY, Deroisy R, Rovati LC, et al. Long-term effects of glucosamine sulphate on osteoarthritis progression: a randomised, placebo-controlled clinical trial. *Lancet* 2001;357:251–6.

25. Pavelka K, Gatterova J, Olejarova M, Machacek S, Giacovelli G, Rovati LC. Glucosamine sulfate use and delay of progression of knee osteoarthritis: a 3-year, randomized, placebo-controlled, double-blind study. *Arch Intern Med* 2002;162:2113–23.

26. Reichenbach S, Sterchi R, Scherer M, et al. Meta-analysis: chondroitin for osteoarthritis of the knee or hip. *Ann Intern Med* 2007;146:580–90.

27. Azad KA, Alam MN, Haq SA, et al. Vegetarian diet in the treatment of fibromyalgia. *Bangladesh Med Res Counc Bull* 2000;26:41–7.

28. Kaartinen K, Lammi K, Hypen M, Nenonen M, Hanninen O, Rauma AL. Vegan diet alleviates fibromyalgia symptoms. *Scand J Rheumatol* 2000;29:308–13.

29. Donaldson MS, Speight N, Loomis S. Fibromyalgia syndrome improved using a mostly raw vegetarian diet: an observational study. *BMC Complement Altern Med* 2001;1:7.

30. Kelman L. The triggers or precipitants of the acute migraine attack. *Cephalalgia* 2007;27:394–402.

31. Marcus DA, Scharff L, Turk D, Gourley LM. A double-blind provocative study of chocolate as a trigger of headache. *Cephalalgia* 1997;17:855–62; discussion 800.

32. Sun-Edelstein C, Mauskop A. Foods and supplements in the management of migraine headaches. *Clin J Pain* 2009;25:446–52.

33. Pall ML. Common etiology of posttraumatic stress disorder, fibromyalgia, chronic fatigue syndrome and multiple chemical sensitivity via elevated nitric oxide/peroxynitrite. *Med Hypotheses* 2001;57:139–45.

34. Bradley LA. Pathophysiologic mechanisms of fibromyalgia and its related disorders. *J Clin Psychiatry* 2008;69 Suppl 2:6–13.

35. Felson DT. Comparing the prevalence of rheumatic diseases in China with the rest of the world. *Arthritis Res Ther* 2008;10:106.

CHAPTER 15: CONTROLLING DIABETES

1. Gerstein HC. Cow's milk exposure and type I diabetes mellitus. A critical overview of the clinical literature. *Diabetes Care* 1994;17:13–9.

2. Dahl-Jorgensen K, Joner G, Hanssen KF. Relationship between cows' milk consumption and incidence of IDDM in childhood. *Diabetes Care* 1991;14:1081–3.

3. Hypponen E, Kenward MG, Virtanen SM, et al. Infant feeding, early weight gain, and risk of type 1 diabetes. Childhood Diabetes in Finland (DiMe) Study Group. *Diabetes Care* 1999;22:1961–5.

4. Norris JM, Scott FW. A meta-analysis of infant diet and insulin-dependent diabetes mellitus: do biases play a role? *Epidemiology* 1996;7:87–92.

5. Shoelson SE, Lee J, Goldfine AB. Inflammation and insulin resistance. *J Clin Invest* 2006;116:1793–801.

6. Knowler WC, Barrett-Connor E, Fowler SE, et al. Reduction in the incidence of type 2 diabetes with lifestyle intervention or metformin. *N Engl J Med* 2002;346:393–403.

7. Klein S, Sheard NF, Pi-Sunyer X, et al. Weight management through lifestyle modification for the prevention and management of type 2 diabetes: rationale and strategies: a statement of the American Diabetes Association, the North American Association for the Study of Obesity, and the American Society for Clinical Nutrition. *Diabetes Care* 2004;27:2067–73.

8. Tonstad S, Butler T, Yan R, Fraser GE. Type of vegetarian diet, body weight, and prevalence of type 2 diabetes. *Diabetes Care* 2009;32:791–6.

9. Halton TL, Liu S, Manson JE, Hu FB. Low-carbohydrate-diet score and risk of type 2 diabetes in women. *Am J Clin Nutr* 2008;87:339–46.

10. Colditz GA, Manson JE, Stampfer MJ, Rosner B, Willett WC, Speizer FE. Diet and risk of clinical diabetes in women. *Am J Clin Nutr* 1992;55:1018–23.

11. Salmeron J, Hu FB, Manson JE, et al. Dietary fat intake and risk of type 2 diabetes in women. *Am J Clin Nutr* 2001;73:1019–26.

12. Meyer KA, Kushi LH, Jacobs DR, Jr, Slavin J, Sellers TA, Folsom AR. Carbohydrates, dietary fiber, and incident type 2 diabetes in older women. *Am J Clin Nutr* 2000;71:921–30.

13. Liu S, Stampfer MJ, Hu FB, et al. Whole-grain consumption and risk of coronary heart disease: results from the Nurses' Health Study. *Am J Clin Nutr* 1999;70:412–9.

14. Villegas R, Gao YT, Yang G, et al. Legume and soy food intake and the incidence of type 2 diabetes in the Shanghai Women's Health Study. *Am J Clin Nutr* 2008;87:162–7.

15. Larsson SC, Wolk A. Magnesium intake and risk of type 2 diabetes: a meta-analysis. *J Intern Med* 2007;262:208–14.

16. Song Y, Manson JE, Buring JE, Liu S. A prospective study of red meat consumption and type 2 diabetes in middle-aged and elderly women: the women's health study. *Diabetes Care* 2004;27:2108–15.

17. Fung TT, Schulze M, Manson JE, Willett WC, Hu FB. Dietary patterns, meat intake, and the risk of type 2 diabetes in women. *Arch Intern Med* 2004;164:2235–40.

18. Jenkins DJ, Kendall CW, McKeown-Eyssen G, et al. Effect of a low-glycemic index or a high-cereal fiber diet on type 2 diabetes: a randomized trial. *JAMA* 2008;300:2742–53.

19. Liese AD, Roach AK, Sparks KC, Marquart L, D'Agostino RB, Jr, Mayer-Davis EJ. Whole-grain intake and insulin sensitivity: the Insulin Resistance Atherosclerosis Study. *Am J Clin Nutr* 2003;78:965–71.

20. Anderson JW, Ward K. High-carbohydrate, high-fiber diets for insulin-treated men with diabetes mellitus. *Am J Clin Nutr* 1979;32:2312–21.

21. Barnard ND, Cohen J, Jenkins DJ, et al. A low-fat vegan diet and a conventional diabetes diet in the treatment of type 2 diabetes: a randomized, controlled, 74-wk clinical trial. *Am J Clin Nutr* 2009;89:1588S-1596S.

22. Franz MJ, Bantle JP, Beebe CA, et al. Evidence-based nutrition principles and recommendations for the treatment and prevention of diabetes and related complications. *Diabetes Care* 2002;25:148–98.

23. Schwingshackl L, Strasser B, Hoffmann G. Effects of monounsaturated fatty acids on cardiovascular risk factors: a systematic review and meta-analysis. *Ann Nutr Metab* 2011;59:176–86.

24. Garg A. High-monounsaturated-fat diets for patients with diabetes mellitus: a meta-analysis. *Am J Clin Nutr* 1998;67:577S-582S.

25. Luchsinger JA, Tang MX, Shea S, Mayeux R. Hyperinsulinemia and risk of Alzheimer disease. *Neurology* 2004;63:1187–92.

26. Esposito K, Maiorino MI, Ciotola M, et al. Effects of a Mediterranean-style diet on the need for antihyperglycemic drug therapy in patients with newly diagnosed type 2 diabetes: a randomized trial. *Ann Intern Med* 2009;151:306–14.

27. Lovejoy JC, Windhauser MM, Rood JC, de la Bretonne JA. Effect of a controlled high-fat versus low-fat diet on insulin sensitivity and leptin levels in African-American and Caucasian women. *Metabolism* 1998;47:1520–4.

28. Vessby B, Uusitupa M, Hermansen K, et al. Substituting dietary saturated for monounsaturated fat impairs insulin sensitivity in healthy men and women: The KANWU Study. *Diabetologia* 2001;44:312–9.

29. Hu FB, van Dam RM, Liu S. Diet and risk of Type II diabetes: the role of types of fat and carbohydrate. *Diabetologia* 2001;44:805–17.

30. Jenkins DJ, Kendall CW, Banach MS, et al. Nuts as a replacement for carbohydrates in the diabetic diet. *Diabetes Care* 2011;34:1706–11.

31. Ros E. Nuts and novel biomarkers of cardiovascular disease. *Am J Clin Nutr* 2009;89:1649S-56S.

32. Paolisso G, Giugliano D. Oxidative stress and insulin action: is there a relationship? *Diabetologia* 1996;39:357–63.

33. Huebschmann AG, Regensteiner JG, Vlassara H, Reusch JE. Diabetes and advanced glycoxidation end products. *Diabetes Care* 2006;29:1420–32.

34. Sims TJ, Rasmussen LM, Oxlund H, Bailey AJ. The role of glycation cross-links in diabetic vascular stiffening. *Diabetologia* 1996;39:946–51.

35. Wu CH, Yen GC. Inhibitory effect of naturally occurring flavonoids on the formation of advanced glycation endproducts. *J Agric Food Chem* 2005;53:3167–73.

36. Lu T, Sheng H, Wu J, Cheng Y, Zhu J, Chen Y. Cinnamon extract improves fasting blood glucose and glycosylated hemoglobin level in Chinese patients with type 2 diabetes. *Nutr Res* 2012;32:408–12.

37. Haddad EH, Berk LS, Kettering JD, Hubbard RW, Peters WR. Dietary intake and biochemical, hematologic, and immune status of vegans compared with nonvegetarians. *Am J Clin Nutr* 1999;70:586S-593S.

38. Waldmann A, Koschizke JW, Leitzmann C, Hahn A. Dietary intakes

and lifestyle factors of a vegan population in Germany: results from the German Vegan Study. *Eur J Clin Nutr* 2003;57:947–55.

39. Jacob S, Rett K, Henriksen EJ, Haring HU. Thioctic acid—effects on insulin sensitivity and glucose-metabolism. *Biofactors* 1999;10:169–74.

40. Jamal GA, Carmichael H. The effect of gamma-linolenic acid on human diabetic peripheral neuropathy: a double-blind placebo-controlled trial. *Diabet Med* 1990;7:319–23.

41. Horrobin DF. Essential fatty acids in the management of impaired nerve function in diabetes. *Diabetes* 1997;46 Suppl 2:S90–3.

42. Knight EL, Stampfer MJ, Hankinson SE, Spiegelman D, Curhan GC. The impact of protein intake on renal function decline in women with normal renal function or mild renal insufficiency. *Ann Intern Med* 2003;138:460–7.

43. Koppes LL, Dekker JM, Hendriks HF, Bouter LM, Heine RJ. Moderate alcohol consumption lowers the risk of type 2 diabetes: a meta-analysis of prospective observational studies. *Diabetes Care* 2005;28:719–25.

44. Jiang R, Manson JE, Stampfer MJ, Liu S, Willett WC, Hu FB. Nut and peanut butter consumption and risk of type 2 diabetes in women. *JAMA* 2002;288:2554–60.

CHAPTER 16: FEELING GOOD:
MANAGING STRESS AND DEPRESSION

1. Kessler RC, Berglund P, Demler O, et al. The epidemiology of major depressive disorder: results from the National Comorbidity Survey Replication (NCS-R). *JAMA* 2003;289:3095–105.

2. Munk-Olsen T, Laursen TM, Pedersen CB, Mors O, Mortensen PB. New parents and mental disorders: a population-based register study. *JAMA* 2006;296:2582–9.

3. Schmidt PJ, Nieman LK, Danaceau MA, Adams LF, Rubinow DR. Differential behavioral effects of gonadal steroids in women with and in those without premenstrual syndrome. *N Engl J Med* 1998;338:209–16.

4. Freeman EW, Sammel MD, Lin H, Nelson DB. Associations of hormones and menopausal status with depressed mood in women with no history of depression. *Arch Gen Psychiatry* 2006;63:375–82.

5. Nolen-Hoeksema S, Larson J, Grayson C. Explaining the gender difference in depressive symptoms. *J Pers Soc Psychol* 1999;77:1061–72.

6. Sheline YI, Sanghavi M, Mintun MA, Gado MH. Depression duration but not age predicts hippocampal volume loss in medically healthy women with recurrent major depression. *J Neurosci* 1999;19:5034–43.

7. McEwen BS. Stress and hippocampal plasticity. *Annu Rev Neurosci* 1999;22:105–22.

8. Saczynski JS, Beiser A, Seshadri S, Auerbach S, Wolf PA, Au R. Depressive symptoms and risk of dementia: the Framingham Heart Study. *Neurology* 2010;75:35–41.

9. McIntyre RS, Konarski JZ, Soczynska JK, et al. Medical comorbidity in bipolar disorder: implications for functional outcomes and health service utilization. *Psychiatr Serv* 2006;57:1140–4.

10. Katon W, Ciechanowski P. Impact of major depression on chronic medical illness. *J Psychosom Res* 2002;53:859–63.

11. Lutgendorf SK, Garand L, Buckwalter KC, Reimer TT, Hong SY, Lubaroff DM. Life stress, mood disturbance, and elevated interleukin-6 in healthy older women. *J Gerontol A Biol Sci Med Sci* 1999;54:M434–9.

12. Ranjit N, Diez-Roux AV, Shea S, et al. Psychosocial factors and inflammation in the multi-ethnic study of atherosclerosis. *Arch Intern Med* 2007;167:174–81.

13. Chiang JJ, Eisenberger NI, Seeman TE, Taylor SE. Negative and competitive social interactions are related to heightened proinflammatory cytokine activity. *Proc Natl Acad Sci U S A* 2012;109:1878–82.

14. Penwell LL, KT. Social support and risk for cardiovascular disease and cancer: a qualitative review examining the role of inflammatory processes. *Health Psychology Review* 2010;4:42–55.

15. Pasco JA, Nicholson GC, Williams LJ, et al. Association of high-sensitivity C-reactive protein with de novo major depression. *Br J Psychiatry* 2010;197:372–7.

16. Gimeno D, Kivimaki M, Brunner EJ, et al. Associations of C-reactive protein and interleukin-6 with cognitive symptoms of depression: 12-year follow-up of the Whitehall II study. *Psychol Med* 2009;39:413–23.

17. Mendlewicz J, Kriwin P, Oswald P, Souery D, Alboni S, Brunello N. Shortened onset of action of antidepressants in major depression using acetylsalicylic acid augmentation: a pilot open-label study. *Int Clin Psychopharmacol* 2006;21:227–31.

18. Pace TW, Negi LT, Adame DD, et al. Effect of compassion meditation on neuroendocrine, innate immune and behavioral responses to psychosocial stress. *Psychoneuroendocrinology* 2009;34:87–98.

19. Kohut ML, McCann DA, Russell DW, et al. Aerobic exercise, but not flexibility/resistance exercise, reduces serum IL-18, CRP, and IL-6 independent of beta-blockers, BMI, and psychosocial factors in older adults. *Brain Behav Immun* 2006;20:201–9.

20. Meier-Ewert HK, Ridker PM, Rifai N, et al. Effect of sleep loss on C-reactive protein, an inflammatory marker of cardiovascular risk. *J Am Coll Cardiol* 2004;43:678–83.

21. Raison CL, Miller AH. Is depression an inflammatory disorder? *Curr Psychiatry Rep* 2011;13:467–75.

22. Motsinger S, Lazovich D, MacLehose RF, Torkelson CJ, Robien K. Vitamin D intake and mental health-related quality of life in older women: the Iowa Women's Health Study. *Maturitas* 2012;71:267–73.

23. Milaneschi Y, Shardell M, Corsi AM, et al. Serum 25-hydroxyvitamin D and depressive symptoms in older women and men. *J Clin Endocrinol Metab* 2010;95:3225–33.

24. Bell IR, Edman JS, Morrow FD, et al. B complex vitamin patterns in geriatric and young adult inpatients with major depression. *J Am Geriatr Soc* 1991;39:252–7.

25. Tolmunen T, Hintikka J, Voutilainen S, et al. Association between depressive symptoms and serum concentrations of homocysteine in men: a population study. *Am J Clin Nutr* 2004;80:1574–8.

26. Savage DG, Lindenbaum J. Neurological complications of acquired cobalamin deficiency: clinical aspects. *Baillieres Clin Haematol* 1995;8:657–78.

27. Skarupski KA, Tangney C, Li H, Ouyang B, Evans DA, Morris MC. Longitudinal association of vitamin B-6, folate, and vitamin B-12 with depressive symptoms among older adults over time. *Am J Clin Nutr* 2010;92:330–5.

28. Appleton KM, Hayward RC, Gunnell D, et al. Effects of n-3 long-chain polyunsaturated fatty acids on depressed mood: systematic review of published trials. *Am J Clin Nutr* 2006;84:1308–16.

29. Lin PY, Su KP. A meta-analytic review of double-blind, placebo-controlled trials of antidepressant efficacy of omega-3 fatty acids. *J Clin Psychiatry* 2007;68:1056–61.

30. Sontrop J, Campbell MK. Omega-3 polyunsaturated fatty acids and depression: a review of the evidence and a methodological critique. *Prev Med* 2006;42:4–13.

31. Kiecolt-Glaser JK, Belury MA, Andridge R, Malarkey WB, Glaser R. Omega-3 supplementation lowers inflammation and anxiety in medical students: a randomized controlled trial. *Brain Behav Immun* 2011;25:1725–34.

32. Steegmans PH, Hoes AW, Bak AA, van der Does E, Grobbee DE. Higher prevalence of depressive symptoms in middle-aged men with low serum cholesterol levels. *Psychosom Med* 2000;62:205–11.

33. Feng L, Yap KB, Kua EH, Ng TP. Statin use and depressive symptoms in a prospective study of community-living older persons. *Pharmacoepidemiol Drug Saf* 2010;19:942–8.

34. Lalovic A, Sequeira A, DeGuzman R, et al. Investigation of completed suicide and genes involved in cholesterol metabolism. *J Affect Disord* 2004;79:25–32.

35. Zhang J. Epidemiological link between low cholesterol and suicidality: a puzzle never finished. *Nutr Neurosci* 2011;14:268–87.

36. Ancelin ML, Carriere I, Boulenger JP, et al. Gender and genotype modulation of the association between lipid levels and depressive symptomatology in community-dwelling elderly (the ESPRIT study). *Biol Psychiatry* 2010;68:125–32.

37. Murphy AJ, Chin-Dusting JP, Sviridov D, Woollard KJ. The anti inflammatory effects of high density lipoproteins. *Curr Med Chem* 2009;16:667–75.

38. Maes M, Smith R, Christophe A, et al. Lower serum high-density lipoprotein cholesterol (HDL-C) in major depression and in depressed men with serious suicidal attempts: relationship with immune-inflammatory markers. *Acta Psychiatr Scand* 1997;95:212–21.

39. Varea V, de Carpi JM, Puig C, et al. Malabsorption of carbohydrates and depression in children and adolescents. *J Pediatr Gastroenterol Nutr* 2005;40:561–5.

40. Ledochowski M, Sperner-Unterweger B, Fuchs D. Lactose malabsorption is associated with early signs of mental depression in females: a preliminary report. *Dig Dis Sci* 1998;43:2513–7.

41. Wurtman RJ, Hefti F, Melamed E. Precursor control of neurotransmitter synthesis. *Pharmacol Rev* 1980;32:315–35.

42. Golden RN, Gaynes BN, Ekstrom RD, et al. The efficacy of light therapy in the treatment of mood disorders: a review and meta-analysis of the evidence. *Am J Psychiatry* 2005;162:656–62.

43. Greer TL, Trivedi MH. Exercise in the treatment of depression. *Curr Psychiatry Rep* 2009;11:466–72.

44. Morita E, Fukuda S, Nagano J, et al. Psychological effects of forest environments on healthy adults: Shinrin-yoku (forest-air bathing, walking) as a possible method of stress reduction. *Public Health* 2007;121:54–63.

45. Tsunetsugu Y, Park BJ, Miyazaki Y. Trends in research related to "Shinrin-yoku" (taking in the forest atmosphere or forest bathing) in Japan. *Environ Health Prev Med* 2010;15:27–37.

46. Boecker H, Sprenger T, Spilker ME, et al. The runner's high: opioidergic mechanisms in the human brain. *Cereb Cortex* 2008;18:2523–31.

47. Dunbar RI, Baron R, Frangou A, et al. Social laughter is correlated with an elevated pain threshold. *Proc Biol Sci* 2012;279:1161–7.

48. Rienks J, Dobson AJ, Mishra GD. Mediterranean dietary pattern and prevalence and incidence of depressive symptoms in mid-aged women: results from a large community-based prospective study. *Eur J Clin Nutr* 2013;67:75–82.

49. Hertzler AA, Anderson HL. Food guides in the United States. An historical review. *J Am Diet Assoc* 1974;64:19–28.

50. Beezhold BL, Johnston CS. Restriction of meat, fish, and poultry in omnivores improves mood: a pilot randomized controlled trial. *Nutr J* 2012;11:9.

51. Baines S, Powers J, Brown WJ. How does the health and well-being of young Australian vegetarian and semi-vegetarian women compare with non-vegetarians? *Public Health Nutr* 2007;10:436–42.

52. Filippi M, Riccitelli G, Falini A, et al. The brain functional networks associated to human and animal suffering differ among omnivores, vegetarians and vegans. *PLoS One* 2010;5:e10847.

INDEX

RECEIPE INDEX